A Practical Guide to
HEMIPLEGIA TREATMENT

A Practical Guide to
HEMIPLEGIA TREATMENT

Ipsit Brahmachari PhD

Physiotherapist

Proprietor
Marg Physiotherapy and Rehabilitation Clinic
Ahmedabad, Gujarat, India

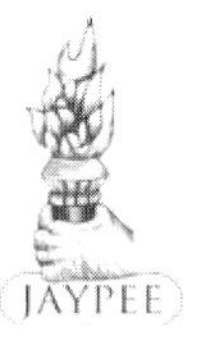

The Health Sciences Publisher

New Delhi | London | Philadelphia | Panama

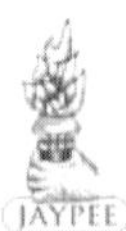 **Jaypee Brothers Medical Publishers (P) Ltd**

Headquarters

Jaypee Brothers Medical Publishers (P) Ltd
4838/24, Ansari Road, Daryaganj
New Delhi 110 002, India
Phone: +91-11-43574357
Fax: +91-11-43574314
Email: jaypee@jaypeebrothers.com

Overseas Offices

J.P. Medical Ltd
83, Victoria Street, London
SW1H 0HW (UK)
Phone: +44 20 3170 8910
Fax: +44 (0)20 3008 6180
Email: info@jpmedpub.com

Jaypee Medical Inc
The Bourse
111 South Independence Mall East
Suite 835, Philadelphia, PA 19106, USA
Phone: +1 267-519-9789
Email: jpmed.us@gmail.com

Jaypee Brothers Medical Publishers (P) Ltd
Bhotahity, Kathmandu, Nepal
Phone: +977-9741283608
Email: kathmandu@jaypeebrothers.com

Jaypee-Highlights Medical Publishers Inc.
City of Knowledge, Bld. 237, Clayton
Panama City, Panama
Phone: +1 507-301-0496
Fax: +1 507-301-0499
Email: cservice@jphmedical.com

Jaypee Brothers Medical Publishers (P) Ltd
17/1-B Babar Road, Block-B, Shaymali
Mohammadpur, Dhaka-1207
Bangladesh
Mobile: +08801912003485
Email: jaypeedhaka@gmail.com

Website: www.jaypeebrothers.com
Website: www.jaypeedigital.com

Inquiries for bulk sales may be solicited at: jaypee@jaypeebrothers.com

A Practical Guide to Hemiplegia Treatment

First Edition: **2015**
ISBN 978-93-5152-412-0
Printed at Rajkamal Electric Press, Plot No. 2, Phase-IV, Kundli, Haryana.

Dedicated to

My Teachers
and
My Patients

Preface

Physiotherapy is a field of science dealing with physical agents and using them to bring about positive changes to the health of the receiver. Hence, it has to be highly objective in nature and its results should be reproducible on application of same treatment techniques on similar conditions. However, it does not hold true in clinical practice. It is observed by every physiotherapist that a similar technique can bring about dissimilar results in patients with similar conditions. This is because of the difference in the skill levels, effort, basic knowledge, dedication, and will of the treatment provider. Thus, execution of the treatment is an art. Physiotherapy is a combination of science and art. Science is the body and art is the soul of physiotherapy. In this light, we can say that physiotherapy is also subjective in nature. This combination of 'objectivity' and 'subjectivity' gives a unique flavor to this profession. Subjectivity, rather than becoming a negative trait, blossoms like a flower when a physiotherapist is treating a patient.

A lot has been written on physiotherapeutic management of a patient suffering from hemiplegia/paresis by developed nations. But, as a matter of fact, the requirement of the patient as well as availability of resources does differ from nation to nation. Our nation too has a different approach to disease, disability and impairment and hence, subtle changes are mandatory and strongly advocated in approach towards the condition and its treatment.

Hemiplegia is not just a neurological or a musculoskeletal dysfunction, but rather is a dysfunction of the personality as a whole. It is extremely difficult for the patient to keep his physical disability and its psychological impact separate. This psychosocial impact on the patient's life spreads its fangs towards their respective family members too, and they become victims of the situation. Thus, there arose a need to address the issue of physiotherapeutic management of hemiplegia in a new light, focusing on needs of our society.

This treatment guide would be beneficial to all the physiotherapy students and fresh graduates who want to make difference in the lives of the patients by doing justice to their profession. This book can become a useful guide for a practicing physiotherapist (undergraduate/postgraduate) working in private setup, government setup, hospitals or as a homecare therapist, for a quick reference and progression of therapy with logical reasoning, as assessment and treatment parts go hand in hand.

For the ease of readers, an attempt has been made to cover all major topics in a nutshell in simple, lucid language with an optimum flow and continuity. The book is divided into various topics ranging from Basic Anatomy and physiology of brain, development of nervous system, to clinical diagnosis, symptomology and detailed assessment. It also deals with essentials of Rehabilitation medicine and approach to treatment. For the ease of quick reference, various exercises and treatment techniques are divided into lying, sitting and standing positions. Topics of orofacial rehabilitation, perception, orthotics, and management of complications are also dealt with. It concludes with homecare program.

I sincerely hope that this book will throw light on the dark path of disability and will help in bringing about improvement in the quality of life of individuals suffering from hemiplegia.

Ipsit Brahmachari

Acknowledgments

Any stream of knowledge is not a discrete entity but rather is a perennial flow which flows from teachers to students over centuries. To claim any creation to be 'self-owned' is erroneous, as present-day creation has its roots in the soil of yesteryears. In bringing out this compilation in the form of a book, I have been highly motivated and influenced by many persons and events, both known and unknown to my conscious mind. Several texts have been instrumental in teaching us the nuances of physiotherapy. To mention a few, Principles of Exercise Therapy by Dena Gardiner, Hemiplegia by Berta Bobath, PNF in Practice by Adler, Beckers and Buck and, Physical Rehabilitation by O' Sullivan, Cash's Textbook of Neurology, and Steps to Follow by Patricia Davies.

I would like to thank all my teachers who have always been guiding force in my life. Some teachers of physiotherapy deserve a special mention; Dr Mina Desai, Dr Sarala Bhatt, Dr Anjali Bhise, Dr Yagna Shukla, and Dr Dilip Patel. I extend my thanks to Dr Roshan Vania and Dr Preeti Shah for initiating me into the teaching of Bobath techniques and neurodevelopment techniques. I sincerely thank Dr Maya Nanavati, an Occupational Therapist for teaching her valuable hands-on skills. I thank Dr Sudhir Shah, a master Neurophysician and a great scholar who extended support, believed in me and allowed me to treat his patients. I thank Dr Amit Bhatt for being always supportive. I extend my thanks to Dr Dhiren Ganjwala (Orthopedic Surgeon) for contributing chapter on Orthopedic Management of Stroke.

I thank my staff and colleagues at Marg Physiotherapy and Rehabilitation Clinic, especially Dr Darshan Rana for photography, coordination, and tolerating me, and Dr Vikas Dhimmar for typing. I also thank Dr Jugal Sherdiwala for his support. I take this opportunity to thank my family Dr Urvi, my wife, Jalormi, my daughter and my parents as pillars of my strength.

I thank Shri Jitendar P Vij (Group Chairman), Mr Ankit Vij (Group President), Mr Tarun Duneja (Director–Publishing), Mr Sharad (Gujarat branch) and all the staff of M/s Jaypee Brothers Medical Publishers (P) Ltd, New Delhi, India, for bringing out this book and believing in me.

Last but not least, I thank all my patients who have lovingly cooperated in this process.

Contents

Basic Anatomy and Physiology of Human Brain

ANATOMY OF THE HEAD

The human *nervous system* consists of the *Central Nervous System* (CNS) and *Peripheral Nervous System* (PNS). The former consists of the brain and spinal cord, while the latter composes the nerves extending to and from the brain and spinal cord. The primary functions of the nervous system are to monitor, integrate (process) and respond to information inside and outside the body. The brain consists of soft, delicate, nonreplaceable neural tissue. It is supported and protected by the surrounding skin, skull, meninges and cerebrospinal fluid.

Skin

The skin constitutes a protective barrier against physical damage of underlying tissues, invasion of hazardous chemical and bacterial substances and, through the activity of its sweat glands and blood vessels, it helps to maintain the body at a constant temperature. Together with the sweat and oil glands, hairs and nails, it forms a set of organs called the *integumentary system*. The skin consists of an outer, protective layer, the *epidermis* and an inner layer, the *dermis*. While the top layer of the epidermis, the *stratum corneum*, consists of dead cells, the dermis is composed of vascularized fibrous connective tissue. The *subcutaneous tissue*, located underneath the skin, is primarily composed of *adipose tissue* (fat) (Figure 1.1).

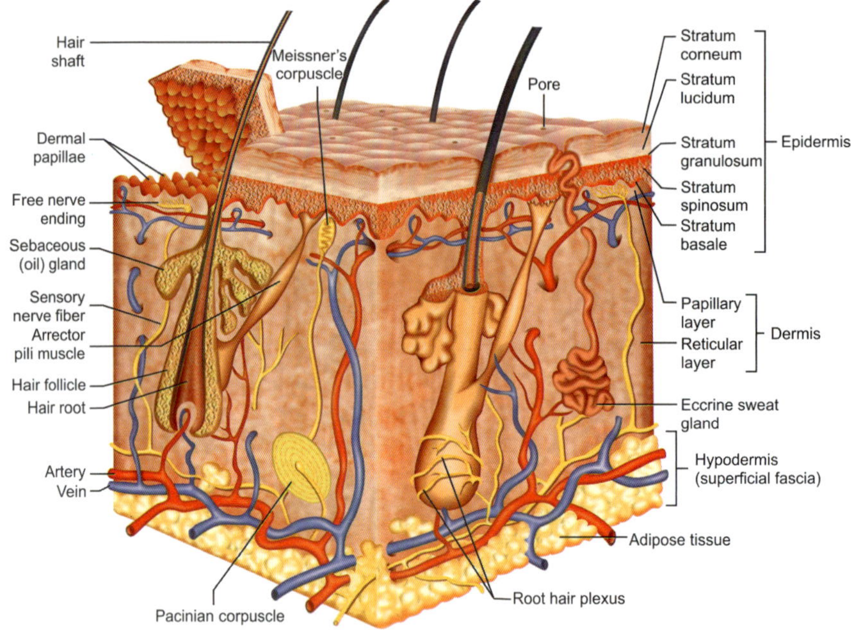

FIGURE 1.1: Layers of skin

Skull

Depending on their shape, bones are classified as long, short, flat or irregular. Bones of different types contain different proportions of the two types of osseous tissue: compact and spongy bone. While the former has a smooth structure, the latter is composed of small needle-like or flat pieces of bone called *trabeculae*, which form a network filled with red or yellow bone marrow. Most skull bones are flat and consist of two parallel compact bone surfaces, with a layer of spongy bone sandwiched in between. The spongy bone layer of flat bones (the diploe) predominantly contains red bone marrow and hence, has a high concentration of blood.

The skull is a highly complex structure consisting of 22 bones altogether. These can be divided into two sets, the *cranial bones* (or *cranium*) and the *facial bones*. While the latter form the framework of the face, the cranial bones form the *cranial cavity* that encloses and protects the brain. All bones of the adult skull are firmly connected by *sutures*. Figure 1.2 shows the most important bones of the skull. The *frontal bone* forms the forehead and contains the *frontal sinuses*, which are air filled cells within the bone. Most superior and lateral aspects of the skull are formed by the *parietal bones* while the *occipital bone* forms the posterior aspects. The base of the occipital bone

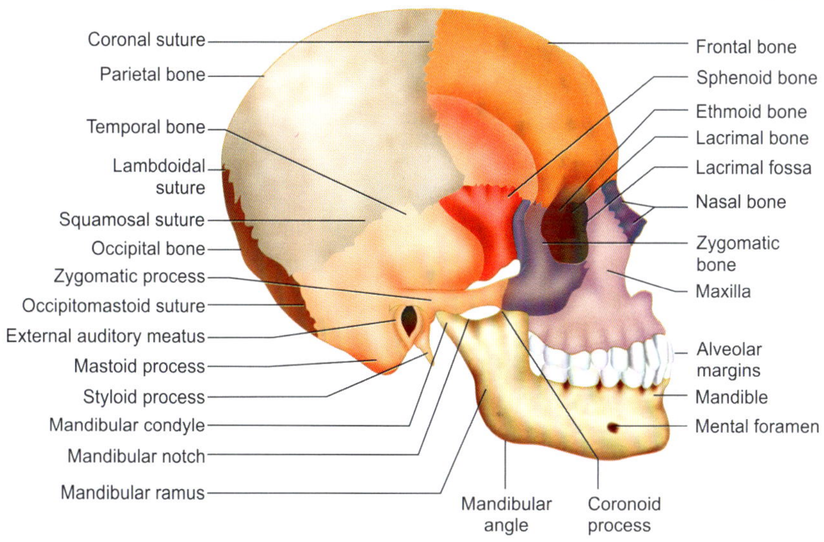

FIGURE 1.2: Bones of the skull

contains the *foramen magnum*, which is a large hole allowing the inferior part of the brain to connect to the spinal cord. The remaining bones of the cranium are the *temporal*, *sphenoid* and *ethmoid bones*.

Meninges

The *meninges* are three connective tissue membranes enclosing the brain and the spinal cord. Their functions are to protect the CNS and blood vessels, enclose the *venous sinuses*, retain the *cerebrospinal fluid*, and form partitions within the skull. The outermost meninx is the dura mater, which encloses the *arachnoid mater* and the innermost *pia mater* (Figure 1.3).

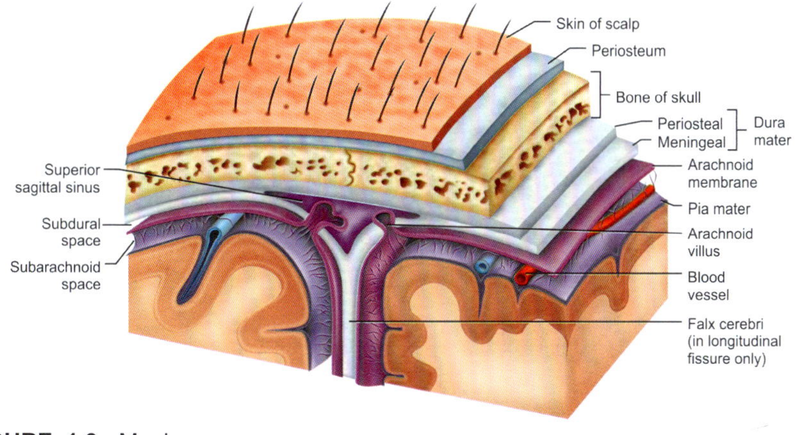

FIGURE 1.3: Meninges

Cerebrospinal Fluid

Cerebrospinal Fluid (CSF) is a watery liquid similar in composition to blood plasma. It is formed in the *choroid plexuses* and circulates through the ventricles into the *subarachnoid space*, where it is returned to the dural venous sinuses by the *arachnoid villi*. The prime purpose of the CSF is to support and cushion the brain and help nourish it. Figure 1.4 illustrates the flow of CSF through the central nervous system.

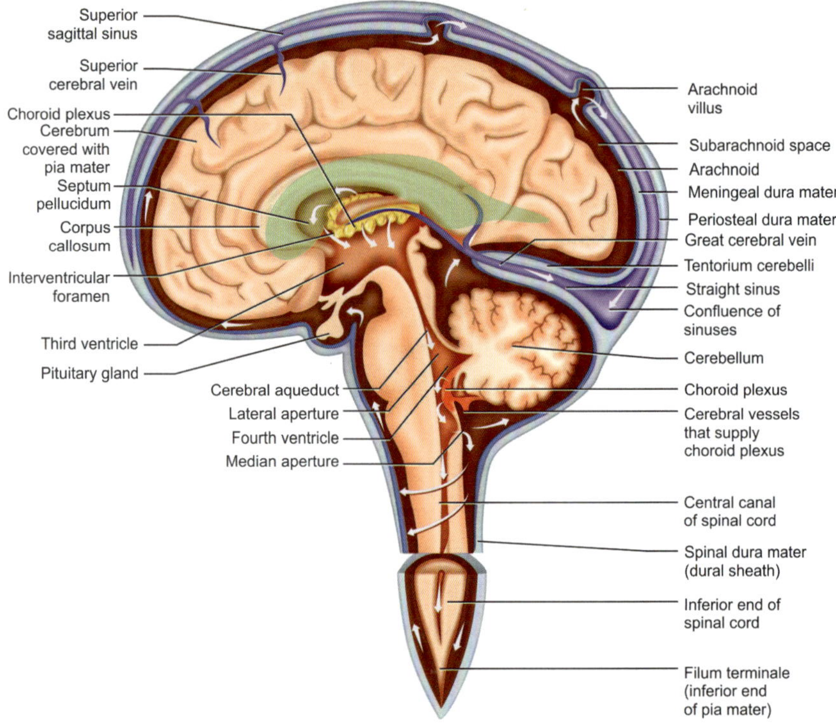

FIGURE 1.4: Cerebrospinal fluid

THE MAJOR REGIONS OF THE BRAIN AND THEIR FUNCTIONS

The major regions of the brain are the *cerebral hemispheres, diencephalon, brainstem* and *cerebellum* (Figure 1.5).

Cerebral Hemispheres

The *cerebral* hemispheres, located on the most superior part of the brain, are separated by the *longitudinal fissure*. They make up approximately 83% of total

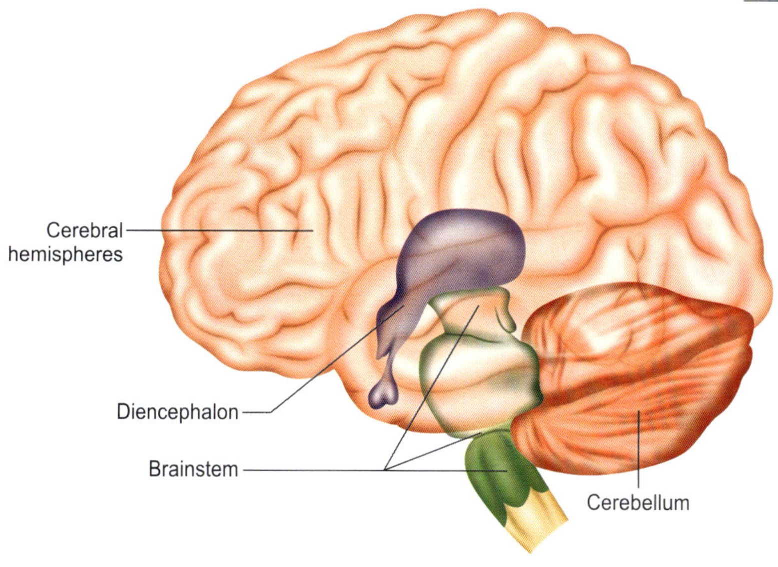

FIGURE 1.5: Major regions of the brain

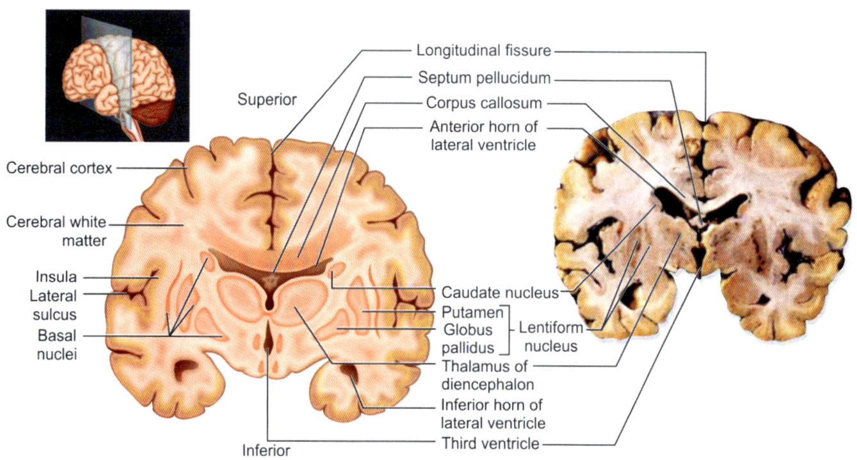

FIGURE 1.6: Cerebral hemispheres

brain mass and are collectively referred to as the *cerebrum*. The *cerebral cortex* constitutes a 2–4 mm thick *gray matter* surface layer and, because of its many convolutions, accounts for about 40% of total brain mass (Figure 1.6).

- Gray matter is responsible for conscious behavior and contains three different functional areas: the *motor areas*, *sensory areas* and *association areas*. Located internally is the *white matter*.

- White matter is responsible for communication between cerebral areas and between the cerebral cortex and lower regions of the CNS, as well as the *basal nuclei* (or *basal ganglia*), involved in controlling muscular movement.

Diencephalon

The *diencephalon* is located centrally within the forebrain. It consists of the *thalamus*, *hypothalamus* and *epithalamus*, which together enclose the third ventricle.

The functions of the thalamus are:
- It acts as a grouping and relay station for sensory inputs ascending to the sensory cortex and association areas.
- It also mediates motor activities, cortical arousal and memories.

The functions of the hypothalamus are:
- By controlling the autonomic (involuntary) nervous system, it is responsible for maintaining the body's homeostatic balance. Moreover, it forms a part of the *limbic system*, the 'emotional' brain.
- The epithalamus consists of the *pineal gland* and the CSF producing *choroid plexus*. Function of the pineal gland is not very well understood.

Brainstem

The brainstem is similarly structured as the spinal cord: it consists of gray matter surrounded by white matter fiber tracts. Its major regions are the *midbrain*, *pons* and *medulla oblongata*.
- The midbrain, which surrounds the cerebral aqueduct, provides fiber pathways between higher and lower brain centers, contains visual and auditory reflex and subcortical motor centers.
- The pons is mainly a conduction region, but its nuclei also contribute to the regulation of respiration and cranial nerves.
- The medulla oblongata takes an important role as an autonomic reflex center involved in maintaining body homeostasis. In particular, nuclei in the medulla regulate respiratory rhythm, heart rate, blood pressure and several cranial nerves. Moreover, it provides conduction pathways between the inferior spinal cord and higher brain centers.

Cerebellum

The *cerebellum*, which is located dorsal to the pons and medulla, accounts for about 11% of total brain mass. Like the cerebrum, it has a thin outer cortex of gray matter, internal white matter and small, deeply situated, paired masses (nuclei) of gray matter. The cerebellum processes impulses received from the cerebral motor cortex, various brainstem nuclei and sensory receptors in order to appropriately control skeletal muscle contraction, thus giving smooth coordinated movements.

THE CEREBRAL CIRCULATORY SYSTEM

Blood Supply to the Brain

Figure 1.7 shows an overview of the arterial system supplying the brain. The major arteries are the *vertebral* and *internal carotid arteries*. The two *posterior* and single *anterior communicating arteries* form the *circle of Willis*, which equalizes blood pressures in the brain's anterior and posterior regions and protects the brain from damage, should one of the arteries become occluded. However, there is little communication between smaller arteries on the brain's surface. Hence, occlusion of these arteries usually results in localized tissue damage.

Cerebral Hemodynamics

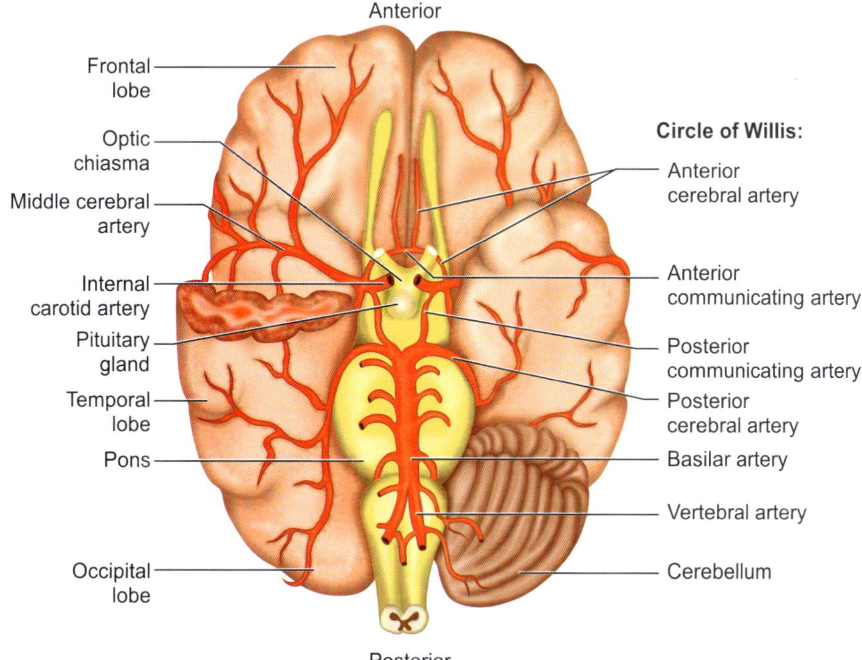

FIGURE 1.7: Cerebral circulatory system

The cardiac output is about 5 L/min of blood for a resting adult. Blood flow to the brain is about 14% of this, or 700 ml/min. For any part of the body, the blood flow can be calculated using the simple formula, blood pressure multiplied by size of the arteries. Pressure in the arteries is generated by the heart, which pumps blood from its left ventricle into the aorta. [Since pressure was historically measured with a mercury manometer, the units are commonly expressed in terms of (mm Hg), although the official SI unit is the Pascal (Pa)]. Resistance arises from friction and is proportional to the following expression (*Vessel Diameter*) divided by (*Vessel Length*). Also, the viscosity of the blood increases the resistance and hence, it decreases the blood flow rate in the arteries as well as the veins. The slow moving and sluggish blood is a breeding ground for the increase in platelet activity and hence, the chances of thrombosis increase. Blood flow is slowest in the small vessels of the capillary bed, thus allowing time for the exchange of nutrients and oxygen to surrounding tissue by diffusion through the capillary walls.

Approximately, 75% of total blood volume is 'stored' in the veins which, because of their high capacity, act as reservoirs. Their walls distend and contract in response to the amount of blood available in the circulation. However, the function of cerebral veins, formed from sinuses in the dura mater, is somewhat different from other veins of the body, as they are noncollapsible.

Autoregulation

Panerai (1998) describes *autoregulation* of blood flow in the cerebral vascular bed as the mechanism by which cerebral blood flow (CBF) tends to remain relatively constant despite changes in cerebral perfusion pressure (CPP). With a constant metabolic demand, changes in CPP or arterial blood pressure, that would increase or reduce CBF, are compensated by adjusting the vascular resistance. This maintains a constant O_2 supply and constant CBF. Therefore, cerebral autoregulation allows the blood supply to the brain to match its metabolic demand and also to protect cerebral vessels against excessive flow due to arterial hypertension. Cerebral blood flow is autoregulated much better than in almost any other organ. Even for arterial pressure variations between 50 and 150 mm Hg, CBF only changes by a few percent. This can be accomplished because the arterial vessels are typically able to change their diameter about 4-fold, corresponding to a 256-fold change in blood flow. Only when the brain is very active, is there an exception to the close matching of blood flow to metabolism, which can raise up to 30–50% in the affected areas. It is an aim of PET, functional MRI, near infrared spectroscopy (NIRS) and possibly, near infrared imaging, to detect or image such localized changes in cortical activity and associated blood flow.

THE NEONATAL BRAIN

The embryonic brain and spinal cord develop from the neural tube, which is formed in the fourth week of pregnancy. The brain grows immensely in both size and complexity, during pregnancy and even soon after birth. Because a membranous skull restricts expansion, the forebrain is bent towards the brainstem and the cerebral hemispheres almost completely envelop the diencephalon and midbrain. Moreover, the spatial restrictions cause the cerebral hemispheres to increase their surface area by becoming highly convoluted such that about two-thirds of its surface is hidden in its folds. The skull bones of the fetus and neonate are soft and the sutures are not yet fused. Hence, the skull is very flexible and deforms under light pressure (Hirschowitz, 1988).

Compared to the adult, neonates have a smaller head size (6–12 cm in diameter), thinner surface tissue, skull and CSF layers, lower scattering coefficients of gray and white matter (due to lesser myelination in the case of white matter), as well as, a comparatively small mismatch between the two.

Arterial and venous hemoglobin saturation values for the fetus in utero are relatively low at 56% and 18% (Rooth, 1963), respectively, compared to about 97% and 67% for adults. This is because there is a gradient in oxygen concentration across the placenta which ensures diffusion of sufficient amounts of oxygen from maternal blood into the fetal bloodstream. A higher oxygen affinity of neonatal hemoglobin compensates for this. Over a period of about 6 months after delivery, the neonatal hemoglobin is gradually substituted by the adult hemoglobin, which has a lower oxygen affinity.

Neurodevelopmental disorders in some *preterm* infants are due to either hypoxic-ischemic damage to the periventricular white matter, or to intra-ventricular hemorrhage and its consequences. The period of highest risk is between 26 weeks and 32 weeks of gestation. In preterm infants, the majority of hemorrhages occur into the ventricles and the surrounding white matter, the periventricular region. Hypoxic-ischemic damage is caused by cerebral under-perfusion, often combined with a global oxygen deficiency due to an impaired lung function. It also affects the periventricular white matter, which is thought to be a result of the following two effects:

1. Increased vulnerability due to high metabolic demands at this phase of the brain development.
2. The area is at a 'watershed' of perfusion from the territories of the posterior and middle cerebral arteries.

Enduring neurodevelopmental disorders can lead to diminished neurological function in later life, and in particular spasticity, since motor fibers run through this region of the white matter. Given the potential of the premature infant's developing brain to repair some damage, spasticity is often restricted to stiff limbs and/or subtle learning disabilities. Cerebral damage in the *mature* infant is most commonly a result of perinatal ('birth') asphyxia, leading initially to cerebral edema (resulting in compressed ventricles and flattening of the convolutions of the brain) and later to tissue necrosis (tissue death) and apoptosis (cell suicide). The subcortical white matter, basal ganglia, cerebellum and brainstem are the areas predominantly affected, frequently leading to learning disabilities or global developmental delay and cerebral palsy.

ASPECTS OF NEUROANATOMY AND PHYSIOLOGY

The Nervous System as a Basic Unit of a Living Being

The nervous system is the basic unit which is used by the living creature in order to be able to react to its environment. The more complex the creature, the more complicated is its nervous system and the more versatile are its reactions. The system is concerned with the physical (sensory, motor and autonomic), intellectual and emotional activities and, in consequence, any disorder may involve any one or all three of these major functions.

Neuron

The nervous system is composed of an enormous number of neurons, connected together and following certain pathways, in order to make functional activity possible. The neuron is the basic unit of the nervous system and comprises of the nerve cell and its processes. Each neuron has a cell body and two types of processes, dendrites and axons. Each ramus carries motor, sensory and autonomic fibers and the sympathetic ganglion communicates with those above and below it in level and also sends fibers to the visceral contents. The corticospinal path represents the pyramidal system and other paths may be considered to be extrapyramidal.

The Synapse

This is the term used to define the area where the process of one neuron links with another. The synapse is the point of contiguity but not of continuity. Synapses may occur between the terminal parts of an axon and the dendrites of another cell or with the cell body. The number of synaptic areas may be very vast in any one neuron. The synapse enables impulses from one neuron to be transmitted to another neuron by virtue of chemical changes taking place which bring about an alteration in membrane potential of receiving neuron. Synapses have certain properties which are of importance. Some of the more important ones are:

- **Synaptic delay:** When an impulse reaches a synapse, there is a brief time lag before a response occurs in the recipient neuron. Consequently, conduction along a chain of neurons is slower than along one single neuron. Thus, monosynaptic pathways conduct more rapidly than polysynaptic routes.
- **One way conduction**: Synapses permit conduction of impulses in one direction only, i.e. from the presynaptic to the postsynaptic neuron.
- **Vulnerability**: Synapses are very sensitive to anoxia and to the effects of drugs. Polysynaptic pathways are very susceptible to anesthesia.
- **Summation:** The effect of impulses arriving at a synapse can be added to by other impulses. For instance, the effect of impulses could be subliminal (insufficient to bring about adequate chemical change for depolarization of the postsynaptic neuron). If, however, another spate of impulses arrives before the effect of the previous one has subsided, then the two effects may complement each other and the total change is sufficient to cause depolarization. Such a phenomenon is called summation. There are two types of summations:
- One is dependent upon the time factor known as temporal summation and
- Other is called spatial summation, which is the result of the adding together of impulses from different neurons, which converge upon the postsynaptic neuron and bring about the depolarization of its membrane.
- **Fatigue**: The synapse is thought to be the site of fatigue in nerve conductivity.
- **Inhibition:** Certain neurons have an inhibitory effect upon the postsynaptic neuron, possibly because they use a different chemical mediator. Thus, the effect of these neurons would be to discourage depolarization of the post-synaptic cell membrane and would be antagonistic to influences exerted by excitatory neurons. These effects can summate in the same way as the excitatory effects. Many interneurons have an inhibitory effect.
- **Post-tetanic potentiation:** This occurs across synapses, which have been subjected to prolonged and repeated activity. The threshold of stimulation of these junctions is thought to be lowered making transmission across it more easily brought about, for a period of several hours. Facilitation of transmission is said to occur and is an elementary form of learning and also forms an important part in the approach to physical treatment of patients with neurological disorders.

■ **Supporting tissue:** Neurons are delicate, highly specialized structures and require support and protection. This is afforded to them in the nervous system by specialized connective tissue called neuroglia. If neurons are damaged and destroyed, their place is filled by proliferation of neuroglial material. The axons are surrounded by a fatty sheath called myelin, which has an important effect on the conduction of impulses. Because of this sheath, bundles of axons give a whitish appearance and form the white matter of the central nervous system.

When the axon and its myelin sheath leave the central nervous system, they become surrounded by a membrane called the neurilemma. This is of vital importance and it should be noted that the neurilemma is absent around the fibers of the brain and spinal cord, whereas it is present, as soon as they leave these areas.

Nerve fibers which are surrounded by the neurilemma may regenerate if they are destroyed. Hence, destruction of fibers in a peripheral nerve does not necessarily mean permanent loss of function, whereas destruction of the fibers in the central nervous system will mean permanent loss of function of those fibers. It should also be noted that the nerve cell is resilient to injury and has recuperative powers but, if it dies, it is incapable of being replaced. Thus, destruction of cell bodies means permanent loss of function.

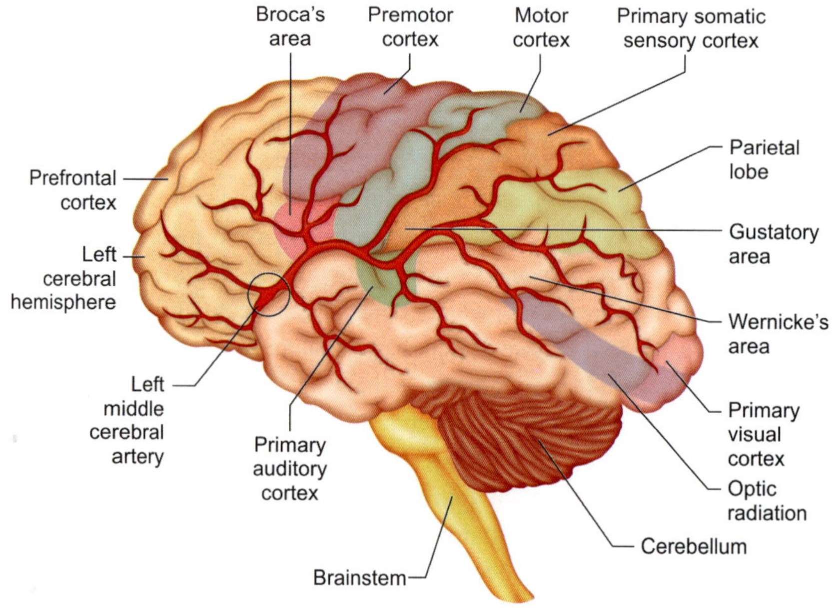

FIGURE 1.8: Areas of brain

TABLE 1.1	Brain structure, function and associated symptoms	
Brain structure	**Functions**	**Associated signs and symptoms**
Cerebral Cortex Ventral view (From bottom)	The outermost layer of the cerebral hemisphere which is composed of gray matter. Cortices are asymmetrical. Both hemispheres are able to analyze sensory data, perform memory functions, learn new information, form thoughts and make decisions	
Left Hemisphere	Sequential analysis: systematic, logical interpretation of information. Interpretation and production of symbolic information: language, mathematics, abstraction and reasoning. Memory stored in a language format	
Right Hemisphere	Holistic functioning: processing multisensory input simultaneously to provide "holistic" picture of one's environment. Visual spatial skills. Holistic functions such as dancing and gymnastics are coordinated by the right hemisphere. Memory is stored in auditory, visual and spatial modalities	

Contd...

Contd...

Brain structure	Functions	Associated signs and symptoms
Corpus Callosum	Connects right and left hemisphere to allow for communication between the hemispheres. Forms roof of the lateral and third ventricles	• Damage to the corpus callosum may result in "Split Brain" syndrome
Frontal Lobe Ventral view (From bottom) Side view	Cognition and memory. Prefrontal area: The ability to concentrate and attend elaboration of thought. The "Gatekeeper"; (judgment, inhibition). Personality and emotional traits Movement: Motor Cortex (Brodmann's): voluntary motor activity Premotor cortex: Storage of motor patterns and voluntary activities Language: Motor speech	• Impairment of recent memory, inattentiveness, inability to concentrate, behavior disorders, difficulty in learning new information. Lack of inhibition (inappropriate social and/or sexual behavior). Emotional lability. • Contralateral plegia, paresis • Expressive/motor aphasia
Parietal Lobe	Processing of sensory input, sensory discrimination Body orientation Primary/secondary somatic area	• Inability to discriminate between sensory stimuli • Inability to locate and recognize parts of the body (Neglect) • Severe injury: Inability to recognize self

Contd...

Contd...

Brain structure	Functions	Associated signs and symptoms
		• Disorientation of environment space • Inability to write
Occipital Lobe	Primary visual reception area Primary visual association area: Allows for visual interpretation	• Primary visual cortex: Loss of vision of opposite field • Visual association cortex: Loss of ability to recognize object seen in opposite field of vision, "flash of light", "stars"
Temporal Lobe	Auditory receptive area and association areas Expressed behavior Language: Receptive speech Memory: Information retrieval	• Hearing deficits • Agitation, irritability, childish behavior • Receptive/sensory aphasia
Limbic System	Olfactory pathways: Amygdala and their different pathways Hippocampi and their different pathways Limbic lobes: Sex, rage, fear, emotions. Integration of recent memory, biological rhythms Hypothalamus	• Loss of sense of smell • Agitation, loss of control of emotion • Loss of recent memory

Contd...

Contd...

Brain structure	Functions	Associated signs and symptoms
Basal Ganglia 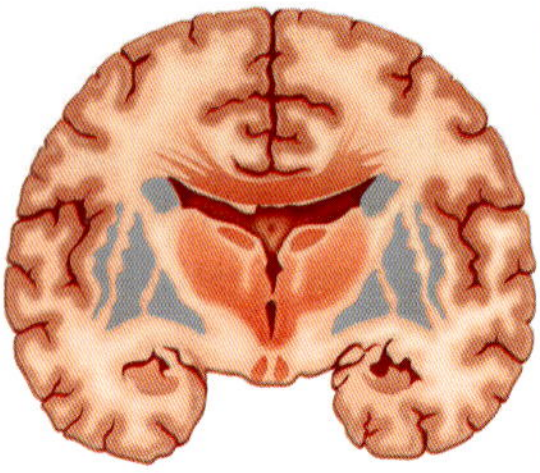	Subcortical gray matter nuclei. Processing link between thalamus and motor cortex. Initiation and direction of voluntary movement. Balance (inhibitory), postural reflexes Part of extrapyramidal system: Regulation of automatic movement	• Movement disorders: chorea, tremors at rest and with initiation of movement, abnormal increase in muscle tone, difficulty initiating movement • Parkinson's symptoms

The Development of Nervous System

INTRODUCTION

The dynamic process of motor structuration in the early stages of infantile development appears to be essentially an interweaving of various patterns which appear and disappear and overlap with each other in their mutual interacting and modulating influence with an orderly integration in the developmental process.

In order to acquire the progressive refinement of selective motor behavior, the massive, gross functional units of reflex patterns have to be broken down into small polyvalent units available for reconstruction of other new patterns for the performance of normal movements (Milani Comperatti, 1994).

DEVELOPMENT OF MOVEMENT, POSTURE AND DEVELOPMENTAL NEUROLOGY

Movement, in its basic performance, is a series of primitive reflex activity. Learning of movements is *"entirely dependent on sensory experiences."*

Sensory input initiates and guides the motor output.

As the central nervous system (CNS) matures and unfolds, the normal child gradually changes, modifies, integrates, conditions and partially inhibits various statokinetic reflex activity to form automatic postural reflex mechanism for:

■ Regulation of body tone
■ Maintenance of balance
■ Performance of skillful, coordinated, goal oriented movements.

The evolution of our erect posture, narrow base and freedom of upper extremities from the function of support to prehension, demands a fully developed and highly complex postural control mechanism (Bobath).

Body tone: The smooth performance of the movement demands normal tones of the entire neuromuscular apparatus. Normal tone permits the movement to flow smoothly without interruption, the limb feels light and when placed in a position, it will momentarily hold before returning to its original resting place. The normal tone must be high enough to maintain us upright against gravity but not too high to impede the movement.

Reciprocal innervation and inhibition for the agonists to perform smooth flow of the movement, the antagonist groups instantly adapts and adjust to their increase in length.

The agonists, antagonists, synergists and fixators come into play in exact well-timed, coordinated order and in precise gradation of contractions for maintenance of balance, posture and movement performance, hence voluntary movements are performed totally against the background of the automatic postural adjustments which are beyond our conscious level and are under subcortical influence. The automatic postural sets precede the voluntary activity. Postural adjustments occur not only as a result of the sensory feedback in respect to unexpected perturbations but also as a result of feed forward in anticipation of expected stimuli which are self-generated perturbations. (For example, When an examiner is going to touch a painful area in the subject).

Voluntary movements have these components:
- Volition
- Purpose
- Awareness
- Effort.

Posture is movement arrested. It is the attitude adopted by the body at rest or in movement and is maintained by neuromuscular activity of muscle groups, for maintenance of balance and performance of various skillful functional movements.

Basic essential for good posture and midline alignment is the stability and mobility of the trunk, because the trunk is the basis for head control, limb functions. Head, neck and limbs are the extensions of the trunk. If one loses trunk control, head and limb movements are lost. The statokinetic patterns of posture interact and reinforce each other for:
- Weight bearing
- Maintenance of balance and equilibrium
- Postural adjustments into gravity: Postural adaptation to gravity and against gravity
- Head neck orientation and postural adjustment of the head to the shift of the body

- Midline orientation: It is the point of references for movement over a base of support; one should be able to stabilize in midline
- To move away and back to midline and to cross over the midline.

Vestibular system plays a critical role in:
- Regulation of the body tone
- Accurate orientation of the body in space
- Development of visuospatial skills.

CNS Functions

Human brain is the most complex system generating both simple and complex behavioral patterns. *Brain is who we are, essence of humanity* (A. N. A 1998). GALEN centuries back stated in his writing, describing the brain to be *the seat of intelligence; movements and sensation.* WALSH (1948) stressed that the *CNS functions as a whole as the integrated sensory motor unit.*

Bobath (1970) said that *the CNS is an organ of reaction rather than action, reacting to various sensory stimuli converting upon it from within and without acting as "coordinating unit" to the multitude of incoming sensory stimuli to produce integrated motor responses adequate to the demands of the environment.*

In the modern day thinking, CNS is looked upon as *a system composed of billions of nerve cells which by virtues of their self-organization, integration, interaction and coordination form a neural network giving rise to how we think, act, decide, remember, perceive, learn, adapt and develop* (Scott Kelso, 1995).

Clinical and experimental evidence indicates that the cortex plays critical role in processing, execution and programming of the normal voluntary motor control on the basis of sensory input signals. Movements are reflex automatic and volitional.

In situation, when speed is paramount to trajectory and accuracy of the movement, the brain abstains from the feedback comparison of the actual with the desired action, like withdrawing finger from a hot burning object and these movements are executed at spinal or subcortical level.

Central nervous system is constantly seeking input for output, for it is continuously perceiving, intending, anticipating, learning and adapting to the environment to form and develop dynamic patterns of function and human behavior (Scott Kelso, 1995).

We are already living in the 21st century but, unfortunately there are therapists who are neglecting the input system and consider only the output of the CNS to improve the motor control or the joint ranges missing out on the CNS function.

Perception signifies our ability to learn, adapt and adjust to the environment. It refers to the activity occurring in the secondary and tertiary sensory association areas of the parietal lobes, which integrates information such as memory, context and experience.

Perception is defined as the ability to interpret various incoming sensory messages so that sensation has meaning. Perception memory and language are described as cognitive skills and are integrated in higher centers in CNS. Affronter and Striker define perception as: "Understanding how the CNS transforms, analyzes, promptly organizes, integrates and structure the various sensory information received from the environment, there is a constant interaction between the individual and environment. Interaction means to be in touch with or contact with, to be in touch with is 'to feel'. In this 'Key Factor' we cannot decide, if we touch the environment or environment touches us."

Newborn baby, at the age of three months, first touches various objects and manipulates, this is through Tactokinesthetic channel. After that, the following develops:

- Eye objects contact through visual channel
- Turning his head in direction of sound through auditory channel.

As we are constantly in touch with one environment, the primary channel of learning is tactokinesthetic. Perceptual processes must have absolutely intact highly developed sensory feedback system. Minutest flaw causes disturbances in perceptual processes as is observed in CNS lesions. Voluntary movement is dependent on the perception of superficial, deep and proprioception sensation and motor power, coordination and tone. Grossly, functions of CNS are:

- Regulation and distribution of muscle tone throughout the body
- Maintenance of posture and balance at rest and in movement
- Orientation of body in space
- Inhibitory control over the undesired movements, to perform goal oriented, selective, skillful movements, reciprocal inhibition and innervation
- Inhibition of undesired movements or activity or overactivity is one of the most important roles of the CNS as a result of the ratio of the inhibitory fibers are far greater in CNS as compared to excitatory fibers in the subcortical and spinal pathways.

Kokte (1978) has stated that every new activity we learn, *"We are surrounded by wall of inhibition."* Inhibition is active at every level of CNS, at spinal levels, it manifests in larger synergic patterns of flexion and extension (flexor withdrawal, extensor thrust). At higher level, inhibition becomes more and more complex, leading to fractionation of the original primitive patterns for the performance of selective motor activity in various combination and skillful, prehensile motor activity. Inhibition is a balance of activity between inhibitory and excitatory fibers and plays important role in the gradation of the movement controlling range, speed and direction of the movement.

Bobath states, "I always think inhibition is a sculpting process, chisels away at the diffuse and rather amorphous mass of excitatory action and gives a more specific form to the neural performance at the every stage of synaptic relay. Removal of inhibition causes excitation by process that is called disinhibition."

The development of the nervous system from conception to maturity is a complex and fascinating process. Development is a concept which implies both growth and maturation. Growth is not just an increase in size, but the development of increasingly more complex interconnections within the brain. The nervous system arises from the neural plate which folds to form the neural tube about the 3rd to 4th week after conception (O' Reilly and Gardner, 1977). The development of a series of flexures then occurs with the different regions of the brain and cerebral hemispheres are visible as paired vesicles at the end of the 5th week.

At birth, the human brain is very well developed; a complex and relatively larger organ than any other animal. The relative size of the brain, 12% of the body mass, is also much larger than at maturity, when it is 2%.

NEONATAL REFLEXES

The neonatal reflexes are responses which can be reproduced readily after a particular stimulus. There are also a number of responses which are patterns of movement regularly seen in the newborn period but which are not elicited after every stimulus.

The neonatal reflexes must be looked at with some circumspection. They are present even in babies with severe abnormality of the brain or even absence of the cortex as in anencephaly. Abnormal reflexes, with asymmetry, or absent or persistent reflexes should be considered significant. Stereotyped responses are particularly significant (Touwen, 1976).

Moro Reflex

The best way to elicit reflex is by the 'head drop' method. The baby is held in supine supported behind the chest and head, the head is allowed to drop about 10°. The arms extend and then flex. The legs also extend and then flex.

The Moro reflex is fully developed in the term infant. It gradually disappears over the first 3–4 months of life, first in the legs, then in the arms.

Absence of the Moro response may signify severe depression of the CNS or marked hypotonia. Persistence of the Moro, particularly an excessive response, occurs in the absence of inhibition. The Moro reflex is probably a vestibular response (Prechtl, 1956), although proprioceptive responses from the cervical vertebrae have also been considered as mediators of the response.

The Asymmetric Tonic Neck Response (ATNR)

A normal posture seen at rest, it may be imposed by the examiner turning the head, between 2 months and 4 months. A strongly imposable reflex after 6 months, or an obligatory response at any age, is the evidence of significant motor handicap.

Palmar Grasp

The infant should be supine with head in the midline; an index finger is placed in the palm of each hand and the palmar surface pressed. A normal response is strong sustained flexion of the fingers for several seconds.

Plantar Grasp

This can be elicited by stimulating the roof of the toes when active flexion will occur.

Rooting Reflex

While the infant supine, head in the midline, each corner of the mouth is stimulated by stroking laterally, the head turns, mouth open and grasps, the lips may curl to the stimulated side.

Sucking Reflex

The index finger is placed in the baby's mouth, pad up and the sucking action noted. A normal reaction is a sustained strong sucking action.

Walking Reflex

The baby is held in a standing position with the chin and head supported by one's fingers; a normal response is discernible steps with knee and hip flexion and a step on each side. The walking response is usually lost within 4 weeks or so of birth and supporting reactions of the legs do not reappear in the infant for several months. Passive extension of the head results in reinforcement of this reflex (Mac Keith, 1964).

The asymmetric tonic neck response (ATNR) is a posture seen frequently in normal babies between 2 months and 5 months. The head is turned to the side, the arm and leg on that side are extended and on the opposite side, they are flexed. This is not an obligatory response except in an abnormal baby, when its persistence and reproducibility indicates pathology.

The disappearance of neonatal reflexes during development occurs as the nervous system matures and the neural mechanisms merge into more complex mechanisms. It is for this reason that infantile response reappears after serious brain damage or in degenerative conditions. It is also for this reason that the reflexes persist in babies who have sustained damage to the nervous system at birth. Although, plasticity in the CNS allows for remodeling of some of the damaged brain, the position of the damage is all-important in the final outcome.

Three types of neural mechanisms, as defined by Touwen (1976), can be distinguished:

1. Primary or basic neural mechanisms, e.g. for visual or acoustic perception and mechanisms for generating adequate muscle tone.
2. Mechanisms which merge into larger and more complex mechanisms or seemingly disappear completely to reappear in another form in a later stage of development, e.g. stepping movements and voluntary walking patterns.
3. Mechanisms which mature more or less independently and become linked together at a particular moment. This process results in differentiated motor patterns, e.g. the development of voluntary grasp ending with a pincer grasp and the development of independent sitting, standing and walking.

DISCUSSION OF DEVELOPMENTAL SEQUENCES AND ITS IMPORTANCE IN TREATMENT PLANNING OF THE PATIENT

Mature movements are complex permutations of the basic flexion and extension synergies. Until the patient can mix flexion and extension components of movements, only mass patterns can be produced. The ability to stabilize the trunk and proximal part of limbs while allowing distal parts to move is important where skilled activity is concerned and cerebellar activity is very important to this. Equally well, the ability to retain a fixed distal extremity while the proximal segments and trunk move over it is also essential. Much of the patient's development progress is related to the ability to produce these two varieties of movement, not only as distinct entities, but going on at the same time.

The Mixture of Flexion and Extension Components

Example 1

When the sitting position is considered:
This requires extension of the vertebral column, but flexion of the hips and knees. If it is impossible to extend the column unless a total extension pattern is used, then the patient is unable to maintain a sitting position.

Example 2

When the lower limbs are considered in the walking synergies:
When the hip and knee flex, the lower limb also abducts and may laterally rotated and the foot dorsiflexes. However, to walk forward we require flexing the hip and knee while adducting the limb. This is followed by extending the knee while dorsiflexing the foot. Here, alone are some interesting synergies. The leg then prepares to take weight it extends at the knee and hip and abducts to prevent a Trendelenburg sign (drop of the pelvis on the nonweight-bearing side). Another mixture of synergy is when the abductors of the weight-bearing limb are working to prevent the pelvis from dropping on the nonweight-bearing side. When the abductors are not working, the pelvis drops into adduction on that side, causing a compensatory lurch of the trunk. This is called a Trendelenburg sign.

The push-off requires more extension of the hip, flexion of the knee and plantar flexion of the foot. This is a very complex series of synergies. The ability is not immediately available. The patient who has recently started walking, flexes and abducts his hip. Only later after proper training, does he keep it adducted as the leg comes forwards.

Proximal Fixation and Distal Freedom and Vice Versa

Example 1

A simple example may be seen when we consider someone in prone lying. When he is able to take weight on one elbow while manipulating an object with the other hand, he is demonstrating distal fixation of the supporting limb with the trunk free to move over it, while the free limb is moving distally against the proximal support of the steady trunk.

Example 2

A more complex example of the same thing occurs with the much more mature pattern of writing. Here, the supporting arm is offering distal stability to the trunk which is free to move over it. The hand which is putting pen to paper is working freely with a more proximal area of stability in the forearm. However, the forearm must also be partly free to move for each word and so movement at the shoulder has to occur. The shoulder is functioning as a stable and mobile structure at one and the same time against the stable background of the trunk which, in turn, is free to move over the other, or supporting limb. This is a very complex synergy. Little wonder that we cannot write at birth!

Many learning processes depend upon the ability to move. We require movement to be able to explore our environment and unless this is possible, our mental processes cannot develop normally. Head control is essential to movement, but is also essential for the ability to make maximum use of the sense of sight. If we cannot control our head position, it is difficult to gain control over our eye activities. The eyes need to have a stable base from which to work. Eye movements are similar to limbs. They can remain stable while the head moves, or they can move while the head stays still, or the two activities may go on at once, none of this is possible if head control is absent. Assessment of spatial relationship depends upon movement. The relationship between hands and eyes depends upon the ability to move and explore, and the perception of depth, space, height, size and shape have all to be learned by experience dependent upon movements of different area of the body. Balance activities basically start by the balance of the head upon the shoulders in prone lying. Progression is then made by balancing the shoulders over the elbows which offers a forward support in prone lying. In sitting, the body is at first inclined forward so that head balance on the shoulders is still an extension activity and the arms are in a supporting forward position, but with extended elbows. Later, the ability to balance with the arms supporting sideways develops and much later the arms may support by being placed behind as when sitting in a backward leaning position. This requires flexor activity the head and neck to maintain the balance of the head on the shoulders. Before the patient is taught to sit with the backward support training for the rotator ability of the trunk should be done, as it is a precursor to more skillful balance activities. Proper balance is said to be gained when upper limbs can carry out skilled activities, while the legs and trunk are dealing with the maintenance of equilibrium. The development of motor skills is not complete until the hands can be used in prehensile activities and much work has been done by various authors on the developments of prehension. The hand activities are inclined to develop from ulnar to radial side. The grasp and release activities of the early stages in development appear to commence with activity of the little finger and radiate out towards the thumb. Gradually, the radial aspect of the hand becomes more dominant and eventually the pincer grasp between thumb and index finger develops while the ulnar side of the hand takes up a more stabilizing function. Much more mature is the 'dynamic tripod' posture described by Wynn Parry in 1966 and explained by Rosen Bloom and Horton (1971). Here the thumb, index and middle fingers are used as a threesome to give fine coordinate movements of the hand. The classic example of the use of this tripod is in writing although it may be seen in other functional activities.

The process of integrating certain reflex mechanisms involved in movement occurs over a period of time and eventually makes controlled purposeful movement possible. The control develops in a cephalocaudal direction. It is closely linked with perception of body image, intellectual and social behavior and, although it is not dependent upon environment factors, these may influence the rate at which perfection develops. Motor development starts with control of the head position in prone, with the upper limbs most able to take weight in a forward or elbow support position. Later development include rolling and supported sitting with the weight supported forwards on the hands at first, and later at the sides and even later behind. Body rotation begins to be perfected as rolling occurs and limb rotation follows trunk rotation as rule. Movements at first follow primitive patterns of synergy, but later the ability to combine flexion-extension patterns to give more complexity of movement should develop. Ultimate maturity of movement is reached when the hands are totally free from an obligation to balance mechanisms, so that they can be freely developed as skillful tools and used in conjunction with visual and other sensory feedback mechanisms.

The patient is always made to experience the normal movement patterns in the actual and factual environment before placing the demand on the developing brain so that the patient will know what exactly to expect while performing a certain task.

Example 3

To sit in a balanced manner, the patient needs to flex at the hips and extend at the trunk. He needs head control and the ability to support himself forwards on his hands. These are minimum requirement. He is prepared for this naturally by the early development of head control; the elbow and hand support prone position and by lying on his back working out on the trunk flexors. The therapist helps him by propping him into a sitting position so that he experiences it prior to achieving it. Help in this manner makes him experiment and he tries to balance when he is put into sitting and in fact learns to do so.

In the meantime, his rolling and rotatory activities are developing. The patient gradually develops the ability to get into sitting after he has learned to balance in that position.

THE CLINICAL VALUE OF KNOWLEDGE OF DEVELOPMENTAL SEQUENCE

When working with handicapped children, hemiplegic patients and, in particular, with the very young, it is easy to see that this information is exceedingly valuable. When treating babies with movement defects, it is important to start as early as possible and to bear in mind the normal sequence of development so that one can, as far as possible, channel the child's reactions along suitable lines and encourage step by step progress without leaving gaps which may lead to abnormality. The earlier the abnormal child is given help the more successful is the treatment likely to be. It is much more difficult to correct abnormal habits than it is to prevent them from occurring. The child's nervous system is very malleable and able to adapt very readily. Consequently, it can be most easily influenced before it is fully matured. It is a great mistake to wait until the child can consciously cooperate. By this time, irretrievable abnormalities will have developed. The skilled physiotherapist is able to exploit the knowledge of the nervous system to stimulate suitable responses in the childe long before he is aware of cooperating.

However, many physiotherapists deal only with adults or, at least the greater bulk of their patient load is adult. Where then does this knowledge have value? The answer is simply that injury or disease to the control nervous system frequently brings about demyelization of certain areas and may damage or destroy the nervous pathways which have been used to control certain activities. The patient frequently shows a regression of motor skills to a more primitive level. Certain of the reflex mechanisms, which have hitherto been integrated into mature movement patterns, may be partly released from cortical control and may exert an excessive influence over the patient, dominating these movement patterns into abnormality or even preventing them from occurring at all. The patient will frequently show absence or disturbance of normal equilibrium reactions, poverty of movement synergy, perception difficulties and diminution of sensory discrimination. If the physiotherapist is going to help the patient to make full use of such nervous connections as are left, he is more likely to be successful if he has knowledge of the way in which more skilled activities develop in the first place so that he can, to some extent, simulate the conditions to facilitate redevelopment. The following example illustrates this point.

A patient with neurological symptoms can often maintain a sitting position but, on attempting to stand, he pulls himself up by placing his hands on a rigid forward support or by pulling on a helper who is standing in from of him. Frequently, the head is flexed forward or, conversely, it may be thrown back so that the nose is pointing upward. In the first instance, the patient is using the symmetrical tonic neck reflex pattern to aid him into standing, and in the second, his legs are making use of the tonic labyrinthine effect. Neither of these is acceptable as the patterns are those of total reflex synergy, and balance in standing will never be achieved using these patterns. Such a patient has his movement excessively influenced by the tonic reflex mechanisms and requires training to modify them and to start early balance activities. He requires help in receiving weight on to his arms in a forward position. Such activities as elbow-support prone lying are suitable, progressing to hand-support forward side sitting, leading to prone kneeling and hand-support forward standing (standing but resting hands on a stool or low support in front of him). He needs to feel the sensation of weight being received forwards instead of pulling back. There are many other facets to this patient's problems which need attention, but the above example makes the point.

Many head injury case regress to an enormous degree and intellectual and social abilities regress also. Motor training along developmental lines is accompanied, in many cases, by a brightening of intellectual activities and the beginning of social communication. The patient may never achieve behavior patterns which are mature, but he is more likely to make balanced progress if a development approach is used.

Clinical Aspects of Stroke: A Major Cause of Hemiplegia

INTRODUCTION

Strokes are, by far, the most common cause of neurological disability in the adult population. They are responsible for about a quarter of all deaths in the developed countries and account for much disability in the elderly. Of patients who suffer a stroke, about a third will die; a third will survive but with severe disability and the remainder will make a good recovery with functional independence. The onset is usually sudden with maximum deficit at the outset, so the shock to patients and relatives is extreme. Stroke or the cerebrovascular accident is the major cause of the residual hemiplegia in the population.

The 1990 global burden of disease (GBD) study provided the first global estimate on the burden of 135 diseases and cerebrovascular diseases ranked as the second leading cause of death after ischemic heart disease. Data on causes of death from the 1990s have shown that cerebrovascular diseases remain a leading cause of death. In 2001, it was estimated that cerebrovascular diseases (stroke) accounted for 5.5 million deaths worldwide, equivalent to 9.6% of all deaths. Two-thirds of these deaths occurred in people living in developing countries and 40% of the subjects were aged less than 70 years. Additionally, cerebrovascular disease is the leading cause of disability in adults and each year, millions of stroke survivors have to adapt to a life with restrictions in activities of daily living as a consequence of cerebrovascular disease. Many surviving stroke patients will often depend on other people's continuous support to survive. Cerebrovascular diseases can be prevented to a large extent and providing an entry point for public health initiatives to reduce the burden of stroke within a population.

DEFINITION

The term 'stroke' is synonymous with cerebrovascular accident or CVA and is a purely clinical definition which, according to the World Health Organization, can be defined as a *rapidly developed clinical sign of a focal disturbance of cerebral function of presumed vascular origin and of more than 24 hours' duration'*. Included within this definition are most cases of cerebral infarction, cerebral hemorrhage and subarachnoid hemorrhage but deliberately excluded are those cases in which recovery occurs within 24 hours. These latter cases are designated 'transient ischemic attacks' (TIA) and because they are often a harbinger of completed stroke, they have received considerable attention over the past two decades. According to the National Stroke Association:

- 10% of stroke survivors recover almost completely
- 25% recover with minor impairments
- 40% experience moderate-to-severe impairments that require special care
- 10% require care in a nursing home or other long-term facility
- 15% die shortly after the stroke
- Approximately 14% of stroke survivors experience a second stroke in the first year following a stroke.

TYPES OF STROKE

Ischemic

The most common cause of stroke is due to obstruction to one of the major cerebral arteries (middle, posterior and anterior, in that order) or their smaller perforating branches to deeper parts of the brain. Brainstem strokes, arising from disease in the vertebral and basilar arteries, are less common. Some 70 to 75 percent of all strokes are due to occlusion, either as a result of atheroma in the artery itself or secondary to emboli (small clots of blood) being washed up from the heart or diseased neck vessels. The patient does not usually lose consciousness but may complain of headache and symptoms of hemiparesis and/or dysphasia develop rapidly. The hemiplegia is initially flaccid but within a few days, this gives way to the typical spastic type. The middle cerebral artery supplies most of the convexity of the cerebral hemisphere and important deeper structures, so there is a dense contralateral hemiplegia affecting the arm, face and leg. The optic radiation is often affected leading to a contralateral homonymous hemianopia and there may be a cortical type of sensory loss. Aphasia can be severe in left hemisphere lesions and there may be neglect of the contralateral side. In right hemisphere lesions, parietal damage can lead to visuospatial disturbances. If the main part of the middle cerebral artery is not affected, but one of its distal branches is, then the symptoms will be less extreme. Thrombotic cerebral infarction results from the atherosclerotic obstruction of large cervical and cerebral arteries, with ischemia in all or part of the territory of the occluded artery. This can be due to occlusion at the site of the main atherosclerotic lesion or to embolism from this site to more distal cerebral arteries.

Embolic cerebral infarction is due to embolism of a clot in the cerebral arteries coming from other parts of the arterial system, for example, from cardiac lesions, either at the site of the valves or of the heart cardiac cavities, or due to rhythm disturbances with stasis of the blood, which allows clotting within the heart as seen in atrial fibrillation. Lacunar cerebral infarctions are small deep infarcts in the territory of small penetrating arteries, due to a local disease of these vessels, mainly related to chronic hypertension. Several other causes of cerebral infarction exist and are of great practical importance for patient management.

Hemorrhagic

About 5 to 10 percent of strokes are caused due to hemorrhage into the deeper parts of the brain. The patient is usually hypertensive, a condition which leads to particular type of degeneration known as lipohyalinosis in the small penetrating arteries of the brain. The arterial walls weaken and as a result small herniations or microaneurysms develop. These may rupture and the resultant hematomas may spread by splitting along planes of white matter to form a substantial mass lesion. Hematomas usually occur in the deeper parts of the brain, often involving the thalamus, lentiform nucleus and external capsule, less often the cerebellum and the pons. They may rupture into the ventricular system and this is often rapidly fatal. The onset is usually dramatic with severe headache, vomiting and, in about 50 percent of cases, loss of consciousness. The normal vascular autoregulation is lost in the vicinity of the hematoma and since the lesion itself may have considerable mass, intracranial pressure often rises abruptly. If the patient survives the initial ictus, then profound hemiplegic and hemisensory signs may be elicited. A homonymous visual field defect may also be apparent. The initial prognosis is grave but those who begin to recover often do surprisingly well as the hematoma reabsorbs, presumably because fewer neurons are destroyed than in severe ischemic strokes. Occasionally, early surgical drainage can be remarkably successful, particularly when the hematoma is in the cerebellum.

Younger, normotensive patients sometimes suffer from spontaneous intracerebral hematoma from an underlying congenital defect of the blood vessels. Such abnormalities are commonly arteriovenous malformations (AVMs);

circumscribed areas of dilated and thin-walled vessels which can be demonstrated angiographically. Patients with AVMs are liable to subsequent rebleeding and surgical excision is undertaken when possible. Spontaneous intracerebral hemorrhages (as opposed to traumatic ones) are mainly due to arteriolar hypertensive disease and more rarely due to coagulation disorders, vascular malformation within the brain and diet (such as high alcohol consumption, low blood cholesterol concentration, high blood pressure, etc.). Cortical amyloidal angiopathy (a consequence of hypertension) is a cause of cortical hemorrhages especially occurring in elderly people and it is becoming increasingly frequent as populations become older.

Subarachnoid Hemorrhage (SAH)

Between 5 and 10 percent of strokes are due to subarachnoid hemorrhage with bleeding into the subarachnoid space, usually arising from a berry aneurysm situated at or near the circle of Willis. The most common site is in the region of the anterior communicating artery with posterior and middle cerebral artery fusions almost as frequent. Congenital factors play some part in the etiology of berry aneurysms but it is not predominantly a disease of the young, since hypertension and vascular disease lead to an increase in aneurysm size and subsequent rupture.

The patient complains of sudden intense headache often associated with vomiting and neck stiffness. Consciousness may be lost and about 10% will die in the first hour or two. Of those that remain, 40% will die within the first 2 weeks and the survivors have a substantially increased risk from rebleeding for the next six weeks or so. A hemiplegia may be evident at the outset, if the blood erupts into the deep parts of the brain and other focal neurological signs may evolve over the first two weeks because there is a tendency for blood vessels, tracking through the bloody subarachnoid space, to go in spasm leading to secondary ischemic brain damage. Early investigation by angiography, followed by a competent neurosurgical procedure to clip the aneurysm and prevent rebleeding offers the best hope for recovery.

LESS FREQUENT CAUSES OF STROKE

Stroke may occasionally occur in the context of a generalized medical disorder which either affects the arteries or the blood going through them. An arteritis or inflammation of the arteries may complicate meningitis, particularly tuberculous and strokes are relatively common in tertiary syphilis. The collagen vascular diseases, particularly systemic lupus erythematosus (SLE) and polyarteritis nodosa, may affect medium and small cranial arteries. Temporal arteritis, an inflammatory condition predominantly affecting the extracranial and retinal arteries in the elderly, may also give rise to stroke by intracranial involvement. Bacterial infection of damaged heart valves (bacterial endocarditis) is sometimes complicated by stroke, either as result of an immune-mediated arteritis or as a consequence of septic emboli impacting in the cranial arteries. Emboli may also arise from left atrium in patients with atrial fibrillation, particularly if there is coincidental mitral stenosis. More recently, an association between mitral valve prolapse (floppy valve), which is a fairly common congenital abnormality and ischemic stroke has been demonstrated. Hematological diseases such as polycythemia rubra vera, thrombocythemia and sickle cell disease can provoke stasis in the intracranial arteries, thus leading to ischemic brain damage. Completed stroke, occasionally, complicates severe migraine if the vessel spasm, which normally produces only temporary symptoms, is of such intensity and such duration that ischemic damage occurs. Finally, there is some evidence that women taking the contraceptive pill, particularly if it has high estrogen content, suffer slightly higher incidence of stroke than those not on the pill. The absolute risk is small but enhanced by cigarette smoking.

THE STROKE-PRONE POPULATION

Once a stroke has occurred, neurons are irreparably damaged but there is a border zone around the infarct where non-functioning neurons may still be viable if an adequate blood supply can be restored. There is no certain way of doing this at present and so much attention has concentrated on trying to define those subjects in the normal population who are at-risk from having a stroke before they show signs of a compromised cerebral circulation. The risk factors might then be amenable to treatment in the hope that the stroke could be prevented from occurring. The most comprehensive epidemiological study to date has been conducted in Framingham, Massachusetts (Kannel and Wolf, 1983) and the first point to emerge is that while the chance of having a stroke increases with age, it should not be considered as a natural concomitant of increasing age. The most significant risk factor to emerge is hypertension, either systolic (>160 mmHg) or diastolic (>90 mmHg.) The risk of stroke increases dramatically with increasing blood pressure and there is good evidence that prophylactic hypertensive therapy alleviates this susceptibility. Patients with diabetes are also much more likely to suffer a stroke than subjects with normal blood glucose. Abnormal blood lipids, smoking and positive family history are independent risk factors but their effect is relatively minor. The 'final common pathway' for all these risk factors is the arterial disease atherosclerosis, a disease of the larger and medium-sized arteries characterized by the deposition of cholesterol and other substance in the arterial wall. The irregular vessel wall provokes clot formation in the lumen of the artery, which may completely occlude the vessel or may dislodge to form emboli. Hypertension and other risk factors, therefore, predispose to ischemic strokes, the most usual cause for intracerebral hematoma is also hypertension and the associated small vessel disease (lipohyalinosis).

RISK FACTORS FOR CEREBROVASCULAR DISEASE

Many risk factors for stroke have been described. They may refer to inherent biological traits such as age and sex, physiological characteristics that predict future occurrence such as high blood pressure, serum cholesterol, fibrinogen; behaviors such as smoking, diet, alcohol consumption, physical inactivity; social characteristics such as education, social class and ethnicity; and environmental factors that may be physical (temperature, altitude), geographical, or psychosocial. In addition, medical factors including previous TIA or stroke, ischemic heart disease, atrial fibrillation and glucose intolerance, all increase the risk of stroke.

At a population level, blood pressure and tobacco use are the two most important modifiable risk factors for stroke due to their strong associations, high prevalence and the possibility for intervention. Epidemiological research has shown that raised blood pressure is the single most important risk factor for ischemic stroke with a population attributable risk of 50%. The risk of stroke rises steadily as blood pressure level rises and doubles for every 7.5 mmHg increment in diastolic blood pressure, with no lower threshold. Treatment with antihypertensive treatment has been shown to reduce stroke risk by about 38%.

Tobacco use increases the risk of ischemic stroke by about two-fold and is furthermore also associated with a higher risk of hemorrhagic stroke. There is a dose-response relationship so that heavy smokers are at a higher risk of stroke than light smokers. Until recently, studies of tobacco use and stroke focused on smoker's risk, however, exposure to environmental tobacco smoking is also an independent risk factor for stroke. This study suggested that previous analyses based on reference groups without differentiating exposure between non-smokers might have led to a general underestimation of the risk of stroke in smokers. While most studies of risk factors for ischemic stroke are based on data from populations in developed countries, there is some evidence from developing countries that many of the risk factors are similar including blood pressure, tobacco use, and obesity. There are estimated 1.2 billion smokers worldwide. In China alone, there are 300 million smokers. A review on obesity from Latin-American countries showed that the prevalence of over-weight people, especially in urban areas, may be as high as the prevalence reported in developed nations. The present knowledge on the prevalence of major risk factors in developing countries is, however, very limited.

Risk factors for stroke:
- Hypertension
- Heredity
- Diabetes mellitus
- Transient ischemic attacks (TIA)
- Cardiac abnormalities
- Carotid bruit
- Hyperlipidemia
- Estrogen contraceptive pill
- Cigarette smoking
- Elevated hematocrit.

CAUSES OF ISCHEMIC STROKE

Thrombosis:
- Atherosclerosis
- Arteritis:
  - Temporal arteritis
  - Granulomatous arteritis
  - Polyarteritis
  - Wegener's granulomatosis
  - Granulomatous arteritis of great vessels (Takayasu's arteritis, syphilis)
- Dissections:
  - Carotid
  - Vertebral
  - Intracranial arteries at the base of the brain (spontaneous or traumatic)
- Hematological disorders:
  - Polycythemia $1°$ or $2°$
  - Sickle cell disease
  - Thrombotic thrombocytopenic purpura, etc.
- Cerebral mass effect compressing intracranial arteries:
  - Tentorial herniations—post cerebral artery
  - Giant aneurysm—middle cerebral artery

- Miscellaneous:
  - Moyamoya disease
  - Fibromuscular dysplasia
  - Binswanger's disease

Vasoconstriction:

- Cerebral vasospasm following SAH
- Reversible cerebral vasoconstriction:
  - Etiology unknown, following migraine, trauma, eclampsia of pregnancy.

Embolism:

- Atherothrombotic arterial source:
  - Bifurcation common carotid artery
  - Carotid siphon
  - Distal vertebral artery
  - Aortic arch
- Cardiac source:
  - Structural heart diseases
- Congenital: Mitral valve prolapse, patent foramen ovale, etc.
- Acquired: Following MI, marantic vegetation, etc.
  - Dysrhythmia, atrial fibrillation, sick sinus syndrome, etc.
  - Infection, acute bacterial endocarditis
- Unknown source:
  - Healthy child or adult
  - Associations
- Hypercoagulable state secondary to systemic disease
- Carcinoma, particularly pancreatic
- Eclampsia of pregnancy
- Oral contraceptive pills
- Lupus
- Anticoagulants
- Factor C deficiency
- Factor S deficiency, etc.

THREATENED STROKE

Transient ischemic attacks (TIAs)

A transient ischemic attack refers to a stroke-like syndrome in which recovery is complete within 24 hours. They are important to recognize because some patients (about 10% per year) will go not to have a complete stroke. The symptoms depend on which part of the brain has been temporarily deprived of blood.

The symptoms evolve rapidly and resolve more gradually, but it is unusual for the whole episode to last more than an hour and there are no permanent neurological deficits. Sometimes the retinal artery is involved, and here; the patient complains of a unilateral visual field disturbance, or blindness, often descending like a curtain across the vision. Within half-an-hour or so (often much more rapidly), the veil lifts vision is restored. This syndrome is known as amaurosis fugax and it is particularly important because observations have been made on patients during the attacks which have thrown light on the mechanism of TIA in general.

By the use of ophthalmoscope, the observer can see the retinal vessel and several authors have reported small platelet and cholesterol plugs, blocking the retinal arteries during an attack of amaurosis fugax (Fisher, 1959). These plugs subsequently disperse, blood flow is re-established and vision recovers. The emboli may come from atherosclerotic plaques in the internal carotid artery, sometimes the heart acts as the source, and it is argued that TIAs characterized by hemispheric disturbances are due to the same process, with emboli ascending to the cerebral rather than the ophthalmic and retinal vessels. Brainstem TIA also occurs with symptoms ranging from transient vertigo to sudden loss of consciousness, and here emboli is thought to arise from the vertebral arteries, aorta and heart. The importance of TIA is that if source of emboli can be defined, then it is sometimes amenable to surgery. For example, carotid endarterectomy or medical treatment with antiplatelet drugs such as aspirin can be useful.

Leaking Aneurysm

About 40% of patients who develop a subarachnoid hemorrhage due to rupture of an aneurysm have preceding symptoms which suggest minor leaks. These usually occur within a month of the major bleed and often go unrecognized by the patient and doctor alike. Symptoms which suggest a minor subarachnoid bleed are sudden headache accompanied by nausea, photophobia and sometimes neck stiffness. The symptoms can resolve rapidly and may be incorrectly attributed to migraine. If a bleed is suspected then it should be confirmed by CT scan and/or lumbar puncture because most of these patients will go on a major bleed with devastating consequences. The operative risk in a healthy subject who has a minor bleed is much less than in the patient who has suffered a major subarachnoid hemorrhage.

Asymptomatic Carotid Bruit

A noise (or bruit) is sometimes heard over the carotid artery during the routine medical examination. The bruit suggests turbulent blood flow due to underlying atherosclerosis and it is referred to as asymptomatic carotid bruit if present in an otherwise healthy individual. Some 5% patients per year who have a bruit will not have a stroke, though not always in the distribution artery.

STROKE MIMICS

Following an ischemic stroke, interventions to bring about reperfusion must be implemented within the recognized timeframe; this means that timely clinical recognition of this condition is vital. The process of diagnosis begins with the initial bedside assessment of the patient to be followed by appropriate imaging studies. However, because reperfusion therapy may be attended by significant adverse consequences and since imaging may be negative for many hours after stroke onset, the clinician must be aware of conditions that mimic cerebral ischemia.

STROKE IN THE YOUNG INDIAN POPULATION

Most of the studies carried out in India have shown that about 10–15% of strokes occur in those below 40 years of age, which is high compared to other countries. This could be due to many local etiological factors. Previously, causes contributing to stroke in the young were reported as meningovascular syphilis in men, puerperal cerebral venous thrombosis in women and rheumatic heart disease in both sexes. A disturbance in the balance of coagulation and fibrinolysis has been suggested in the etiopathology of non-embolic cerebral infarction in the young. Other studies have incriminated subacute tubercular meningitis, leading to arteritis or autoimmune angiitis, as an important risk factor in India. More recently reported risk factors among the young include viper envenomation, elevated lipoprotein (a) and elevated anticardiolipin antibodies. A recent Indian study suggests that the squatting posture adopted in the toilet could be an important triggering factor for stroke in Indians, by the mechanism of raising the blood pressure.

OTHER UNUSUAL CAUSES OF STROKE IN CHILDREN

Stroke is always a consideration when a previously healthy child or infant suddenly develops focal neurological disturbance. Half of these cases are of ischemic etiology and half are non-traumatic intracerebral and subarachnoid hemorrhages arising from vascular malformation. In children, ischemic stroke may be precipitated by a hemoglobinopathy (e.g. sickle cell anemia), hypercoagulable state, congenital and rheumatic heart disease, trauma, vasculitis, and vasculopathies such as MELAS (mitochondrial myopathy, encephalopathy, lactic acidosis, and stroke-like episodes). Nonvascular causes of focal neurological disturbances include alternating hemiplegia, migraine, seizures, Kawasaki disease, trauma and space occupying lesions.

STROKE WITH ATYPICAL PRESENTATION

Strokes with atypical presentations that take on the appearance of other disease process may change and evolve with time. The clinician is left with the daunting problem of discovering the unusual manifestation of an uncommon clinical process. A seemingly infinite number of unusual clinical syndromes have been attributed to ischemic stroke after thorough investigation. The presence of historical risk factors for cerebrovascular disease and the abrupt onset of symptoms may be the best clues available to the emergency physician to detect these unusual stroke syndromes. A few that are of clinical importance are briefly summarized:

- Most strokes present as a deficit or loss of function. Uncommonly, movement disorders will present due to a focal lesion such as an ischemic stroke or hemorrhage. Acute hemiballismus or unilateral dyskinesias often result from acute vascular lesions in the subthalamic nucleus or connections. The movements may vary from wild flinging movements to mild uncontrollable unilateral movements. The key to diagnosis is the abrupt onset of symptoms and the presence of risk factors for cerebrovascular disease. A review note that any kind of dyskinesias, hypokinetic as well as hyperkinetic, may be found from lesions at many different levels in the frontal motor cortical and subcortical regions.

- Confusional states, agitation, and delirium have all been reported as a consequence of focal neurologic injury; structures involving the limbic cortex of the temporal lobes and the orbitofrontal regions are commonly involved. These states must be distinguished from the neglect syndromes and fluent aphasias in which patients are often reported as confused but careful examination demonstrates a clear focal deficit. In syndromes of visual neglect especially, testing for visual fields will reveal a dramatic field cut that the patient cannot report since he or she is unaware of the deficit.

■ Sensory complaints of either unusual sensations or loss of sensation are common in parietal and thalamic strokes. At times, the sensory manifestation of a stroke may take on the characteristics of another clinical condition. Chest pain and limb pain that mimicked that of myocardial infarction were reported in a small series of patients; most had thalamic strokes but one had a lateral medullary infarct. Sensory symptoms may occur with lesions in many places in the central nervous system. Cortical involvement is usually accompanied by other neurologic deficits such as hemiparesis, aphasia, hemineglect, or visual field abnormalities.

■ Cortical blindness is unusual but may occur; it can be distinguished from bilateral ocular disease by the normal pupillary light responses and normal optic disks. As many as 10% of patients with cortical blindness deny visual symptoms (Anton's syndrome); at times, there is an element of 'blind sight,' with patients retaining some residual visual ability in their blind areas. For example, patients with blind sight may make correct 'guesses' about movements or colors of objects in the visually deficient areas, demonstrating some remnant perception of which they are not consciously aware.

Clinical Diagnosis of Neurological Condition

INTRODUCTION

As in other branches of medicine, the art of the neurologist consists of making a diagnosis from the patient's own account of his illness and from a physical examination aided by appropriate radiographic or laboratory tests. Once the diagnosis has been reached, suitable treatment can be given and the outlook predicted. What distinguishes neurology from its sister specialties, is the degree of attention to detail in taking the medical history and in examining the patient. This quest detail, so mysterious to the non-neurologist, is linked to a wealth of knowledge of nervous anatomy, physiology and pathology, accumulated over more than a century, the application of which at the bedside often enables a precise diagnosis to be made. Now that computerized tomography (CT-scanning) and magnetic resonance imaging (MRI) have become generally available, the brain can be X-rayed as readily as the chest, resulting in a trend toward simpler clinical neurological assessment.

BEDSIDE ASSESSMENT OF STROKE

Simultaneous to the process of confirming the diagnosis of stroke, there needs to be an ongoing assessment at the bedside. The initial evaluation of a potential stroke patient is similar to that of other critically ill patients: Stabilization of airway, breathing and circulation (ABC). This is quickly followed by a secondary assessment of the neurological deficits and possible comorbidities. The overall goal is not only to identify patients with possible stroke but also to exclude stroke mimics, identify other conditions requiring immediate intervention and determine potential causes of the stroke for early secondary prevention. A good history and a thorough physical examination to elicit the associated signs may help in differentiating stroke from the common mimics.

NEUROLOGICAL CASE HISTORY

For the neurologist, a complete and accurate history is essential. Very often a precise diagnosis can be made from the history, and examination is simply confirmatory; the converse, a physical examination which provides signs not predicable from the history, tends to come as a surprise. Although it may not be absolutely accurate, some early historical data and clinical findings may direct the physician toward a diagnosis of another cause for the patient's symptoms. Alteration of mental status or loss of consciousness, in the absence of lateralizing symptoms or signs, points towards metabolic or other causes of encephalopathy. March of symptoms or positive symptoms is indicative of increased brain activity as seen in seizures. Headache, as the presenting symptom in the appropriate (young) age-group, is more likely to represent, migraine, though, it is also a feature seen commonly in stroke.

In addition to the historical aspects of the symptoms, it is important to ask about risk factors for atherosclerosis and cardiac disease in all patients, as well as any history of cigarette smoking, migraine, seizure, infection, trauma, or pregnancy. Historical data necessary for deciding the eligibility of the patient for therapeutic interventions in acute ischemic stroke are equally important. Bystanders or family witnesses should be asked for information about onset time and historical issues, especially when patients are unable to speak or provide history. A list of the patient's medications, or the medication containers themselves, should be sought, with particular attention paid to identifying any anticoagulant (both oral and injectable), anti-platelet and antihypertensive drug use.

The description of the tempo of the illness—acute or chronic, coming on slowly or abruptly, steadily progressive or remitting, often suggests the type of pathological process. Vascular problems are usually of acute onset, tumor symptoms and tend steadily to progress, demyelinating disease may remit. The characterization of symptoms is then attempted, the neurologist assisting the patient with suitable questions. 'Headaches', 'dizziness' and 'fainting' are three of the most frequent problems dealt with in neurological clinics. It is the task of the neurologist to decide if the patient's headaches are from a brain tumor or simply from muscular tension or from migraine. Dizziness may signify disease of the balance mechanisms in the ear and brainstem. Faints may or may not mean neurological disease: Epilepsy may resemble fainting attacks and careful enquiry with specific questions is often needed to obtain a clear picture of such episodes. Other symptoms of special significance to the neurologist include disturbances of memory or concentration; loss of vision; double vision; facial pain or weakness; difficulty with speech or swallowing; weakness, wasting, pain or numbness in a limb; abnormal movements; trouble with walking; and disturbance of bladder control. Each of these symptoms, described by the patient, has a range of possible cause which needs to be considered, thus, it will set in train a particular process of enquiry as the neurologist attempts on the basis of the information given by the patient — to form a clear image of the nature and localization of the underlying neurological disorder.

THE NEUROLOGICAL EXAMINATION

To a certain extent, neurological examination begins from the moment the patient enters the consulting room. Gait, mental attitude, alertness and speech may all give important diagnostic clues. However, the formal examination of the nervous system follows completion of history-taking.

- Testing of the head, trunk and limbs for motor and sensory function is preceded by an evaluation of mental state and intellectual level.
- The patient's overall appearance and behavior, mood, orientation, thought processes memory and intelligence may be affected in many brain diseases and need to be assessed.
- A disturbance of speech may point to a disorder of the dominant cerebral hemisphere or of motor control.
- The carotid arteries are felt and listened to in the neck to check on arterial blood flow to the brain, neck movement is tested and the skull is felt and listened to for abnormal sounds.
- Functions of the cranial nerves are then examined in turn. Sense of smell (olfactory nerves); visual fields, visual activity, optic fundi—using the ophthalmoscope (optic nerves); examination of the pupils (oculomotor nerves) and of eye movement (oculomotor, trochlear and abducent nerves); facial sensation, corneal sensation and reflexes, jaw movement (trigeminal nerves); facial movement (facial nerves); hearing (auditory nerves); palatal sensation and movement (glossopharyngeal and vagus nerves); movement of sternomastoid and trapezius muscles (spinal accessory nerves); and tongue movement (hypoglossal nerves) are the major cranial nerve functions assessed in a full neurological examination. Abnormalities observed in any of these will suggest the anatomical basis of the patient's complaint.

■ The systematic examination of the trunk and limbs includes both motor and sensory testing; the patient's symptoms should suggest which of these is carried out first, since either can be tiring. In order to decide if muscle function is normal or abnormal, the doctor must first carefully look at the limbs for signs of muscle wasting, abnormality of posture (suggesting muscular imbalance), involuntary movement (which may be a sign of extrapyramidal disease) and fasciculation (often a sign of damage to motor nerve cells). The neurologist then evaluates the tone of the limb musculature (the state of tension in the muscles, which may be increased or decreased under abnormal conditions), assesses power systematically, muscle group by muscle group, looks for signs of incoordination of movement and tests the tendon reflexes (which can reveal derangement of function at or above or below the spinal segments each represents).

■ Sensation from different zones of skin is conveyed to the nervous system via different spinal nerves and spinal cord segments, while distinct forms of skin sensation (e.g. pain and touch) have separate pathways in the nervous system. Clearly, careful sensory testing can also be of great localizing value. In practice, the neurologist will often test pain sensation with a pin, touch with a piece of cotton wool and joint position sense by carefully moving a finger or toe. He makes much use of the vibration of a tuning fork as an overall test of sensory function.

PHYSICAL EXAMINATION

■ The general physical examination continues from the original assessment of the airway, breathing and circulation (ABC) and should include pulse oximetry and body temperature.

■ Examination of the head and neck may reveal signs of trauma or seizure activity (e.g. contusions or tongue biting), carotid disease (bruits), or congestive heart failure (jugular venous distension).

■ The cardiac examination focuses on identifying concurrent myocardial ischemia, valvular conditions and irregular rhythm and, in rare cases, aortic dissection, which could precipitate a cardioembolic event.

■ The respiratory and abdominal examinations seek to identify other co-morbidities.

■ Examination of the skin and extremities may also provide insight into important systemic conditions such as hepatic dysfunction, coagulopathies, or platelet disorders (e.g. jaundice, purpura, or petechia).

NEUROLOGICAL EXAMINATION AND STROKE SCALE SCORES

The emergency physician's neurological examination should be brief but thorough. It is enhanced by use of a formal stroke score or scale, such as the NIH Stroke Scale (NIHSS). It enables examiners to rapidly detect focal neurological deficits. In addition, it may help quantify the neurological deficit resulting from a stroke and is useful in monitoring progress with stroke treatment such as thrombolysis. The scale can be used by a broad spectrum of non-neurological healthcare providers. Use of a standardized examination helps to ensure that the major components of a neurological examination are performed in a timely fashion. These scores not only help to quantify the degree of neurological deficit but also facilitate communication between healthcare professionals, identify the possible location of vessel occlusion, provide early prognosis and help to identify patient eligibility for various interventions and the potential for complications. It may also have some predictive value in detecting stroke mimics. Several studies have demonstrated that emergency physicians committed to stroke care may correctly identify and safely treat stroke patients, especially with the use of such standardized scales. Access to neurological expertize when required may benefit care of the stroke patient.

DIAGNOSTIC TESTS

Diagnostic tests should be performed routinely in patients with suspected ischemic stroke to identify systemic conditions that may mimic or cause stroke or that may influence therapeutic options. Neuroimaging in the form of CT and MRI are critically important. While non-contrast CT scan is useful in distinguishing hemorrhagic from ischemic stroke, it is of limited diagnostic value in differentiating stroke from stroke mimics. It may remain normal up to 24 hours from symptoms onset in ischemic stroke patients. Contrast CT, including CT perfusion (CTP) and CT angiogram (CTA), can contribute significantly to this differentiation. An abnormal CTP or CTA will not only aid in confirming the diagnosis of ischemic stroke, but also enable detection of contrast-enhancing lesions such as tumor and abscess. MR diffusion-weighted imaging has been found to have a high sensitivity and specificity in the early diagnosis of ischemic stroke. Perfusion-weighted imaging, which requires MR imaging with contrast, may be a useful adjunct to non-contrast DWI in confirming the diagnosis of ischemic stroke.

In addition to the neuroimaging modalities, blood tests are useful in the diagnosis of the stroke mimics. These tests include blood glucose measurement, complete blood count with platelet count, prothrombin time, activated partial thromboplastin time, international normalized ratio and renal function studies. Hypoglycemia may cause focal symptoms and signs that mimic stroke and hyperglycemia is associated with unfavorable outcomes. Determination of the platelet count and, in patients taking warfarin or with liver dysfunction, the prothrombin time/international normalized ratio is important. Because time is critical, it is advocated that thrombolytic therapy should be started for stroke patients while awaiting the results of the prothrombin time, activated partial thromboplastin time, or platelet count; therapy with thrombolytic drugs is withheld in absence of these test results, if a bleeding abnormality or thrombocytopenia is suspected, if the patient has been taking warfarin and heparin, or if there is any uncertainty regarding anticoagulation use.

FURTHER TESTS

Radiographs

These are invaluable for disease affecting the bones of the skull and the spine. However, they cannot show the soft tissue contained inside. For these to be seen, it is necessary either to inject into the blood vessels of the brain or cord a substance which is opaque to X-rays (angiography) or to outline the nervous tissue by defining the fluid spaces within and outside them, using air or an opaque medium (pneumoencephalography or ventriculography for the brain; myelography for spinal cord). The selective uptake of radioactive isotopes by diseased nervous tissue can be used to produce images of the brain (isotope scans).

The CT scanner, mentioned earlier, gives in many cases a definitive structural diagnosis. Its principle is the detection of minute changes of tissue density from point to point inside the head. In this way, radiography of the brain itself, and not just the skull, can be assembled.

Electrodiagnostic Tests

- These involve the amplification and recording of the electrical activity of nervous tissue and have certain diagnostic applications. Electro-encephalography (EEG) is useful in the investigation of some epileptic patients, in some cases of coma and in certain forms of encephalitis.
- Electromyography is an essential part of the evaluation of patients with neuromuscular disease. Measurement of sensory and motor nerve conduction is equally essential in the study of lesions of the peripheral nervous system.

Cerebrospinal Fluid Tests

These are important in neurological diagnosis. Lumbar puncture is the usual technique for obtaining a sample. It is a necessary procedure where meningitis or subarachnoid hemorrhage is suspected and it may give useful information in certain inflammatory diseases of brain tissue. Examination of the cerebrospinal fluid is indicated if the patient has symptoms suggestive of subarachnoid hemorrhage and a CT scan does not demonstrate blood.

Other Tests

- A clinical cardiovascular examination, measurement of serum levels of cardiac enzymes, and a 12-lead ECG may be performed in all stroke patients. Cardiac abnormalities are common among patients with stroke and the patient can have an acute cardiac condition that mandates urgent treatment. For example, acute myocardial infarction can lead to stroke and acute stroke can lead to myocardial ischemia.
- In addition, cardiac arrhythmias can occur among patients with acute ischemic stroke. Atrial fibrillation, an important potential cause of stroke, can be detected in the acute setting. Cardiac monitoring should be conducted routinely after an acute cerebrovascular event to screen for serious cardiac arrhythmias.
- Although CT scan is more sensitive than MRI in detecting subarachnoid blood in the acute phase, in the subacute phase, MRI sequences, in particular gradient-echo T2 images followed by fluid-attenuated inversion recovery (FLAIR) images, are considered to be the most sensitive. The clinical features of subarachnoid hemorrhage differ considerably from those of ischemic stroke. Cerebrospinal fluid analysis may be of additional value when CNS infection needs to be excluded as the cause for the stroke-like presentation.
- Electroencephalography may be helpful for evaluating patients in whom seizures are suspected as the cause of the neurological deficits or in whom seizures could have been a complication of the stroke. Seizure in the absence of imaging confirmation of acute ischemia is a relative contraindication for the use of rt-PA in acute ischemic stroke.
- Additional tests may be performed as indicated by the patient's history, symptoms, physical findings, or comorbidity. A toxicology screen, blood alcohol level, arterial blood gas and pregnancy test should be obtained if the physician is uncertain about the patient's history or if suggested by findings on examination.

In summary, bedside assessment is important in distinguishing stroke from stroke mimics. Blood tests and brain imaging are often useful adjuncts to bedside assessment. The latter may play critical roles in identification of stroke, decision to treat and prioritization of tests, in view of the fact that thrombolytic therapy carries the risk of bleeding and is often limited by a narrow time window of opportunity. Despite recent advances in stroke therapy, the majority of stroke patients do not seek immediate medical attention. Even in developed countries like USA, UK and France, there is a lack of knowledge among stroke patients about warning symptoms and risk factors. In a multicenter survey in USA, over one-half of the patients at increased risk for stroke were unaware of their risk factors. This study reveals the importance of the need of research in India. Intravenous (IV) recombinant tissue plasminogen activator (rt-PA) is being used for acute ischemic stroke in India. Knowledge about stroke warning symptoms and risk factors is essential for the patients to effectively utilize the thrombolytic therapy for acute stroke. In country like India, studies regarding stroke patients' knowledge about warning symptoms and risk factors should be carefully evaluated for prompt treatment and hence reduction in overall disability.

5

Symptoms of Brain Damage

CNS DISORDERS AND BRODAL'S PASSAGE

Anatomist Brodal (1973)

A Norwegian anatomist named Brodal, suffered stroke and reports his own experiences.

The patient had found that destruction of even a minor part of the brain causes changes in number of functions, which are difficult to study objectively. They were, however, very obvious to him. They are what one might call general deficits of the brain.

- Loss of concentration power
- Reduced short-term memory
- Reduced initiative
- Incontinence of movements of emotional expression and other phenomena.

It has also been astonishing to note how long it takes for these symptoms to improve visibly. Even after ten months, if the patient seems to be as he was, apart from his slight remaining paresis, he is *painfully aware* that this is not so.

CNS Disorders

CNS lesions or stroke produces sudden and devastating trauma to the entire personality. Main problems arising from the "functional disturbances" are very complex:

- Somatosensory
- Motor
- Speech and language
- Visuospatial
- Cognitive

- Perceptual
- Behavioral.

These disturbances are frequent causes of disability ranging from moderate-to-severe depending upon the *side, site* and *area of lesion.* The stroke divides the body into two separate halves, distorting the body symmetry and image and causing *alien arm syndrome* in left hemiplegics. The cortex is subject to faulty sensory input misinformation resulting in derangement of entire normal postural reflex mechanism causing:

- Weakness (hemiparesis) or paralysis (hemiplegia) on one side of the body that may affect the whole side or just the arm or leg; the weakness or paralysis is on the side of the body opposite the side of the brain affected by the stroke
- Spasticity, stiffness in muscles and painful muscle spasms
- Problems with balance and/or coordination
- Problems using language, including having difficulty understanding speech or writing (aphasia); and knowing the right words but having trouble saying them clearly (dysarthria)
- Being unaware of or ignoring sensations on one side of the body (body neglect or inattention)
- Pain, numbness or odd sensations
- Problems with memory, thinking, attention or learning
- Being unaware of the effects of a stroke
- Trouble in swallowing (dysphagia)
- Problems with bowel or bladder control
- Fatigue
- Difficulty controlling emotions (emotional liability)
- Depression
- Difficulties with daily tasks.

Spasticity

The concepts and origins of spasticity are also changing; it has always become a controversial subject with the neurophysiologist. Earlier believed to be due to overactivity of the myotatic stretch reflex of the muscle spindle and loss of inhibitory cortical control, is today believed to be due to hyperactivity of long tracts—corticospinal, vestibular spinal and reticulospinal. This is the outcome of the recent studies of spindle activity by neuroelectrodes of selected nerve trunks which did not correlate well with the hyperactive tendon reflex.

Sensations

Impairments result in distorting information from the self and environment affecting:

- Superficial sensations
- Joint position sense
- Perceptual: This refers to activity occurring in secondary and tertiary sensory associated areas of the cortex which integrate information such as memory, context and experience.

Lesions in parietal lobes disturb sensory integration:

- Neglect
- Hemianopia
- Unawareness of the body parts, distorted body image and left-right disorientation
- Inability to localize body parts
- Alien-arm syndrome
- Bizarre statements regarding body parts and position of their limbs
- Referring to paralyzed limbs with different names
- Inattention and increased fatigue
- Lack of concentration and initiative
- Emotional liability
- Reduced short-term memory
- Speech without context
- Underestimating the gravity of the disability
- Studies of lesions in CNS have shown that:
  - Corticospinal and rubrospinal tracts are important for distal muscle control and function
  - Vestibular reticulospinal tracts are more critical for maintenance of posture and postural adjustments, balance, position of head in space, body righting, ocular stability and proximal motor control
  - Basal ganglia and cerebellum and vestibular system are critical for balance and postural adjustment and most important for ensuring harmonious, coordinated and most precise performance of movements.

Successful rehabilitation depends on:

- Amount of damage to the brain
- Skill on the part of the rehabilitation team
- Cooperation of family and friends. Caring family/friends can be one of the most important factors in rehabilitation

■ Timing of rehabilitation—the earlier it begins, the more likely survivors are to regain lost abilities and skills.

The goal of rehabilitation is to enable an individual who has experienced a stroke to reach the highest possible level of independence and be as productive as possible. Because stroke survivors often have complex rehabilitation needs, progress and recovery are unique for each person. Although a majority of functional abilities may be restored soon after a stroke, recovery is an ongoing process.

■ Hospital programs: In an acute care facility or a rehabilitation hospital.

■ Long-term care facility with therapy and skilled nursing care

■ Outpatient programs

■ Home-based programs.

Preventing Another Stroke

Stroke

People who have had a stroke are at an increased risk of having another one, especially during the first year following the original stroke.

The following factors increase the risk of having another stroke if they do not modify their previous lifestyle:

■ High blood pressure (hypertension)

■ Cigarette smoking

■ Diabetes

■ Having had a TIA (transient ischemic attack)

■ Heart disease

■ Older age

■ High cholesterol

■ Obesity

■ Sedentary lifestyle.

Although some risk factors for stroke cannot be changed (e.g. age), others such as high blood pressure and smoking can be altered. Patients and families should seek guidance from their physician about lifestyle changes to help prevent another stroke.

SITES OF LESION AND CLINICAL MANIFESTATION (TABLE 5.1)

Hemiplegia that spares cranial musculature may be caused by a lesion in the lateral column of the spinal cord at cervical level. Usually, the symptoms

TABLE 5.1	Sites of lesion and clinical manifestation
Site of lesion	**Clinical manifestation**
Cerebral cortex, cerebral white matter, internal capsule	Weakness or paralysis of face, arm, and leg in the contralateral side
Cortical or subcortical	Convulsive seizures, aphasia, astereognosis, two point discrimination loss, anosognosia
Small discrete lesion in posterior horn of internal capsule, cerebral peduncle, or medullary pyramids	Pure motor hemiplegia affecting the face, arm and leg
Corticospinal, corticobulbar tracts in upper brainstem	Paralysis of face, arm, and leg in contralateral side, cranial nerve deficit on same side
Brainstem syndrome	Paralysis of oculomotor nerve on same side with contralateral limb paresis is known as Weber's syndrome
Low pontine lesions	Same sided abducent or facial palsy combined with contralateral limb paresis is known as Millard Gubler syndrome
Medulla	Affect the tongue, sometimes pharynx and larynx on one side and arm and leg on the other side
Basis pontis	Ataxic hemiplegia with or without dysarthria

are bilateral and hence, result in quadriplegia. Homolateral paralysis, if combined with a loss of vibratory and position sense on the same side and contralateral loss of pain and temperature is known as *Brown-Séquard Syndrome.*

Muscle atrophy of minor degree is often associated with hemiplegia but never reaches the proportions seen in diseases of the lower motor neurons. The reason for this is the disuse of the affected part. There is an important exception in this rule: when the motor cortex and adjacent parts of the parietal lobe are damaged in infancy or childhood, the normal development of the muscles and the skeletal system in the affected limbs is retarded and the palsied limbs and even the trunk on one side are small. If hemiplegia occurs after reaching the puberty, the skeletal system and hence, the size of the body parts are not affected.

SIGNS AND SYMPTOMS AND STRUCTURES INVOLVED

See Table 5.2.

TABLE 5.2	Signs and symptoms and the structures involved

Signs and symptoms	Structures involved
Paralysis of the contralateral face, arm and leg, sensory impairment over the same area	Somatic motor area for face and arm and the fibers descending from the leg area to enter the corona radiata and corresponding somatic sensory system
Motor aphasia	Motor speech area of the dominant hemisphere
Central aphasia, word deafness, anomia, jargon speech, sensory agraphia, acalculia, alexia, finger agnosia, right-left confusion (Last four- Gerstmann syndrome)	Central, suprasylvian speech area and parietooccipital cortex of the dominant hemisphere
Conduction aphasia	Central speech area (parietal operculum)
Apractognosia of the minor hemisphere (amorphosynthesis), anosognosia, hemiasomatognosia, unilateral neglect, agnosia for the left half of external space, dressing apraxia, constructional apraxia, distortions of visual coordinates, inaccurate localizations in the left field, impaired ability to judge distance, upside down reading, visual illusions	Nondominant parietal lobe, loss of topographic memory is usually due to a nondominant lesion, occasionally to a dominant one
Homonymous hemianopia	Optic radiation deep to 2nd temporal convolution
Paralysis of conjugate gaze to opposite side	Frontal contraversive field of fibers projecting there from
Paralysis of opposite foot and leg	Motor leg area
A lesser degree of paresis of opposite arm	Arm area of cortex, or fibers descending to corona radiata there from
Urinary incontinence	Sensory motor area in paracentral lobule
Cortical sensory loss over toes, foot and leg	Sensory area for foot and leg

Contd...

Contd...

Signs and symptoms	Structures involved
Contralateral grasp reflex, sucking reflex, gegenhalten (paratonic rigidity)	Medial surface of the posterior frontal lobe, supplemental area
Abulia (akinetic mutism), slowness, delay, intermittent interruptions, lack of spontaneity, whispering, reflex distraction to sight and sound	Uncertain localization—probably cingulate gyrus and medial inferior portion of frontal, parietal, and temporal lobes
Impairment of gait and stance (gait apraxia)	Frontal cortex near leg motor area
Dyspraxia of left limbs, tactile aphasia in left limbs	Corpus callosum
Homonymous hemianopia	Calcarine cortex or optic radiation
Bilateral homonymous hemianopia, cortical blindness, awareness or denial of blindness, tactile naming, achromatopsia (color blindness), failure to see to-and-fro movements, inability to perceive objects not centrally located, apraxia of ocular movements, inability to count or enumerate objects, tendency to run into things which the patient sees and tries to avoid	Bilateral occipital lobe with possibly the parietal lobe involvement
Verbal dyslexia without agraphia, color anomia	Dominant calcarine lesion and posterior part of corpus callosum
Memory defect	Hippocampal lesion bilaterally or on the dominant side only
Topographic disorientation and prosopagnosia	Nondominant calcarine and lingual gyrus
Simultagnosia, hemivisual neglect	Dominant visual cortex, contralateral hemisphere
Unformed visual hallucinations, peduncular hallucinosis, meta-morphopsia, teleopsia, illusory visual spread, irreminiscence, palinopsia, distortion of outlines, central photophobia	Calcarine cortex

Contd...

Contd...

Signs and symptoms	Structures involved
Complex hallucinations	Usually nondominant hemisphere
Thalamic syndrome: Sensory loss (all modalities), spontaneous pain and dysesthesias, choreoathetosis, intention tremor, spasms of hand, mild hemiparesis	Posteroventral nucleus of thalamus, involvement of the adjacent subthalamus body or its afferent tracts
Thalamoperforate syndrome: Crossed cerebellar ataxia with ipsilateral third nerve palsy (Claude's syndrome)	Dentothalamic tract and issuing third nerve
Weber's syndrome	Third nerve and central peduncle
Contralateral hemiplegia	Cerebral peduncle
Paralysis or paresis of vertical eye movement, skew deviation, sluggish papillary responses to light, slight miosis and ptosis, (retraction nystagmus and tucking of the eyelids may be present)	Supranuclear fibers to third nerve, interstitial nucleus of Cajal, nucleus of Darkschewitsch, and posterior commissure
Contralateral rhythmic, ataxic action tremor, rhythmic postural or holding tremor	Dentothalamic tract
Medial medullary syndrome (occlusion of vertebral artery or branch of vertebral or lower basilar artery) 1. *On side of lesion*: Paralysis with atrophy of half the tongue 2. *Opposite side of lesion*: Paralysis of arm and leg sparing face, impaired tactile and proprioceptive sense over half side of the body Lateral medullary syndrome (occlusion of any of the five vessels may be responsible—vertebral, posterior inferior cerebellar, superior, middle, or inferior lateral medullary arteries)	Ipsilateral 12th nerve Contralateral pyramidal tract and medial lemniscus

Contd...

Contd...

Signs and symptoms	Structures involved
On the side of lesion: • Pain, numbness, impaired sensation over half the face • Ataxia of limbs, falling to side of lesion • Nystagmus, diplopia, oscillopsia, vertigo, nausea, vomiting • Horner's syndrome: miosis, ptosis, anhydrosis • Dysphagia, hoarseness, paralysis of palate, paralysis of vocal cord, diminished gag reflex • Loss of taste • Numbness of ipsilateral arm, trunk or leg *On side opposite to lesion:* Impaired pain and thermal sense over half the body, sometimes face	Descending tract and nucleus fifth nerve. Uncertain. Vestibular nucleus. Descending sympathetic tract Issuing fibers 9th and 10th nerve Nucleus and tractus solitarius Cuneate and gracile nuclei Spinothalamic tract
Totally unilateral medullary syndrome	Combination of medial and lateral syndromes
Lateral pontomedullary syndrome Occlusion of vertebral artery	Combination of lateral medullary and lateral inferior pontine syndromes
Basilar artery syndrome	A combination of various brain stem syndromes plus those arising in posterior cerebral artery distribution
Bilateral long tract signs, sensory and motor, cerebellar and peripheral cranial nerve abnormalities	Bilateral long trace, cerebellar and peripheral cranial nerves
Paralysis or weakness of all extremities, plus all bulbar musculature	Corticobulbar and Corticospinal tracts bilaterally
Medial superior pontine syndrome (Paramedian branches of upper basilar artery) *On side of lesion*: Cerebellar ataxia	Superior and/or middle cerebellar peduncle

Contd...

Contd...

Signs and symptoms	Structures involved
Internuclear ophthalmoplegia Myoclonic syndrome, palate, pharynx, vocal cords, respiratory apparatus, face, oculomotor apparatus, etc. *On opposite side lesion:* Paralysis of face, arm and leg Rarely touch, vibration, and position are affected	Medial longitudinal fasciculus Localization uncertain Corticobulbar and Corticospinal tracts Medial lemniscus
Lateral superior pontine syndrome (syndrome of superior cerebellar artery) *On side of lesion:* Ataxia of limbs, and gait, falling to side of lesion Dizziness, nausea, vomiting, horizontal nystagmus Paresis of conjugate gaze-ipsilateral. Skew deviation Horner's syndrome *On side opposite to lesion:* Impaired pain and thermal sense on face, limbs and trunk Impaired touch, vibration and position sense, more in leg than arm. There is a tendency to incongruity of pain and touch deficits	Middle and superior cerebellar peduncles, superior surface of cerebellum, dentate nucleus Vestibular nystagmus Pontine contralateral gaze Uncertain Descending sympathetic fibers Spinothalamic tract Medial lemniscus (lateral portion)
Medial midpontine syndrome (Paramedian branch of midbasilar artery) *On side of lesion:* Ataxia of limbs and gait, predominantly in bilateral involvement. *On side opposite to lesion:* Paralysis of face, arm, and leg	Pontine nuclei Corticobulbar and Corticospinal tract

Contd...

Contd...

Signs and symptoms	Structures involved
Variable impaired touch and proprioception when lesion extends posteriorly	Medial lemniscus
Lateral midpontine syndrome (short circumflex artery) *On side of lesion*: Ataxia of limbs Paralysis of muscles of mastication Impaired sensation over side of face *On side opposite to lesion*: Impaired pain and thermal sense on limbs and trunk	Middle cerebellar peduncle Motor fibers or nucleus of fifth nerve Sensory fibers or nucleus of fifth nerve Spinothalamic tract
Medial inferior pontine syndrome (occlusion of Paramedian branch of basilar artery). *On side of lesion*: Paralysis of conjugate gaze to side of lesion (preservation of convergence) Nystagmus Ataxia of limbs and gait Diplopia on lateral gaze *On opposite side of lesion*: Paralysis of face, arm and leg Impaired tactile and proprioceptive sense over half of the body	"Center" for conjugate lateral gaze Vestibular nucleus Middle cerebellar peduncle Abducent nerve Corticobulbar and Corticospinal tract in lower parts Medial lemniscus
Lateral inferior pontine syndrome (occlusion of anterior inferior cerebellar artery) *On side of lesion*: Horizontal and vertical nystagmus, vertigo, nausea, vomiting, oscillopsia Facial paralysis Paralysis of conjugate gaze to side of lesion Deafness, tinnitus	Vestibular nerve or nucleus 7th nerve Center for conjugate lateral gaze. Auditory nerve or cochlear nucleus.
Ataxia Impaired sensation over face.	Middle cerebellar peduncle and cerebellar hemisphere. Descending tract and nucleus 5th nerve.

Contd...

Contd...

Signs and symptoms	Structures involved
On side opposite to lesion: Impaired pain and thermal sensation over half the body may include face.	Spinothalamic tract.

SEQUENTIAL STAGES

During the early stages of stroke, flaccidity with no voluntary movements is common. Usually, this is replaced by the development of spasticity, hyper-reflexia and mass patterns of movement, termed synergies. These are not selective motor movements but are abnormal reflex activity patterns. Muscles involved in synergy patterns are often so strongly linked together that isolated movements outside the mass synergistic patterns are not possible. As recovery progresses, spasticity and synergies begin to decline and advanced movement patterns become possible. Bobath et al. described these recovery patterns comparing it to the normal development sequences of a normal baby from birth to three years of age.

General pattern of recovery was described in detail by Twitchell and Brunnstrom, who elaborated the process in to six stages:

Brunnstrom Classification

- **Stage 1:** Recovery from hemiplegia occurs in a stereotyped sequence of events that begins with a period of flaccidity immediately following the acute episode.
  No movement of the limbs can be elicited.
- **Stage 2:** As recovery begins, the basic limb synergies or some of their components may appear as associated reactions, or minimal voluntary movement responses may be present.
  Spasticity begins to develop.
- **Stage 3:** Thereafter, the patient gains voluntary control of the movement synergies, although full range of all synergy components does not necessarily develop.
  Spasticity has further increased and may become severe.
- **Stage 4:** Some movement combinations that do not follow the paths of either synergy are mastered, first with difficulty, then with more ease.
  Spasticity begins to decline.

- **Stage 5:** If progress continues, more difficult movement combinations are learned as the basic limb synergies lose their dominance over motor acts. *Motor movements begin to develop in a normal activity pattern.*
- **Stage 6:** With the disappearance of spasticity, individual joint movements become possible and coordination approaches normal. From here on, as the last recovery step, normal motor function achieved, but this last stage is not achieved by all, for the recovery process can plateau at any stage. *This is the last recovery stage which may plateau at any stage.*

Bobath Classification

Bobath collapsed the sequence into three main recovery stages:

- The initial flaccid stage
- The stage of spasticity
- The stage of relative recovery.

Additional investigators have confirmed this pattern of motor recovery following stroke. Motor recovery occurs in a relatively predictable pattern. The recovery stages are viewed as sequential, although variability in the clinical picture at each stage is possible. Not all patients recover fully. Patients may plateau at any stage, depending upon the severity of their involvement and their capacity for adaptation. Finally, recovery rates differ among patients. Also, the recovery of lower limbs is more spontaneous whereas the upper limb functions and fine motor functions are difficult to achieve for the patient as well as the treating physiotherapist. Importance of the trunk in influencing the recovery was ably worked upon by Kabat, B Bobath and Patricia Davies. Presently, the basis of neurorehabilitation lies in early activation of the stabilizers of the trunk, to minimize the synergistic patterns and to develop and aid in near normal selective motor activity. Development of various associated problems and complications delay or modify the amount and quality of the recovery as well as patient's personality is a major factor in determining the overall recovery.

ALTERATIONS IN TONE OF THE MUSCLES

Recognition of the tonal changes is of vital importance in management of the patient with stroke. The clinical therapist should understand the difference between the changes in the tone and synergistic patterns and they should know the relationship between the two. Flaccidity is usually present immediately after the stroke and is generally short-lived, lasting hours, days, weeks. Spasticity emerges in about 90 percent of cases and tends to occur in predictable muscle groups, commonly the antigravity muscles. The effects of spasticity include restricted movements and posturing of the limbs.

■ In the upper extremity, spasticity is frequently strong in:
  Scapular retractors; shoulder adductors, depressors and internal rotators; elbow flexors and forearm pronators; and wrist and finger flexors.

■ In the lower extremity, spasticity is often found in:
  Pelvic retractors; hip adductors and internal rotators; hip and knee extensors; plantar flexors and supinators; and toe flexors.

■ Automatic postural tone: The automatic adjustment of muscle tension that occurs normally in preparation for and during a movement or task may also be impaired.

Thus, patients with stroke may lack the ability to stabilize proximal joints and trunk appropriately, with resulting mal-alignment of body segments and in longstanding cases, fixed musculoskeletal impairments. The loss of automatic postural adjustment will require the patient to give constant conscious effort for the maintenance of the posture and hence, would produce large energy expenditure. Fear of falling off to the ground from sitting and standing position is common. Few patients are fearful of turning in the bed too. This fear of falling will increase the protective tone in all the muscles of the body but the muscles in which the tone is already high due to lesion, will become more spastic and hence, will further more be difficult for the patient to adjust and align different body segments to each other.

Effort, stress, fears, emotional state, consciousness of the people watching, newer places and pain increases tone.

LOSS OF SELECTIVE MOVEMENT

The degree and quality of voluntary control is recorded carefully. Although many patients with hemiplegia appear able to move all parts of their bodies, they may be unable to move one part in isolation without other muscles acting simultaneously, in a stereotyped mass pattern of movement. These synergies are stereotyped because the muscles that participate in the patterned motion and the strength of their responses are the same for every effort, regardless of demand. This primitive pattern response is a voluntary act, initiate when the patient wishes to perform a task (Perry, 1969). For example, he may be able to grip only while the elbow flexes and the shoulder adducts, or stand up with the hip and knee extended and the foot planter flexed. Similarly, dorsiflexion of the foot may only be possible when the hip and knee are flexed.

The therapist must remember that not only are the arm and leg affected but the whole side, and therefore, the trunk will be similarly affected. Movement does not become effective unless and until the undesired components of movement is these reflex patterns can be inhibited, at the same time, the desired components are excited (Kottke, 1980).

SYNERGY PATTERNS

Synergy patterns of the extremities are stereotyped, primitive movement patterns associated with the presence of spasticity. They may be elicited either reflexly, as associated reactions, or as voluntary movement patterns. There are two basic synergies of each extremity: a flexion synergy and an extension synergy including the Latissimus dorsi, Teres major, Serratus anterior, Finger extensors and Ankle evertors.

These muscles, therefore, are generally difficult to rehabilitate and represent important functional limitations for many patients in their activities and in gait. Loss of isolated movement patterns also has important functional implications. Usually, upper limbs have dominant flexor synergy, while, lower limbs will have predominantly extensor synergy. It seems that the nature has taken care with the development of synergies in a sense that extensor synergy helps the knee joint to remain in extension and thus, is available for weight bearing in standing. This may be a very gross activity but nonetheless, in absence of therapy, the patient can at least stand. In few patients with gross arthritis in knee joint or in patients with flexor spasms in lower limbs, maintaining knee extension during getting up from sitting and in standing and walking is extremely difficult, resulting in delayed rehabilitation. Thus, we can thank nature in a way that gross walking can be achieved post hemiplegia even in absence of proper therapy.

REFLEXES

Reflexes are altered and vary according to the stage of recovery. Initially, stroke results in hypotonia and areflexia. During the middle stages of recovery when spasticity and synergies are strong, hyperreflexia emerges. Stretch reflexes become hyperactive and patients typically demonstrate clonus and the clasp-knife reflex. Cutaneous reflexes (positive Babinski) may be present. Primitive or tonic reflex patterns may appear in a readily identifiable form. Some of the clinically important reflexes are documented below.

Tonic Neck Reflexes

Movement of the head elicits an obligatory change in resting tone or movement of the extremities. Flexion of the neck results in flexion of the arms and extension of the legs; extension of the neck produces the opposite responses (symmetric tonic neck reflex-STNR). Head rotation to the left cause extension of the right arm and leg (jaw limbs) with flexion of the right arm and leg (skull limbs); head rotation to the right causes the reverse pattern (asymmetric tonic neck reflex-ATNR).

Tonic Labyrinthine Reflexes

Supine positioning produces an increase in extensor tone, while prone positioning increases flexor tone (symmetric tonic labyrinthine reflex-STLR).

Tonic Lumbar Reflexes

Rotation of the upper trunk, with respect to the pelvis, influences movement of the extremities. Rotation towards the hemiplegic side results in flexion of the hemiplegic upper extremity and extension of hemiplegic lower extremity. Rotation toward the uninvolved side produces the opposite responses (tonic lumbar reflex-TLR).

Positive Supportive Reactions

Pressure on the bottom of the hemiplegic foot may produce a strong co-contraction response of lower extremity extensors and flexors, resulting in a rigidly extended and fixed limb (positive supporting reaction).

Associated Reactions

Associated reactions are also commonly present. These consist of abnormal, automatic responses of the involved limb resulting from action occurring in some other part of the body, either by voluntary or reflex stimulation (e.g., yawning, sneezing, coughing, stretching). They are easier to elicit in the presence of spasticity and frequently interact with tonic reflexes. Generally, although this is not true in every case, associated reactions elicit the same direction of movement in the contralateral upper extremity (i.e., flexion evokes flexion), while in the lower extremity opposite movements are elicited (i.e., flexion of one lower extremity evokes extension of the other). Newer studies have proven that this fact is clinically feasible. Therapy for hand and scapular functions, in which bilateral movement patterns are used, is gaining fast popularity with good results. Specific associated reactions have also been identified. Elevation of the hemiplegic arm above the horizontal may elicit an extension and abduction response of the fingers *(Souques' phenomenon)*. Resistance to abduction or adduction produces a similar response in the opposite limb (adduction elicits adduction) in both the upper and lower extremities *(Ramiste's phenomenon)*. Homolateral limb synkinesis is the term used to describe the mutual dependency that exists between hemiplegic limbs (flexion of the arm elicits flexion of the leg on the hemiplegic side).

Higher level balance reactions like righting, equilibrium and protective extension reactions are frequently impaired or absent. Patients may be unable to maintain their head in its normal upright alignment: face vertical with the mouth in a horizontal position in response to a change in body position or movement. Impaired righting reactions are also evident when rotation of either the head or trunk within the body axis fails to produce a log rolling: trunk moving as one unit; or segmental rolling: head, upper trunk and then lower trunk pattern. Lack of equilibrium reactions may cause the patient to lose balance and fall in response to a change of the center of the mass over the base of support. Protective extension of either hemiplegic limb, in response to falling, is also commonly impaired or absent.

Majority of the associated reactions are treated with strong stimulation and active fixation of the body parts by the patients themselves. Strong stimulation includes tactile, verbal and visual biofeedback.

Associated movement occurs in the normal person during strenuous activity, but with hyper-tonicity, they appear as associated reactions in abnormal stereotyped patterns which inhibit functions. Example of associated movement in normal subject is the movement of left hand in a painter who is painting with his right hand. Many such examples can be sited for the associated movements.

WEAKNESS

Paresis or weakness is a common finding. Patients with spastic hemiparesis are unable to generate normal levels of force necessary for initiating and controlling movement or for maintaining posture. Specific changes occur in both the motor neuron and muscle. The number of functioning agonist motor units is decreased, by as much as 50 percent at 6 months in some patients with stroke. The recruitment order of motor units may be altered and firing rates decreased. Thus, patients have increased difficulties trying to maintain a constant level of force production. Denervation potentials are common, as a result of denervation changes in the corticospinal tracts. Changes in muscle include atrophy of muscle fibers with a greater loss of fast-twitch fibers. Contraction time is increased with increased fatigability noted in paretic muscle. Patients consistently report that increased effort produces less than maximum muscular force.

Active restraint arising from antagonist muscles can influence agonist strength. Bobath has suggested that spasticity of antagonist muscles is a major factor in the agonist weakness. Some investigators demonstrated a correlation between paresis and spasticity in agonist muscles but not with antagonist spasticity. Inappropriate co-activation of agonist-antagonist muscles is another form of active restraint and may be more of a factor than spasticity, especially in rapid and reciprocal contractions. Passive restraint secondary to abnormal mechanical changes in the soft tissues can also affect agonist strength. Loss of strength in either of the fast and slow twitch fibers can produce either loss of optimum force production or loss of optimum sustainability of contraction.

Not all muscle groups are affected equally. The amount of paresis experienced by the patient may also vary according to specific situational contexts. Thus, a patient may appear stronger in some functional tasks than in others. Paresis on the "supposedly normal" unaffected side has also been reported. As a matter of fact, body segments of each right and left half has influence on each other via crossing tracts and they work in unison, especially in stabilizing functions. This rhythm is lost and hence, even the strength of the uninvolved side seems to be decreased due to the lack of the force couple and lack of stabilization.

INCOORDINATION

Incoordination can result from cerebellar or basal ganglia involvement, from proprioceptive losses, or from motor weakness. Ataxia of the extremities or trunk is common in patients with cerebellar lesions. Reciprocal interaction with graded control of agonist-antagonists muscle pairs and synergistic activation may be impaired. The stretch reflex responses that allow automatic adaptation of muscles to changes to posture and movement, are commonly abnormal.

DYSTONIA

Dystonia is a variant of hypertonicity in which there is an increased tone in a group of muscles, especially during activity. The antagonist muscle group also contracts during the activity of the agonist group instead of relaxing and hence, wrying movement occurs. The limbs move as if tied up tightly. Even with patients having sufficient motor activity, the limbs would not become functional as the patients have tremendous difficulty in carrying out smooth and coordinated movements.

MOTOR PROGRAMMING DEFICITS

Hemispheric differences have been reported in the area of movement control.

- The left hemisphere has a primary role in the sequencing of movements. Thus, patients with left CVA (right hemiplegia) have increased difficulty initiating and performing sequences of movements, and may take longer time to learn a task. They also demonstrate slower movements overall, with more positioning errors.
- The right hemisphere, on the other hand, may have an increased role in sustaining a movement or posture. Thus patients with right CVA (left hemiplegia) characteristically demonstrate motor impersistence (inability to sustain a movement or posture).
- Patients with left hemisphere lesions are also more likely to present with apraxia. Apraxia is defined as an inability to perform purposive movements although, there is no sensory or motor impairment. Problems exist in performing previously learned movements, gestures, and sequences of movements. Two categories of apraxia are:
  - *Ideomotor,* where movement is not possible upon command but may occur automatically, and
  - *Ideational,* where purposeful movement is not possible, either automatically or on command.

Thus patients with left hemisphere damage are more likely to present with motor programming deficits than are patients with right hemisphere damage. In study of motor programming differences, Light and co-workers, found support for these conclusions and in both, involved and uninvolved arms of patients with left CVA.

FUNCTIONAL ABILITIES

Functional ability skills following stroke are mostly impaired or absent and differ considerably from patient to patient. In general, rolling, sitting up, transfers, standing up and walking pose significant problems for the moderately to severely involved patient with acute stroke. Basic ADL skills such as feeding and dressing are also compromised. The ability to perform functional tasks is influenced by a number of factors. Motor, sensory and perceptual impairments have the greatest impact on functional performance, but other limiting factors include disorientation, communication disorders, decreased cardiorespiratory endurance and lack of motivation.

SPEECH AND LANGUAGE DISORDERS

Patients with lesions involving the parieto-occipital cortex of the dominant hemisphere (typically, the left hemisphere) demonstrate speech and language impairments. Aphasia is the general term used to describe an acquired communication disorder caused by brain damage and characterized by an impairment of language comprehension, formulation and use. Aphasia has been estimated to occur in up to 40 percent of all stroke patients. There are many different types of aphasias; major classification categories are fluent, nonfluent and global.

- In *fluent aphasia*, speech flows smoothly, with a variety of grammatical constructions and preserved melody of speech. Auditory comprehension is impaired.
- In *nonfluent aphasia,* the flow of speech is slow and hesitant, vocabulary is limited and syntax is impaired. Articulation may be labored. Comprehension is good.
- *Global aphasia* is a severe aphasia characterized by marked impairments of the production and comprehension of language. It is often an indication of extensive brain damage.
- Patients with stroke may also present with *Dysarthria*. This term refers to a category of motor speech disorders caused by impairment in parts of the central or peripheral nervous system that mediate speech production. Respiration, articulation, phonation, resonance, and/or prosody may be affected.
- Volitional and automatic actions, for example, chewing and swallowing: *Dysphagia*; and movement of the jaw and tongue may also be impaired. In patients with stroke, dysarthria can accompany aphasia, complicating the course of rehabilitation.

PERCEPTUAL DEFICITS

It is important to be aware of any reduction in sensory input although accurate testing is frequently difficult. Proprioception and stereognosis is noted in addition to superficial and deep sensation and temperature. Information about disturbance of body image and unilateral neglect is also recorded.

There may be disturbance of awareness of parts of the body in relation to each other or their position in space. Loss of sensation impairs the patient's ability to move and balance normally. In many cases, deficit can be attributed to inattention towards the affected side rather than actual loss of feeling. Impairment of sensation can be improved with treatment and there would seem to be many exceptions to the traditional belief that impaired sensation precludes functional recovery and that the loss is greater in the arm than the leg.

Lesions of the parietal lobe of the nondominant hemisphere can produce perceptual deficits. These are discussed in great detail in subsequent chapters. To enumerate, these may include visuospatial distortions, disturbances in body image and unilateral neglect. Patients with visuospatial impairments may not be able to judge distance, size, position, rate of movement, form, or the relation of parts to the whole. Thus, the patient may consistently bump the wheelchair in to the door frame and is unable to get through the doorway. With topographical disorientation, the patient consistently gets lost going from one place to another. Patients may also experience difficulties in distinguishing figure-ground relationships. The brakes on a wheel chair may be indistinguishable from the rest of the parts of the wheelchair. Problems in the perception of verticality, especially in dimly lit areas, may also occur. This may be manifested by a patient who is constantly leaning over to one side. Body scheme (a postural model of the body and the relationship of its parts) and body image (a visual and mental image of one's body) may be distorted. Patients, with unilateral neglect, are generally unaware of what happens on the hemiplegic side. A severe form (anosognosia) includes frank denial of the presence or severity of one's disability. Sensory losses and hemianopsia frequently contribute to this perceptual problem.

COGNITIVE AND BEHAVIORAL CHANGES

Patients with stroke differ widely in their approach to processing information and in their behavioral styles.

- Those with left hemisphere damage (right hemiplegia) demonstrate difficulties in processing information in a sequential, linear manner. They are frequently described as negative, anxious and depressed. They are likely to be slower, more cautious, uncertain and insecure. This makes them more hesitant when performing tasks and increases the need for more frequent feedback and support. They tend, however, to be realistic in their appraisal of their existing problems.

■ Patients with right hemisphere damage (left hemiplegia), on the other hand, demonstrate difficulty in grasping the whole idea or the overall organization of a pattern or activity. These patients are frequently described as indifferent, quick and impulsive and euphoric. They tend to over stimulate their abilities while minimizing or denying their problems. Safety is, therefore, a far greater issue with left hemiplegia, where poor judgment is common. These patients also require a great deal of feedback when learning a new task. The feedback should be focused on slowing down the activity, checking each component part and relating it to the whole task. The patient with left hemiplegia frequently cannot attend to visuospatial cues effectively, especially in a cluttered or crowded environment.

Cognitive deficits may exist across a wide area of function. Deficits in orientation, attention, information, processing speed, conceptual abilities, executive functioning, memory and learning can occur. They may be primary impairments resulting from the stroke, or premorbid changes associated with pathologic aging. The patient with stroke typically has a short retention span, remembering only the first few bits of information in a series of commands. Immediate and short-term memory is often impaired, while long term memory remains intact. Thus, the patient cannot remember the instructions for a new task given only 30 seconds ago but can remember things done 30 years ago. The patient may also have difficulties in generalizing information. Thus, information learned in one setting cannot be transposed to other situations.

The patient with stroke may demonstrate an emotional dysregulation syndrome termed emotional lability. It is characterized by pathologic laughing and weeping in which the patient changes quickly from laughing to crying with only slight provocation. Such a patient is typically unable to inhibit the expression of spontaneous emotions. Frequent crying may also accompany depression. Thalamic lesions are usually responsible for the same.

Sensory losses coupled with an unfamiliar hospital environment and inactivity following acute stroke can lead symptoms of sensory deprivation such as irritability, confusion, restlessness and sometimes psychosis, delusions, or hallucinations. Night time may be particularly problematic. Positioning the bed with the affected side towards the door, limits social interaction and may increase the patient's disorientation. Some patients with diminished capacity are equally unable to deal with a sensory overload, produced by too much stimulation. Altered arousal levels are implicated. Sometimes, as in cases with the hemineglect, the problem manifolds as there are diminished sensory inputs from the affected side.

Dementia can result from multiple infarcts of the brain, termed multi infarct dementia. It is characterized by a generalized decline in higher brain functions and typified by faulty judgments, impaired consciousness, poor memory, diminished communication and behavioral or mood alterations. These changes are often associated with episodes of cerebral ischemia, focal neurologic signs, and hypertension. The patient may fluctuate between periods of impaired function and periods of improved or normal function.

Epileptic seizures occur in a small percentage of stroke patients and are slightly more common in occlusive carotid disease than in MCA disease. Seizures also occur at the onset of cerebral hemorrhage in about 15% cases. They tend to be of the partial motor type and in some patients may occur as the initial presenting symptom. Convulsions during the recovery stages disturb the patient as most of them feel that there is a re-stroke. Weakness in the muscles and deterioration of the functions for a period of few hours to few weeks is also common.

BLADDER AND BOWEL DYSFUNCTION

Urinary incontinence may require the temporary use of an indwelling catheter. Generally, this problem improves quickly. Early removal of a catheter is desirable to prevent the development of infection. Patients are frequently impacted and may require stool softeners and low residue diets to resolve this problem. Bladder and bowel functions tend to improve with the improvement in overall general awareness.

OROFACIAL DYSFUNCTION

Swallowing dysfunction, dysphagia, is a common complication after stoke. It occurs in lesions affecting the medullary brainstem (cranial nerves 9 and 10) as well as in acute hemispheric lesions. In patients referred for detailed evaluation of dysphagia, the most frequent problem seen is delayed triggering of the swallowing reflex followed by reduced pharyngeal peristalsis and reduced lingual control. Poor jaw and lip closure, altered sensation, impaired head control and poor swallowing difficulties can be seen. Most demonstrate multiple problems that result in drooling, difficulty ingesting food, aspiration, dysarthria, and asymmetry of the muscles of facial expression. Decreased nutritional intake may require the temporary use of a nasogastric tube for feeding. These problems have tremendous social implications, for the patient frequently feels humiliated and frustrated by their presence.

PATTERNS OF BEHAVIOR IN RIGHT AND LEFT BRAIN

See Table 5.3.

TABLE 5.3	Patterns of behavior in right and left brain	
Behavior	**Left hemisphere**	**Right hemisphere**
Cognitive style	Processing information in a sequential, linear manner observing and analyzing details	Processing information in a simultaneous, holistic, or gestalt manner Grasping overall organization or pattern
Perception/cognition	Processing and producing language	Processing nonverbal stimuli Visual–spatial perception Drawing inferences, synthesizing information
Academic skills	Reading: sound-symbol relationships, word recognition, reading comprehension Performing mathematical calculations	Mathematical reasoning and judgment Alignment of numerals in calculations
Motor	Sequencing movements Performing movements and gestures to command	Sustaining a movement or posture
Emotions	Expression of positive emotions	Expression of negative emotions Perception of emotion

SECONDARY IMPAIRMENTS

Psychological Problems

The patient who has had a stroke is often frustrated by changes in the ability to sense, move, communicate, think, or act as he or she did before. Non acceptance of the present condition is the prime reason for the same. Common psychologic reactions include anxiety, depression, or denial. Additionally, the patient's behavior may be influenced by cognitive deficits that leave him or her irritable, inflexible, hypercritical, impatient, impulsive, apathetic, or over dependent on others. These behaviors along with a poor social perception of one's self and environment may lead to increasing isolation and stress. Depression is extremely common, occurring in about one third of the cases. Most patients remain significantly depressed for many months, with an average time of 7 to 8 months. The period from six months to 2 years after CVA is the most likely time for depression to occur. Depression occurs in both mildly and severely involved patients and thus, is not significantly related to the degree of impairment. Patients with lesions of the left hemisphere may experience more frequent and more severe depression than patients with right hemisphere or brain stem strokes. These findings suggest that post-stroke depression may not be simply a result of psychological reaction to disability but rather a primary impairment directly related to the CVA.

Decrease in Range of Movement, Contracture and Deformity

Decrease in range of movement (ROM), contracture and deformity may result from loss of voluntary movements and immobilization. Flexibility of connective tissue is lost and muscles experience disuse atrophy. As contractures progress, edema and pain may develop and further restrict attempts to gain motion. In the upper extremity, limitations in shoulder motions are common. Patients also frequently develop contractures of the elbow, wrist and finger flexors, and forearm pronators. In the lower extremity, plantar flexion contractures are common. Alterations in alignment coupled with decreased efficiency of muscles may lead to increased energy expenditure, altered patterns of movement and excessive effort.

Deep Venous Thrombosis

Deep venous thrombosis (DVT) and pulmonary embolism are potential complications for all immobilized patients. Common symptoms of DVT include calf pain or tenderness, calf pain, swelling and discoloration of the leg. About 50% of the cases do not present with clinically detectable symptoms and can be identified by Doppler or other noninvasive techniques. Anti-coagulants and anti-platelet agents are the primary medical treatments, along with bed rest, graded and guarded mobilization and elevation of the affected limb.

Pain

Patients with lesions affecting the thalamus may initially experience a contra-lateral sensory loss. After several weeks or months, this may be replaced by a severe burning pain, generalized on the hemiplegic side (thalamic syndrome). Pain is increased by stimuli or contact with that side. Thalamic syndrome is extremely debilitating and the patient generally has a poor functional outcome.

Pain may also result from muscle imbalances, improper movement patterns, musculoskeletal strain, osteoporosis and poor alignment. For example, knee pain is a common finding with prolonged or severe hyperextension during gait. The sequelae of pain are reduced function, impaired concentration, depression and decreased rehabilitation potential.

Shoulder Dysfunction

Shoulder subluxation and pain

Shoulder pain is extremely common following stroke, occurring in 70 to 84 percent of patients. Pain is typically present with movement and, in more severe cases, at rest. Several causes of shoulder pain have been widely proposed. In the flaccid stage, proprioceptive impairment, lack of tone and muscle paralysis, reduce the support and normal seating action of the rotator cuff muscles, particularly the supraspinatus. The ligaments and capsule, thus, become the shoulder's sole support. The normal orientation of the glenoid fossa is upward, outward and forward, so that it keeps the superior capsule taut and stabilizes the humerus mechanically. Any abduction or forward flexion of the humerus, or scapular depression and downward rotation reduces this stabilization and causes the humerus to sublux. Initially, the subluxation is not painful, but mechanical stresses resulting from traction and gravitational forces produce persistent malalignment. Glenohumeral friction-compression stresses also occur between the humeral head and superior soft tissues during flexion or abduction movements in the absence of normal simultaneous rotation of the arm and normal scapulohumeral rhythm. In the spastic stage, abnormal muscle tone contributes to subluxation and restricted movement. Secondary tightness in ligaments, tendons and joint capsule quickly develops. Adhesive capsulitis is a common finding. Poor handling and positioning of the hemiplegic arm have also been implicated in producing joint micro-trauma and pain. Activities that traumatize the shoulder include passive range of motion (PROM) without adequate mobilization of the scapula pulling on the arm during a transfer, or using reciprocal pulleys.

Pain develops in a typical pattern. Patients at first report sharp end-range pain with movement and can easily pinpoint the location of the pain. If the causative factors are not addressed, pain increases to include pain on all movement, particularly with shoulder flexion and abduction. Increasing pain may also be experienced in certain positions, for example, lying in bed at night. Eventually, the patient complains of intense pain and does not tolerate any movement of the arm. At this point, the pain is diffuse and not easily localized. Pain may extend in to arm and hand. Long standing cases may also have osteoporosis in the humeral head.

Reflex Sympathetic Dystrophy

Reflex sympathetic dystrophy (RSD) also occurs in approximately 12 to 25% of the cases. The patient experiences swelling and tenderness of the hand and fingers along with shoulder pain. Elbow joint is usually spared. Sympathetic vasomotor changes are evident and include warm, red and glossy skin. Trophic changes of the finger nails develop. The patient experiences increasing pain with movement and further immobilization leads to increased stiffness, contracture and atrophy of muscle. In the late stages, the skin is typically cool, cyanotic and damp. The hand typically contracted in metacarpophalangeal (MP) extension and interphalangeal (IP) flexion, similar to the "intrinsic minus hand". There is marked atrophy of thenar and hypothenar muscles with flattening of the hand. Osteoporotic changes become evident on radiographs. Early diagnosis and treatment are critical in preventing or minimizing the late changes of RSD. Because of close daily contact with the patient, the therapist is frequently one of the first to recognize and report early signs and symptoms. Radionuclide bone scans can be used to reliably confirm early symptoms of RSD. Many times, the patient's symptoms progress up to the entire arm and hence, all the movements of the entire upper extremity become painful and restricted. When this is coupled with the thalamic pain syndrome, the condition takes a long time to recover.

Deconditioning

Patients who suffer a stroke as a result of cardiac disease may demonstrate impaired cardiac output, cardiac decompensation and serious rhythm disorders. If these problems persist, they can directly alter cerebral perfusion and produce additional focal signs (e.g., mental confusion). Cardiac limitations in exercise tolerance may restrict the patient's rehabilitation potential and require diligent monitoring and careful exercise prescription by the physical therapist. Deconditioning is a common finding in older adults with limited activity levels and may have been present prior to the stroke. Age related changes in the cardiorespiratory systems and musculoskeletal systems all affect activity tolerance and endurance levels. Prolonged bed rest during the acute stroke phase further diminishes rehabilitation potential, decreases energy reserves and increases activity intolerance. Activity tolerance may also be related to depression, a common finding in stroke.

RECOVERY FROM STROKE

Mortality for initial strokes varies considerably with an overall rate ranging from 22 to 37% at 3 weeks to 1 month, 25 to 50% at one year, and 68 to 72% at 5 years. At ten years, only 35% of patients are still alive. The type of stroke is significant in determining survival. Patients with intra-cerebral hemorrhage account for the largest number of deaths following an acute episode flowed by subarachnoid hemorrhage and thrombo-emobolic stroke. Survival rates are dramatically lessened by a number of medical conditions and comorbities, including age, hypertension, heart disease and diabetes. Loss of consciousness at stroke onset, lesion size, persistent severe hemiplegia, multiple neurologic deficits and history of previous stroke are also important predictors of mortality. Most patients suffer recurrent episodes of stroke, usually of the same type and these are influenced by the same risk factors influencing survival.

Recovery from stoke is fastest in the first few weeks after onset, with most measurable neurologic recovery occurring in the first three months. Patients may continue to make functional gains for longer periods, up to six months or a year after insult. A few patients may demonstrate remarkable and unexpected recovery with improvements occurring over a period of years. Rates of improvement will vary across management categories: patients suffering minor stroke may rapidly recover with few or no residual deficits, while patients with severe stroke may demonstrate limited recovery. An important finding is that recovery has been demonstrated even in patients with extensive central nervous system (CNS) damage and advanced age due to a process called neuroplasticity. So it becomes a general unwritten rule for the rehabilitation specialist to try and try till the full functional recovery.

Early recovery is generally thought to be result of resolution of local vascular and metabolic factors. Thus the reduction of edema, absorption of damaged tissue and improved local circulation allows intact neurons that were previously inhibited to regain function. Central nervous system plasticity is thought to account for continuing recovery. In the presence of cell death, functional reorganization of the CNS may occur. A number of different mechanisms have been identified, including collateral sprouting and unmasking. Sprouting involves synaptic reclamation of a denervated region by nearby intact neurons. Unmasking refers to the release of previously inactive neurons, which then take over function of the damaged neurons. These processes are thought to occur both locally and at brain areas remote from the lesion. The redevelopment of adequate CNS inhibitory mechanisms may underline the emergence of selective movement control inhibition mass movements and pathologic reflexes. Results from animal studies also suggest that environment plays an important part in recovery. Brain injured rats raised in "enriched conditions" did considerable better than rats raised in "impoverished conditions".

Essentials of Assessment

PHYSICAL THERAPY ASSESSMENT

A thorough assessment of each patient's problems is essential if the treatment is to be successful. The therapist needs to observe the patient closely while he moves against gravity and performs but also in other instance which occur during his daily life. At first, these may be only in and around his bed, but later it will be mandatory to observe how he moves when he walks outside, is confronted by other people, climbs the stairs or sits down to eat. Observation alone does not provide sufficient information as to why the patient has difficulties. The therapist needs to feel the difficulties as well. Therapist must use one's hands to feel muscle tone and the resistance it offers, while the patient is moving. With the hands one can feel the ease with which he transfers his weight and maintains his balance. To understand what is observed and felt, the therapist needs to remember that the inability to move normally is due to disturbed tone and reciprocal innervations, not to actual muscle weakness. That is the reason why physiotherapy is considered a combination of art and science by many. A physiotherapist requires scientific mind to diagnose the problem and treat it and an artistic mind to understand the requirements of the patient and designing the approach and the techniques of the treatment (Figure 6.1).

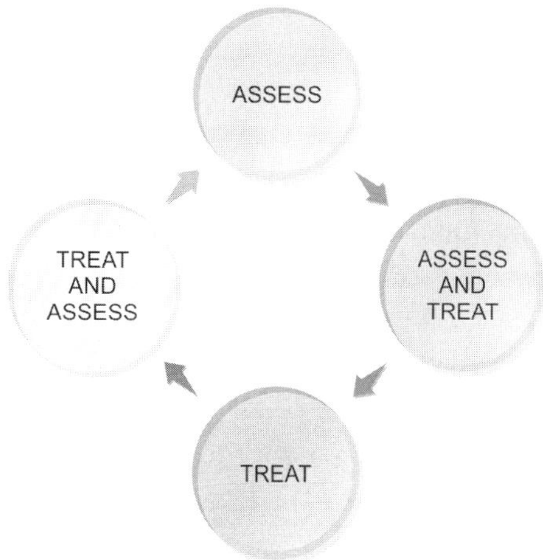

FIGURE 6.1: Physical therapy assessment

Assessment is continuous process as even during one therapy session, changes will occur and treatment must be adjusted accordingly. When assessing the problems, the therapist is constantly comparing the way in which the patient moves to the way in which the same movement would normally be performed. In the treatment, the therapist will try to facilitate normal patterns of movement. It is essential that there is knowledge of how each movement sequence should be carried out and how balance is maintained.

The physical therapy assessment will be determined by each patient's unique needs and problems. Comprehensive assessment of the patient with neurologic impairments may include entire physical assessment, assessment of the higher brain functions, assessment of the functional status of the body parts, assessment of the synergistic patterns and associated reactions, in detail. Physiotherapy and assessment usually go hand in hand and the therapist would constantly assess, treat and modify the treatment strategy, whenever and wherever applicable.

Mental Status

It is important to assess cognitive function first, since it may affect the results of other assessments. An evaluation of level of consciousness, memory (immediate recall, short- and long-term), orientation (to person, place, time), ability to follow instructions (one, two and three level commands), higher cortical functions (calculation ability, abstract reasoning) and attention span should be included, as well as an investigation of behavioral and emotional responses. Learning deficits including retention and generalization deficits can significantly impede rehabilitation efforts and should be identified early.

Communication Ability

Communication deficits severely limit the validity of other assessments; patient comprehension should be fully ascertained before proceeding with these evaluations. Close collaboration with the speech pathologist will be important in making an accurate determination of the patient's communication deficits. Impairments in receptive language (word recognition, auditory comprehension, reading comprehension) and/or expressive language function (word finding, fluency, writing and spelling) should be noted. Education of the staff members in communication with the patient would ensure a smooth understanding between the two parties and misunderstanding created by taking to understand the patient would be minimized. A quick assessment to check an individual's level of understanding can be performed by saying one thing to the patient and gesturing another (e.g. "it's not here" and putting on a shirt). The functional deficits of dysarthria and dysphagia should be carefully examined. Alternated forms of communication should be well-established before additional testing begins. Help from the immediate family members can be taken if needed.

Common Assessment Format (Table 6.1)

TABLE 6.1	Assessment for neurologically impaired patients

- Demographic information
- History
- Patient's chief complaint
- Mental status
- Communication ability
- Sensation
- Perception
- Joint mobility
  - Range of motion(ROM)
  - Joint play
  - Soft tissue compliance
- Joint stability
- Skin condition
- Edema
- Motor control
  - Muscle tone
  - Reflexes/reactions
  - Strength
  - Voluntary movement patterns
  - Coordination
  - Balance
- Functional mobility skills
  - Bed mobility
  - Transfers
  - Wheelchair
  - Gait
- Endurance/cardiorespiratory status
- Discharge planning
  - Environmental assessment
  - Equipment needs

Sensation

A sensory examination should include superficial, proprioceptive and combined sensations. Deficits may be apparent in one sensory modality and not in others. Differences can also be expected between the hemiplegic extremities.

Comparisons with the intact side can be made, but the therapist should be cognizant that deficits may exist in the supposedly "normal" extremities secondary to effects of comorbid conditions or aging. The visual system should be carefully investigated, including tests for acuity, peripheral vision, depth perception, and hemianopsia. Hearing status should be determined.

Perception

Significant information on sensory and perceptual deficits will be provided by close collaboration with the occupational therapist. Many tests and formalized test batteries have been developed to assess body scheme, body image, spatial relations, agnosia, and apraxia. Since the patient with left hemiplegia may behave in ways which overestimate this patient's ability to perform, whereas verbal cues (either the therapist's or the patient's) may permit success. Carefully structuring the environment will also improve patient performance (Discussed in detail in subsequent chapters).

Joint Mobility

An assessment of joint mobility should include an evaluation of range of motion (ROM), joint play, and soft-tissue compliance. Problems with spasticity may result in inconsistent ROM findings, since alterations in tone may exist from one testing session to the next. Thus tonal abnormalities should be noted at the time of examination. Active ROM tests may be invalid since synergy dominance may influence performance and preclude movement in standard active range of motion (AROM) tests. Fixed contracture and developing deformity should be carefully documented. Passive range of motion (PROM) tests should be also performed to check the joint stiffness or contractures of muscles and other soft tissues. All the movements must be checked firstly in lying for the ease of the patient as he or she would feel fully supported and the tone of the muscles would be minimum. Secondly, the same assessment should be carried out in functional position also and the difference between the two should be aptly noted, the reason being, the synergistic patterns are position and velocity dependent and any assessment in a single layer would prove to be misleading. Goniometric assessment is done where applicable and any change in the ROM is noted after comparing to the 'normal side'.

Motor Control

Motor control assessment is a qualitative assessment in case of hemiplegia and hence any attempt to quantify creates a vague picture of the patient's condition. Also, if the assessment is carried out qualitatively, taking into consideration the overall motor ability, the treatment planning would be obvious to a clinical practitioner.

Voluntary movement patterns should be examined for synergy dominance and selective movement control (in synergy or out of synergy). Those movements with selective control should be examined closely for coordination and timing deficits. Strength should be examined. In the early recovery stages, traditional manual muscle tests may be invalid in the presence of significant problems of spasticity, reflex, and synergy dominance. An estimation of strength can alternately be made from observation of performance during functional tasks. An assessment of the strength of key muscles for upper extremity function and lower extremity function (hip flexion, knee extension, ankle dorsiflexion) has been weighted to yield a motoricity index score. This index can be rapidly administered and has proved to be reliable in assessing motor impairment after stroke. The examination should also include an investigation of motor planning abilities, postural control and balance.

Specific hemiplegic assessments tools like that of Brunnstrom and Bobath have been developed that are adapted. The Brunnstrom assessment is based upon sequential recovery stages, and carefully plots the emergence, dominance, and variation of the motion synergies. Both synergy and isolated movements are assessed in terms of the active ROM completed. Gross sensory changes and tone alterations associated with specific stages of recovery are also determined. Later-stage control is assessed by timed tasks in which the patient is asked to complete test items as quickly as possible. This test also presents a quantitative analysis of hand function and lower extremity control in sitting, standing and walking.

Fugl-Meyer and co-workers expanded on the work of Brunnstrom to develop the Fugl-Meyer assessment (FMA) of physical performance. They used many of the Brunnstrom test items organized in to five sequential recovery stages. Their test improvements consisted of the development of a three point ordinal scale with grades ranging from 0 (item cannot be performed) to 2 (item can be fully performed). Specific subtests with subtest scores are available. The cumulative test score for all components is 226.

The Bobath assessment is based upon a qualitative assessment of postural and movement patterns in early, middle, or late recovery stages. Tonal abnormalities are assessed during both passive and active movements. The therapist may place the limbs in various positions and observe the patient's responses during attempts to hold the position. Tests for active movements are divided in to two groups: advanced movement combinations progressing from easiest to most difficult, and tests for balance and/or automatic postural responses. Individual assessment items can also be used as a basis for treatment using this approach since they represent an advanced recovery progression. Since, the central state and general function of patients may vary considerably from one treatment session to the next, frequent reassessments are recommended.

The motor assessment scale (MAS) was developed by Carr and Shepherd to measure functional capabilities of the patient with stroke. This scale uses eight items of motor function, including movement transitions, balanced sitting, walking, upper-arm function, hand function and advanced hand function. The ninth item evaluates general tonus. Each item is scored on a seven-point scale. The scale has been shown highly reliable (r = 0.87–1.0) with high concurrent validity. *Please refer to the chapter of scales and scores for a variety of assessment batteries.*

Videography, nowadays, is a cheap and effective tool for recording the observations initially and later to compare the outcome of rehabilitation.

Gait

Gait is usually altered following stroke, due to a number of factors, including impairments in sensation and perception and motor control. Some of the common problems in hemiplegic gait and their causes are shown in the Table 6.2.

Assessment of gait may be done using a subjective rating system and/or objective measures. Individual rating systems may bias the examiner to identify problems in specific areas. For example, the Brunnstrom form assesses independence from synergies, based on a normal recovery sequence; the Bobath assessment stresses qualitative control and balance reactions; while the Barthel index stresses functional independence and endurance. The accuracy of rating scales for observational gait analysis is highly dependent upon the skill of the examiner and the consistency and endurance of the patient; these latter may be limited following a stroke. Videography, which allows the permanent recording of gait pattern is currently the best tool for analyzing the minor nuances of the gait. The therapist can then replay the tape and re-examine gait deficits without tiring the patient.

Functional Assessment

At varying stages of recovery, functional mobility skills (bed mobility, movement transitions, transfers, locomotion, stairs), basic ADL skills (feeding, hygiene, dressing) and instrumental ADL skills (communication, home chores) should be carefully assessed. Functional testing frequently serves to evaluate outcomes of stroke rehabilitation and determine long-term placement. The Barthel index

TABLE 6.2	**Gait analysis format**

STANCE PHASE
- Trunk/pelvis
  - Unawareness of affected side: Poor proprioception
  - Forward trunk: Weak hip extension
  - Flexion contracture
- Hip
  - Poor hip position: Poor proprioception
  - Trendelenburg limp: Weak abductors
- Knee
  - Flexion during forward progression
  - Flexion contracture combined with weak knee extensors and/or poor proprioception
- Ankle dorsiflexion range past neutral, combined with weak hip and knee extension or poor proprioception at knee and ankle
  - Weakness in extension pattern or in selective pattern or in selective motion of hip and knee extensors and plantar flexors
  - Slow contraction of knee extensors/knee remains flexed 20°–30° during forward progression
  - Plantar flexion contracture past 90 degrees
  - Impaired proprioception: Knee wobbles or snaps back in to recurvatum
  - Severe spasticity in quadriceps
  - Weak knee extensors: Compensatory locking of knee in hyperextension
- Ankle/foot
  - Equinus gait (heel does not touch the ground); spasticity or contractures of gastroc-soleus
  - Varus foot (patient bears weight on the lateral surface of the foot): Hyperactive or spastic anterior tibialis, post tibialis, toe flexors and soleus
  - Unequal step lengths: Hammer toes caused by spastic toe flexors prevent the patient from stepping forward onto the opposite foot because of pain/weight-bearing on flexed toes
  - Lack of dorsiflexion range on the affected side (approximately 10 degrees is needed)

SWING PHASE
- Trunk/pelvis
  - Insufficient forward pelvic rotation (pelvic retraction): Weak abdominal muscles
  - Inclination to sound side for foot clearance: Weakness of flexor muscles
- Hip
  - Inadequate flexion
  - Weak hip flexors, poor proprioception, spastic quadriceps, abdominal weakness, hip abductor weakness of opposite side

Contd...

Contd...

- Abnormal substitutions include circumduction, external rotation/adduction, backward leaning of trunk/dragging toes; momentum uncontrolled swing
- Exaggerated hip flexion: Strong flexor synergy
• Knee
  - Inadequate knee flexion
  - Inadequate hip flexion and poor foot clearance; spastic quadriceps
  - Exaggerated but delayed knee flexion: Strong flexor synergy
  - Inadequate knee extension at weight acceptance: Spastic hamstring or sustained total flexor pattern
  - Weak knee extensors or poor proprioception
• Ankle/foot
  - Persistent equinus and/or equinovarus: Plantar flexor contracture or spasticity; weak dorsi flexors, delayed contraction of dorsi flexors/toes drag during midswing
  - Varus: Spastic anterior tibialis, weak peroneals and toe extensors
  - Equinovarus: Spasticity of post-tibialis and/or gastroc-soleus
  - Exaggerated dorsiflexion: Strong flexor synergy pattern

is one of the more reliable and widely used scales to measure stroke outcomes. Granger et al. reported that score of 60 out of possible 100 was pivotal in determining the attainment of assisted independence. Patients with stroke having scores below this level, demonstrated marked dependence, while scores below 40 demonstrated severe dependence. These patients typically had longer rehabilitation stays and were less likely to have successful outcomes. Outcome studies using other functional scales (e.g., the functional independence measure or FIM) are also available. All the functional scores can be individualized for a specific patient and the nature of his environment at home and at the workplace according to the socioeconomic conditions and patient's needs and preferences. For clinical implications, customized assessment for functional aspect is strongly advocated rather than following preprogrammed scores which are not very useful in India.

ASSESSMENT OF NORMAL POSTURAL REFLEX MECHANISM

To assess and treat the problems of the hemiplegic patients, the factors underlying normal movement must be understood. The normal postural reflex mechanism which provides a background for movement has two types of automatic reaction: righting reactions and equilibrium reactions.

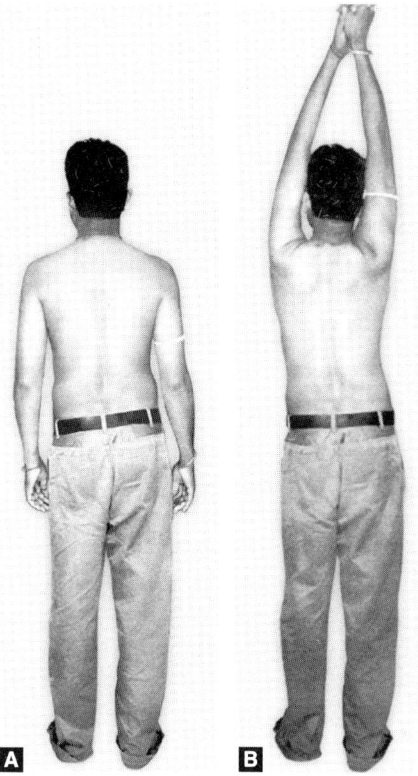

FIGURES 6.2A AND B: Standing posture from behind, right hemiplegia

- Righting reactions allow the normal position of the head in space and in relation to the body and normal alignment of trunk and limbs (Bobath, 1978). They give the rotation within the body axis which is necessary for most activities (Figures 6.2A and B).
- Equilibrium reactions maintain and regain balance. More complex than the righting reaction, they may be either visible movements or invisible change of tone against gravity. Basic patterns of movement evolve from the righting reaction of early childhood, which later become interacted with the equilibrium reaction. (Fiorentino, 1981).

The brain is continuously receiving sensory impulses from the periphery, is informing it of the body's activities. All movement is in response to these sensory stimuli and is monitored by proprioceptors (in muscles and joints), exteroceptors (in skin and subcutaneous tissue) and telereceptors (the eyes and ears); without sensation human beings do not know how to move or how to react to various situations, but in the conscious state intention may govern these reactions. Normal function of the body depends on the efficiency of the central nervous system as an organ of integration. Every skilled movement depends on:

Normal Postural Tone

Postural tone, which is variable, provides the background on which movement is based and is controlled at a subcortical level. It must be high enough to resist gravity yet still permit movement. Hypertonia is loss of dynamic tone, giving stability without mobility. Hypertonia precludes the stable posture necessary for movement. With each movement, posture changes and cannot be separated from it.

Normal Reciprocal Innervation

Reciprocal Innervations allows action between agonists and antagonists (Bobath, 1974). Proximally, the interaction results in a degree of co-contraction which provides fixation and stability. Distally, skilled movements are made possible by a greater degree of reciprocal inhibition.

Normal Patterns of Movement

Movement takes place in the patterns that are common to all although there are slight variations in the way different people perform the same activity. Normally, the brain is not aware of individual muscles, only of patterns of movement produced by the interaction of groups of muscles. This is Sherrington's principle.

SHORT ASSESSMENT AND TREATMENT PLANNING FOR ADULT HEMIPLEGIA (BOBATH ASSESSMENT FORM)

PATIENT'S NAME:

ADDRESS:

DIAGNOSIS:

DATE OF ONSET:

- General impression of patient:
  Seemingly younger or older than chronological age. Cooperation, indifference, emotional release, depression, negativism, aggression, euphoria, instability

- State of health:

    (How careful one has to be). Hypertension; heart insufficiency; respiration, giddiness, weakness, etc.

- What can the patient do?

    Does she use her trunk for balance? Does she use her normal side for every activity?

    Could she function with less compensation?

- What can she not do?

    Does she really need a tripod? An elbow crutch? A stick? A brace? A sling?

    Could she learn to walk with or even without an ordinary walking stick? With or without a brace?

- Is there potential on the affected side? Arm? Hand? Leg? Foot?

- Is she still within the period of spontaneous recovery?

- How is her balance in:

    Sitting:

    Standing:

    Walking:

- Can she use her affected arm?

- Her affected hand?

- Has she got associated reactions?

- Can she speak?

- Does she understand language?

- Can she read or write?

- The sensory state:

    (This is very important because of the effect of sensory deficit on movement, muscle power and prognosis)

    To test:

    Deep sensation (proprioception): of arm and leg. Position sense. Appreciation of movement (Both to be tested separately)

    Arm:

    Leg:

    Tactile sensation: On arm and leg. Discrimination of light touch. Pressure, stereognosis, temperature, dermatographia.

- Tonus

    Test reactions to being moved on arm and leg. Test in supine and sitting.

    Spasticity: Gives abnormal resistance or exaggerated assistance.

    Flaccidity: Uncontrolled full weight of limb.

There may be a mixture of both.

Leg:

Arm:

1. What is the most important and first aim in treatment?
2. Which function should the patient be prepared for at this stage?
3. What may be your final limitations?
4. What can you make the patient do with little help?
5. What will you do in treatment?

Tests for the Quality of Movement Patterns

Patterns to be Tested

Tests for arm and shoulder girdle (to be tested separately in supine, sitting and standing, as the result will be different in these positions.)

Grade 1

   i. Can he hold extended arm in elevation after having it placed there?
     With internal rotation?
     With external rotation?

  ii. Can he lower the extended arm from the position of elevation to the horizontal plane and back again to elevation?
     Forward-downwards?
     Sideway-downwards?
     With internal rotation?
     With external rotation?

 iii. Can he move the extended abducted arm from the horizontal plane to the side of his body and back again to the horizontal plane?
     With internal rotation?
     With external rotation?

Grade 2

   i. Can he lift his arm to touch the opposite shoulder?
     With palm of hand?
     With back of hand?

  ii. Can he bend his elbow with his arm in elevation to touch the top of his head?
     With pronation?
     With supination?

 iii. Can he fold his hands behind his head with both elbows in horizontal abduction?
     With wrist flexed?
     With wrist extended?

Grade 3

Can he supinate his forearm and wrist?

Without side-flexion of trunk on the affected side?

With flexed elbow and flexed fingers?

With extended elbow and extended fingers?

Can he pronate his forearm without adduction of arm at shoulder.

Can he externally rotate his extended arm?

In horizontal abduction?

By the side of his body?

In elevation.

Can he bend and extend his elbow in supination to touch the shoulder of the same side? Starting with:

- Arm by the side of his body?
- Horizontal abduction of the arm?

Tests for Wrist and Fingers

Grade 1

Can he place his flat hand forward down on table in front?

Can he do this sideways, when sitting on plinth?

With fingers and thumb abducted?

Grade 2

Can he open his hand to grasp?

With flexed wrist?

With extended wrist?

With pronation?

With supination?

With adducted fingers and thumb?

Grade 3

Can he grasp and open his fingers again?

With flexed elbow?

With extended elbow?

With pronation?

With supination?

Can he move individual fingers?

Thumb?

Index finger?

Little finger?

2nd and 3rd finger?

Can he oppose fingers and thumb?
  Thumb and index finger?
  Thumb and 2nd finger?
  Thumb and little finger?

Tests for Pelvis, Leg and Foot (Prone)

Grade 1
Can he bend his knee without bending his hip?
  With foot in dorsiflexion?
  With foot in plantar flexion?
  Foot inverted?
  Foot everted?

Grade 2
Can he lie with both legs externally rotated and extended, feet dorsiflexed and everted, heels touching?
Hold position when placed?
Turn affected leg out again to touch heel of sound leg after it has been internally rotated by therapist?
Perform internal and external rotation unaided?

Grade 3
Can he keep his heels together and touching while bending both knees to right angle?
  Affected foot inverted?
  Affected foot everted?
Can he hold knee of affected leg flexed at right angle and alternately dorsiflex and plantiflex ankle?
  Foot inverted?
  Foot everted?
  Without moving his knee?

Tests for Pelvis, Leg and Foot (Supine)

Grade 1
Can he bend affected leg?
  With sound leg flexed, foot off support?
  With sound leg extended?
  Without bending affected arm?
Can he bend hip and knee with foot remaining on the support from the beginning of extension until the foot is near his pelvis?
Can he extend his leg by degrees, his foot remaining on the support?

Grade2

Can he lift his pelvis without extending his affected leg, both feet on the support?

Can he keep his pelvis up and lift his sound leg?

Without dropping pelvis on the affected side?

Can he keep pelvis up and adduct and abduct knees?

Grade3

Can he dorsiflex his ankle?

Can he dorsiflex his toes?

   With flexed leg, foot on the support?

   With extended leg?

   With foot inverted?

   With foot everted?

Can he bend his knee when he lies near the edge of plinth, his leg over side of plinth? (Hip extended)

Sitting Tests on Chair

Grade1

Can patient adduct and abduct affected leg, foot on ground?

Can he adduct and abduct affected leg, foot lifted off ground?

Grade 2

Can he lift affected leg and place foot on sound knee? (Without use of hand to lift leg)

Can he draw affected foot back under chair, heel on the floor?

Can he stand up with sound foot in front of affected one? (Without use of hand?)

Standing Tests

Grade 1

Can he stand with parallel feet, feet touching?

Grade 2

Can he stand on affected leg, lifting sound one?

Can he stand on affected leg, sound one lifted and bend and extend standing leg?

Can he stand in position, sound leg forward with weight on it, affected leg behind and bend knee of affected leg without taking toes off ground?

Grade 3

Can he stand in step position, weight forward on sound leg, affected leg behind and lift foot without bending hip of affected leg?

Foot in inversion?

Foot in eversion?

Can he stand on affected leg and transfer weight over it to make step with sound leg?

Forward?

Backward?

Can he stand on sound leg and make steps forwards with affected leg without hitching pelvis up?

Can he stand on sound leg and make step backwards with affected leg without hitching pelvis up?

Can he stand on affected leg and lift his toes?

Tests for Balance and Other Automatic Protective Reactions

Balance Reactions
- Support and balance reactions on the affected forearm or on the affected extended arm when he lifts his sound arm and turns over from prone lying on his side.
- Balance reactions of the trunk and legs in sitting without the use of his sound hand, weight on the affected hip.
- Balance reactions in four-foot kneeling.
- Balance reactions in kneel-standing.
- Balance reactions in half-kneeling.
- Balance reactions in standing, feet parallel.
- Balance reactions in standing, feet in step position.
- Balance reactions on affected leg when making steps with sound leg.
- Balance reactions standing on the affected leg, the sound leg lifted.

Protective Extension and Support on Affected Arm
- In being moved forward towards table or wall.
- On being moved sideways to affected side towards table or wall.
- To protect face with affected arm and hand against ball or pillow thrown against.

Balance Reactions
- His shoulder girdle is pushed towards affected side. Does he remain supported on affected forearm?

- His sound arm is lifted forward and up, as when reaching out with one hand.

  Does he immediately transfer his weight towards the affected arm?

- His sound arm is lifted and moved backwards and he is turned to his side, support on affected arm.

  Does he remain supported on affected arm?

  Patient sitting on the plinth, his feet would be unsupported.

- He is pushed towards the affected side. Does he stay upright?

  Does he laterally flex his head towards the sound side?

  Does he abduct his sound leg?

  Does he use the affected forearm for support?

  Does he use the affected hand for support?

- He is pushed forward.

  Does he bend affected hip and knee?

  Does he extend his spine?

  Does he lift his head?

- Both his legs are lifted up by the therapist, knees flexed.

  Does he stay upright?

  Does he move affected arm forward?

  Does he support himself backwards with affected arm?

  Patient in four-foot kneeling

- His body is pushed towards the affected side.

  Does he abduct the sound leg?

  Does he remain on all fours?

- His sound arm is lifted and held up by the therapist.

  Does he keep affected arm extended?

- His sound leg is lifted.

  Does he keep affected leg flexed and transfer weight on to it?

- His sound arm and affected leg are lifted.

  Does he keep affected arm extended?

- His affected arm and his sound leg are lifted.

  Does he remain on affected flexed leg?

- His sound arm and leg are lifted.

  Does he transfer his weight towards the affected side and maintain position.

  Patient in kneel standing.

- He is pushed towards the affected side.

  Does he abduct the sound leg?

  Does he bend head laterally towards the sound side?

  Does he use his affected hand for support?

- He is pushed towards the sound side.
  Does he abduct the affected leg?
  Does he extend the affected arm sideways?
- He is pushed backwards and asked not to sit down.
  Does he extend the affected arm forwards?
- He is pushed gently forwards, his sound arm held backwards by the therapist.
  Does he use affected arm and hand for support on the ground?
  Does he lift affected foot off the ground?
  Patient half kneeling, sound foot forwards. (He should not use sound hand for support)
  His sound foot is lifted up by the therapist.
  Does he remain upright?
  Does he keep affected hip extended?
- His sound foot is lifted by the therapist and placed sideways.
  Does he remain upright?
  Does he show balance movements with his affected arm?
- His sound foot is placed from the above position back to kneel-standing.
  Does he keep upright?
  Does he keep affected hip extended?
  Patient standing, feet parallel, standing base narrow.
- He is tipped backwards and not allowed to make step backwards with sound leg. (Therapist puts her foot on his sound one to prevent step.)
  Does he step backwards with affected leg?
- He is tipped backwards and not allowed to make steps with either leg.
  Does he dorsiflex toes of affected leg?
  Big toe only?
  Dorsiflex ankle and toes of affected leg?
  Does he move affected arm forwards?
- He is tipped towards sound side.
  Does he abduct affected leg?
  Does he abduct and extend affected arm?
  Does he make steps to follow with affected leg across sound leg?
  Patient standing on affected leg only. (He is not allowed to use sound hand for support.)
- His sound foot is lifted by the therapist and moved forwards as in making a step, extending his knee.
  Does he keep the heel of affected leg on the ground?
  Does he keep the knee of the affected leg extended?
  Does he assist weight transfer forward over affected leg?

- His sound foot is lifted by the therapist and held up while he is pushed gently sideways towards the affected side.
  Does he follow and adjust his balance, moving the foot of the affected leg sideways by inverting and everting his foot alternately?
  The same maneuver is done pulling him towards the affected side.
  Does he follow and adjust his balance by moving his foot as above?

Tests for Protective Extension and Support of the Arm

When testing these reactions, the patient's sound arm should be held by his hand so that he cannot use it. It is advisable to hold the sound arm in extension and external rotation because this facilitates the extension of the affected arm and hand.

- The patient stands in front of a table or plinth. His sound arm is held backwards, he is pushed forwards towards the table.
  Does he extend his affected arm forward?
  Does he support himself on his fist?
  On the palm of his hand?
  His thumb adducted?
  His thumb abducted?
- The patient stands facing a wall, at a distance, which allows him to reach it with his hand. He is pushed forward against the wall, his sound arm held backwards.
  Does he lift his affected arm and stretch it out against the wall?
  Does he place his hand against the wall, fingers flexed, thumb adducted?
  Fingers open, thumb abducted?
- The patient is sitting on the plinth. His sound arm is held sideways by the therapist. He is pushed towards the affected side.
  Does he abduct the affected arm and support himself on his forearm?
  On his extended arm?
  Does he support himself on his fist?
  On his open palm?
  Thumb and fingers adducted?
  Thumb and fingers abducted?
- The patient stands sideways to a wall, at a distance which allows him to reach it with his affected hand.
  Does he abduct and lift the affected arm?
  With flexed elbow?
  Does he reach out for the wall with extended elbow?
  With his open hand?
  With adducted thumb and fingers?
  With abducted thumb and fingers?

■ The patient lies on the floor on his back. His sound hand is placed under his hip so that he cannot use it. The therapist takes a pillow and pretends to throw it towards his head.

Does he move his affected arm to protect his face?

With flexed elbow?

With internal rotation?

With external rotation?

With fisted hand?

With open hand?

Can he catch the pillow?

SUMMARY

The foregoing suggested tests should be used during treatment as well as for the initial assessment of the patient's need. They are not intended to be used as a test battery on every patient, one test after another before treatment is begun. Testing in this way gives the therapist not only constant information about the patient's ability and disability and about improvement achieved or not achieved, but it also gives a guide for necessary changes of treatment and for the way in which treatment should be progressed.

The importance of a closed link between assessment and treatment has been presented, together with three groups of detailed tests specifically designed to assist the hemiplegic patient's motor patterns. The results of the test will give the therapist a guide to the planning of treatment and information about patient's recovery.

While treating a patient having hemiplegia, the physiotherapist should always be focused on the assessment of the condition rather than the prototype exercise program. The treatment is never commenced before a thorough and stringent assessment protocol. The assessment comprises of the evaluation of the physical, mental, medical, emotional, social and other aspects which affect a person, as required and all these parameters are used in designing the 'exercise program' for the patient. The assessment and the treatment always go parallel to each other and an experienced physiotherapist would agree that all the treatment or therapy sessions are truly assessment sessions and vice versa. If a detailed and dedicated attempt is made towards the evaluation, the treatment program becomes evident and self-revealing. For the beginners, it is recommended that all the evaluation parameters should be written down and hence, it would become easier to design a perfect program for the patient. An experienced mind will gel both the assessment and therapy sessions with ease and hence, a lot of time saving on the part of the patient as well as the therapist is saved and the sessions become more effective.

Many scientists and clinicians of repute have taken great pains to divide the total recovery of the hemiplegic patient in to sequences as described before. A working knowledge of all these stages is recommended for an overview of the progression of the patient's condition.

Management and Rehabilitation Medicine

MEDICAL MANAGEMENT

Medical management includes the identification and control of risk factors. Primary prevention strategies may include:

- Regulation of blood pressure
- Dietary adjustments: Reduced intake of saturated fats and control of hypercholesterolemia and sodium and potassium intakes
- Cessation of smoking
- Platelet-inhibiting therapy: Use of platelet anti-aggregates, or anticoagulants
- Control of associated diseases (e.g. diabetes, heart disease)
- Surgery (carotid or vertebrobasilar endarterectomy, angioplasty)
- Spasticity management
- Critical care management in early stages
- Control of the complications and their management.

Medical management of acute cerebral infarction and progressing stroke generally includes strategies to:

- Restore fluid and electrolyte balance
- Maintain adequate airway and pulmonary function.

Patients in the acute stage may require suctioning but rarely intubation or assisted ventilation. Oxygen therapy may improve clinical signs of hypoxia but is not normally indicated.

- Maintain sufficient cardiac output. If the causes of stroke are cardiac in origin, medical management focuses on control of arrhythmias and cardiac decomposition
- Prevent hypoxia and control blood pressure. Hypotension is managed with volume expanders. Hypertension agents may be used but have the added risk of inducing hypotension and decreasing cerebral perfusion

- Prevent hypoglycemia or hyperglycemia
- Control seizures and infections
- Control intracranial pressure and uncal herniation using antiedema agents. Ventriculostomy may be indicated to monitor and drain cerebrospinal fluid (CSF).

Additional strategies currently under intense investigation include:

- Administration of clot-dissolving enzymes (fibrinolysins such as tissue plasminogen activator (TPA or streptokinase), with rapid referral to neurologic services
- Strategies aimed at increasing cerebral perfusion (hemodilution) and interrupting the cytotoxic chain of events (e.g., glumate receptors blockers, calcium channel blockers, barbiturates, or naloxone).

Neurosurgery may be indicated in cases where intracranial bleeding or compression cause elevated intracranial pressures, since death may result from brain herniation and brainstem compression. Generally superficial or lobar lesions (subdural hematoma, aneurysm, subarachnoid hemorrhage and arteriovenous malformation) are more amenable to neurosurgery than large, deep lesions.

Comprehensive services for the patient with stroke can best be provided by a team of rehabilitation specialists including the physician, nurse, physical therapist, occupational therapist, speech pathologist and medical social worker. Additional disciplines may also include a neuropsychologist, audiologist, dietician, or ophthalmologist. One of the critical aspects of communication with team members is the development of an integrated plan of care with collaborative goals and treatments that are mutually reinforced in all therapies.

PHILOSOPHY OF REHABILITATION MEDICINE

Hope, acceptance of the disability, goal setting, persistent efforts and reaching the goal.

Rehabilitation medicine means to make the disabled person "independent" and "self-sufficient" in all aspects of life.

Mahatma Gandhi, the father of nation has given many life philosophies which are well-recognized and honored by the people all over the world. The philosophy

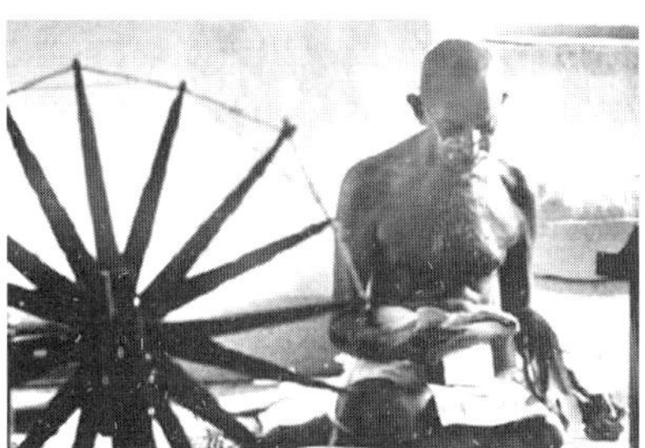

FIGURE 7.1: Gandhian philosophy of vocational self-sufficiency

of "self-sufficiency" and "independence" is the prime focus of the rehabilitation medicine professionals (Figure 7.1).

Need of Rehabilitation Medicine

Once the person becomes disabled (minor or major disability), the person is dependent for his activities of daily living (communication, self-care, mobility, feeding and earning for their livelihood). If proper measures are not taken for the rehabilitation of these disabled, they will become a burden to themselves, their family, society and the nation at large; hence, rehabilitation of a disabled person is an important thing not only for the person, but for the family and society and the nation.

Principles of Rehabilitation Medicine

Treatment
- It is a nondrug treatment program
- Natural physical agents are used for this treatment viz:
    - Heat
    - Cold
    - Light
    - Sunrays
    - Electricity
    - Therapeutic exercises
    - Supportive and assistive gadgets
    - Human support
    - Mind of the patient
    - Team work.

Patient is the most important person of the rehab medicine team. He is not a passive recipient of the treatment but also an active achiever of the goal. Rehabilitation medicine is not just restoration of the lost body functions but the final aim is to place the disabled person back to the family and to integrate the person in the work place and to provide a meaningful altered life style.

The goals of medical sciences are:
- To promote health
- To preserve health
- To restore health.

These goals are embodied in the word "prevention."

1. **Primary prevention:**

   It can be defined as "Action taken prior to the onset of disease, which removes the possibility that a disease will ever occur." It can be achieved through vaccines, hygiene, good nutritive food, cleanliness, hygiene, good habits, balance between activity and rest, exercises and education about potent threat to the health. The diseases and trauma are prevented and a good health is maintained.

2. **Secondary prevention:**

   It can be defined as "Action which halts the progress of a disease at its incipient stage and prevents complication". The specific interventions are early diagnosis and adequate treatment-means treating it before irreversible changes have taken place. The health programs initiated by the government are at the level of secondary prevention.

3. **Tertiary prevention:**

   It can be defined as "All measures available to reduce or limit impairments and disabilities, minimize the sufferings caused by existing departures from good health and to promote the patient's adjustments to irremediable conditions". Once the recovery and the restoration of the lost body functions is reached to the plateau—the disabled person is trained to maximize the available potentials and to retrain him "For return to living" back in the family, society and at work place by rehabilitation. Rehabilitation has been defined as "The combined and coordinated use of medical, social, individual to the highest possible level of functional ability." Rehabilitation medicine involves disciplines such as physical medicine or physiotherapy, occupational therapy, speech therapy and audiology, psychology, special education, social work, vocational guidance, etc.

AREAS OF REHABILITATION

The following areas of concern in rehabilitation have been identified:

- **Medical rehabilitation**—Restoration of lost function.
- **Physical rehabilitation**—Restoration of lost physical functions.
- **Vocational rehabilitation**—Restoration of the capacity to earn a livelihood.
- **Social rehabilitation**—Restoration of family and social relationships.
- **Psychological rehabilitation**—Restoration of personal dignity and confidence.
- **Sexual rehabilitation**—Hemiplegic patients are taught and trained about their sexual problems, sexual needs and how to find out sexual options for the sexual gratifications and sexual rehabilitation.

ASPECTS OF REHABILITATION

Physical rehabilitation has four aspects are given below:

Institution-based Rehabilitation (IBR)

The rehabilitation measures takes place in the institution, where ideal therapy takes place. It is provided by the high standard professionals. It is costly to use high technology. In the institution, lots of interactive learning takes place with other medical professionals. Medical education and research work also takes place.

Community-based Rehabilitation (CBR)

Here, proper study and the assessment of the community are done where the patient is going to live. The resources are found out from within the community (i.e. persons and materials). Persons are trained by professionals and low-cost appliances are used to help the disabled person.

Outreach-based Rehabilitation (OBR)

The rehabilitation medicine teams reach out in the community from the IBR and provide necessary assessment, treatment and guidance through camps, touring the patient's area program, etc.

Community Approach to Handicap in Development (CAHD)

Generally, the people in the society have a low level image for the disabled person. Some of these misconceptions are that the disabled cannot perform many tasks; he needs only custodial care and the person has to live a vegetative life, etc. Instead of giving sympathy, these people are to be considered as *differently abled* and empathy is to be provided to them, in their resettlement. Necessary mass education is needed to be given through media, handouts etc. to increase awareness about disability and its management and also to provide support to the disabled by the abled ones.

IMPAIRMENT, DISABILITY AND HANDICAP

The World Health Organization's International Classification of Impairments, Disabilities and Handicaps (ICIDH–2) defines these terms as follows:

Impairment

Any loss or abnormality of physiological, psychological, anatomical structure or function. Examples—loss of a finger, loss of conduction of impulse in the heart, or loss or certain chemicals in the brain leading to Parkinsonism. Not all impairments lead to disability, for example, loss of pinna of ear would not lead to loss of hearing but merely results in cosmetic deficiency.

Disability

Any restriction or loss of ability to perform an activity in the manner or within the range considered normal for a human being resulting from impairment, for example, difficulty in walking after lower limb amputation. To be considered disabled, a person should not be able to perform day to day activities, considered normal for his age, sex or physique.

Handicap

A disadvantage for a given individual in his or her social context, resulting from impairment or a disability that limits or prevents the fulfillment of a role that is normal for that individual. Many socioeconomic factors like family background, skills achieved and financial stability come into play while determining handicap. Impairment is a manifestation of a problem at the tissue or organ level, disability at the level of individual, while handicap is the translation of the problem at the social level.

REHABILITATIVE MANAGEMENT

General Considerations

- Rehabilitation, begun early in the acute stage, optimizes the patient's potential for functional recovery.
- Early mobilization prevents or minimizes the harmful effects of deconditioning and the potential for secondary impairments.
- Functional reorganization is promoted through use of the affected side.
- Maladaptive patterns of movement and poor habits may be prevented.
- Mental deterioration can be reduced through the development of a positive outlook and an early, organized plan of care that stresses resumption of normal, everyday activities.
- In the acute care setting, patients may be referred for rehabilitation services or may be admitted to a specific stroke rehabilitation unit, if such a kind

of unit is functioning in the vicinity of the patient's residence. Both groups have consistently demonstrated significantly improved functional outcomes when compared to patients not receiving those services.

■ Patients with moderate to severe residual deficits generally require intensive rehabilitation services to assist functional recovery. Optimal timing of rehabilitation based upon individual patient readiness is also important consideration.

■ A number of factors appear to be related to rehabilitation readiness, including the side of the lesion. There is some evidence to suggest that patients with right hemiplegia may respond more favorably to earlier comprehensive rehabilitation efforts. Patients with left hemiplegia, who suffer more cognitive perceptual deficits and generally have longer rehabilitation stays, may benefit from the additional preadministration time to allow for cognitive and perceptual motor reorganization.

■ Equally important factors that might influence the timing of rehabilitation efforts include medical stability, motivation, patient endurance, stage of recovery and ability to learn and last but not the least, the support from the immediate family members and financial considerations.

THE REHABILITATION TEAM

■ Family physician
■ Neurophysician
■ Neurosurgeon
■ Physician-rehabilitation medicine
■ Physiotherapist
■ Occupational therapist
■ Speech therapist and audiologist
■ Orthotist and prosthetist
■ Rehabilitation specialist nurses
■ Clinical psychologist
■ Medical social worker
■ Vocational guide
■ Recreational expert
■ Relatives of the patient.

The role of each member of the rehabilitation team is as important as other at different stages of the rehabilitation process. Each one of them has got a specific, well-defined work cutout for them in an ideal condition.

Family Physician

Family physician or a family doctor as we call them in India, is the backbone of the total medical care that the patient receives. They are the coordinators of the overall process. The patient usually goes to the family physician on the start of the symptoms. After carrying out primary clinical neurological examination, the patients are then referred to the specialists. Even during patient's hospital stay, they communicate with the specialist and with the relatives of the patient in a bilateral talk and become a bridge between the two. They carry forward the same job throughout the process of rehabilitation. From time to time, they also tackle the minor health related issues and mostly tackle all the queries imposed by the patient and their relatives. They always address to the psychological aspect of the patient and their immediate family. Thus, their role in the rehabilitation is of immense value and they therefore, influence directly on the final outcome of the patient suffering from hemiplegia. They are the primary caretakers in the rehabilitation team along with the neurophysicians, neurosurgeons and the physicians. In a typical Indian setup, they are of utmost importance.

Neurophysician–Neurosurgeon

They diagnose the patient's condition with various clinical, radiological, pathological and other tests and come to a proper conclusion. This in turn leads them to starting of the medical treatment through which, the patient's life is saved and the post disease disability is minimized. The intervention of the other rehabilitation personals is duly prescribed by them and the entire treatment protocol is set up. Time to time, the patient's condition is accessed and changes in the treatment are made if necessary. They diagnose the problem, by integrating the information obtained from the various clinical, pathological, radiological tests. After promptly diagnosing the problem, various treatment programs are started immediately and the services of other professionals are taken if required. Assessment of the condition is done by them from time to time and the treatment is duly changed and modified.

Rehabilitation Medicine Expert

There are these kinds of professionals in some of the countries which only deal with the rehabilitation medicine. However, in India, we do not have such kind of professionals in most of the places. They take over from the medical experts after the initial health and the general condition of the patient improves. In our country, this work is jointly done by the neurophysicians and the enlightened physiotherapists. Together as a team, they carry out the essentials of the rehabilitation process.

Physiotherapists

Physiotherapists or the physical therapists as they are widely known in the world today are arguably one of the most important members of the rehabilitation team, who are gaining acceptance world over in managing the treatment of the hemiplegic patients. They assess the physical condition of the patient and find out the areas of concern and help in accurate physical diagnosis of the condition of the patient. After the assessment, they plan out the therapy program most suitable for the individual and start the program, continue it and regularly modify the strategy of the same till the patient becomes self-sufficient, self-reliant and independent to carry out the lifestyle of choice.

Occupational Therapists

As the name suggests, the occupational therapists are the ones who actually prepare the patients to jump back to the vocation of the premorbid state. With various techniques and designs, they ensure that the environment becomes user-friendly. They work on the ergonomic level of the patient as well as the environment. They work on the perception of the patient so that the patient has a conducive environment for other rehabilitation members to work upon.

Speech Therapists and Audiologists

The speech therapists assess, diagnose and treat various disorders of speech, language and comprehension. They train them to become expressive and communicate with the fellow men clearly.

Orthotists and Prosthetists

These are the professionals who make the artificial devices to keep the limbs of the patient in a desired position. Along with the physiotherapists, they design and develop a befitting device which can be worn by the patient and which will assist profusely in speedy recovery. The splints can be either static or dynamic in nature. The commonly used splints are enumerated below. Cock up splint, ankle foot orthosis, knee support, shoulder subluxation strap, night splints and pneumatic splints are few of the most useful splints. The exact functions of these splints would be discussed in detail elsewhere.

Special Rehabilitation Nurses

As such, nursing is of paramount importance to any patient. But, the hemiplegic patients require some special attention on the part of the nursing staff. Initially, when the patient is totally bedridden, he will require special attention towards the hemiplegic side. Hygiene, on the affected side, may be low if not properly taken care of due to unwanted spastic patterns of motor activity, e.g. clenched fist. Also, there may be a combination of hypotonia as well as hypertonia which needs special attention while turning the patient during sponging or toilet training. Special nurses know the importance of giving all the kind of sensory inputs from the hemiplegic side, so that the motor response may be adequate. Problems like subluxated shoulder joint or stiff shoulder joints can be prevented right from the beginning by ensuring up to the mark nursing care. Thus, the nursing staff which is trained in dealing with the neurological patients in particular help in the speedy recovery of the patient.

Clinical Psychologists

Preparing the patient for the difficult times ahead so that the disturbed mind of the patient does not interfere in the rehabilitation process but in fact helps in the process, is the main aim of all the patients going through the routine of psychological orientation program. Clinical psychologists assist them to cope up with the real life situational problems post-hemiplegia. Not all the patients require an intervention of a psychiatrist, most of the patients respond well to the sessions given by the clinical psychologists. Here in India, this work is mainly done by the relatives of the patients in accordance with almost all the members of the rehabilitation team. This is a double-edged sword, because unscientific input given by untrained relatives may cause more psychological impairment rather than helping patient. Severe cases of behavioral problems may be well-referred to the psychiatrists. Many cases require support of the medicines like antidepressants or mood elevators.

Medical Social Worker

Medical social workers are the ones who create a social structure or framework for the patient so that the patient can get reasonably adjusted back in the society. We are today living in the 21st century which is very advanced society, but, unfortunately the disability is looked down upon by the so called able population. In such circumstances, the medical social worker will strive hard to put the patient back to the social life once again despite of the disability status. He will ensure that the resources which are present for the disabled, given by either government or charitable trusts, etc., reach the patient in totality and are used by the patient judiciously.

Vocational Guide

Not all the patients go back to the vocation of the premorbid state. They are now differently abled and hence, may not be able to function as efficiently as their prediseased state. That is why, they will require some other occupation for their livelihood. The vocational guide will help to tap the patient's potential to a greater extent and arrange for the same.

Recreational Therapists

These types of professionals may not exist in developing nations, but in some countries like Australia they do function in the rehabilitation hospices. They bring the recreation and fun back into the lives of the patients. They make the patients play games and modified sports activities. In some hospitals, these activities are carried out by the staff of the hospital. These activities look very simple but amazingly they are highly refreshing and energizing for the patients. They should be incorporated into the weekly routine of the patient's rehabilitation program. A sense of healthy competition motivates the patients to achieve the desired goal in a playful manner. Playing or sports of any kind would improve the quality of the movement of the body and will facilitate secretions from the brain which would be relaxing and mood elevating.

Relatives of the Patient

India is a country with strong traditional values and cultural ethos. Here, most of the work of the rehabilitation is carried out by the close relatives of the patient right from the acute condition to the final stages of the rehabilitation program. Coordination, integration, support, nursing, recreation, vocational guidance, carrying out exercises, all aspects of the treatment is duly carried out by the relatives and mostly very actively and with pleasure. This is the beauty of India and Indian culture. But, unfortunately as the country is growing and moving towards bigger cities, the nuclear families are at an increase and the support of the relatives is diminishing fast especially in bigger cities. In this scenario, the coordination of the rehabilitation team is vital, as it is the only support for the immediate family of the patient. We, as physiotherapists routinely see that nowadays, numbers of care takers for the patient are decreasing. The patients and the immediate family members are willing to carry out the optimum for the recovery, but they do not get enough support. For an example, the patient has started walking and can attend the physiotherapy department for the treatment. But, he will require transportation and help to reach the department. This is difficult to get and hence, the therapy is compromised. This leads to inadequate treatment and the disability is higher and the time of recovery is prolonged, or even, the recovery is denied.

It should be understood that providing only the facility will not ensure that the patient is receiving it, there should be an effort for ensuring that the patient is actually able to utilize the same.

ETHICAL VALUE SYSTEM IN PATIENT CARE

In our country, traditionally, the value system was always strong. But, nevertheless, strong competition in all fields and depletion of resources has forced some of the young to modify their moral values. But, in case of patient care, if any decrease in moral standard would directly affect the outcome of the recovery of the patient and there would be a breach in the trust between the patient and the treatment provider. Thus, in all faith, strong value system on both the sides would ensure a healthy environment.

A Systematic Approach to Treatment

APPROACH TO TREATMENT

The Unilateral Approach

It is generally accepted today that patients who have suffered from hemiplegia need not spend the rest of their lives in bed, but it was not so with the traditional methods. They were directed towards gaining independence by strengthening and training the sound side to compensate for the affected side. Many disadvantages are inherent in such methods:

- The resultant one-sidedness accentuates the lack of sensation and awareness.
- Relying on a tetrapod or stick for balance not only increases spasticity and abnormal associated reactions, but prevents use of the unaffected hand for functional tasks (the hand being solely involved in maintaining the patient in an upright position).
- One-sidedness requires increased effort to perform and function, making movement tiring and difficult. Consequently, spasticity increases and movement becomes more abnormally in a self-perpetuating manner.
- Progressive spasticity in the lower limb demands increasingly complex appliances which are difficult, if not impossible, for the patient to apply himself and which may ultimately fail to control the position of the foot.
- Increased tone in the upper limb leads to a distressingly obvious deformity, which hinders mobility and everyday activities including washing and dressing.
- The patient has no means of maintaining his balance or saving himself when he falls toward the hemiplegics side or backward as the stick or tetrapod would leave the floor, He is, therefore, very afraid walking or moving while standing.

- Strengthening only the sound side will further accentuate the hemineglect of the affected side and even the natural process of recovery is hindered.
- Over stimulation of the sound side along with the strengthening will produce biomechanical faults and this 'out of line' posture will be hazardous to the entire musculoskeletal system.

The Bilateral or Symmetrical Approach

- The bilateral approach is self-explaining term in which importance is given to both the sides and the therapy is aimed to gain movements of both the sides, which are biomechanically correct.
- Thus, this approach is also known as the symmetrical approach.
- Preferable methods stress the need to re-educate movement throughout the body, realizing that as the quality of movement improves, function will automatically improve.
- They aim to normalize tone and to facilitate normal movement, thus providing the sensorimotor experience on which all learning is based. If the patients are allowed to move in an abnormal manner with abnormal muscle tone, such experience of movement will be all he knows and correction afterwards will be more difficult.
- Everyone, regardless of age, should be treated in a way which gives the opportunity to develop maximum potential (Adler et al, 1980). Even if dramatic motor recovery is not achieved, each patient will be able to function better and live more normally.
- For those who have not reached complete independence, at least they will feel safer and move more freely and therefore will be easier to help.
- All treatment should be directed towards obtaining symmetry with normal balance reactions throughout the body.
- The affected side should be bombarded with every form of stimulation possible to make the patient aware of himself as a whole person again.
- Re-education of bilateral righting and equilibrium reactions in the head and trunk are vital for regaining independent balance. Importance of the trunk, as a base for the normal movements in space, is beyond question.
- *The recovering brain will learn whatever is presented to it, just like a child up to few years grasps even the complex concepts.* Thus, right from the initial stages of the treatment, patient is moved in normal patterns of activity.
- From the beginning, the patient must be discouraged from using the good arm to assist every movement as this reduces stimulation of the normal postural reflex mechanism and could prevent retune of control on the affected side.

- The patient should never struggle to perform an activity which is too advanced for him. Any movement he is unable to manage himself should be assisted to make the action smooth and easy without being passive. Excess effort induces abnormal tone and unwanted associated reactions (Brunnstrom, 1970)
- Assistance should be gradually lessened, until the patient performs the movement unaided
- Repetition re-establishes a memory of the feeling of normal movement
- Assistance does not mean that the therapist should replace the patient's effort. Assistance is given only to augment the active effort on patient's part. Even while carrying out passive movements in initial stages, patient is always told to produce some effort along with and in the direction of the movement
- When and if movement returns to the limbs it will be in abnormal patterns. It is most important to make the patient very aware of unwanted abnormal movements or associated reactions; such stereotyped patterns must be firmly corrected at once to prevent those becoming established habits (Kottke, 1980). It is vital to teach the patient to inhibit such reaction by self, e.g. to learn to stop the arm flexing up or the leg shooting into extension, each time, anything is done
- It is important that the fight against the hemiplegic posture be carried out on a 24-hours basis and not only by the intermittent therapy session (Ruskin, 1982). Thus, the therapy sessions do not end with the therapist leaving the patient but he should make sure that vital information is taught to the patient as well as the caretakers for the follow-up throughout the day

If everyone in contact with the patient reinforces the approach from the start, hours of physiotherapy time will be saved, easier and quicker learning is facilitated and the final result will be far more satisfactory. Because it is an overall management of the patient, the patient is never 'too ill to treat.'

Let us now consider few important techniques for treating a hemiplegic patient one by one. First let us consider the Bobath technique.

Bobath Concept for the Treatment of Adult Hemiplegia

The main concept of the treatment protocol designed by Berta Bobath is: *It is impossible to superimpose normal patterns on abnormal ones, so the abnormal patterns must be suppressed.* This is to inhibit spasticity at their "key points" of control to change the tone and facilitate:

- As near normal patterns of posture.
- To teach specific voluntary control.

The aim of the treatment is to reduce spasticity and facilitate more selective movement patterns both voluntary and automatic in preparation for functional activities, maintenance of posture and balance reaction.

- **Shunting**: By shunting, it means that the afferent impulses from muscle and joints influence the excitatory and inhibitory state (i.e. the synaptic pathways) of the spinal centers of the CNS. Shunting makes it possible to direct efferent impulses into predictable channels (the desired muscle groups) by positioning the body parts in various shunts—synaptic chains.
- **Inhibition**: it is the ability to refrain from one action in favor of another. This includes normal reaction to stimulus, i.e. the reaction in proper relation to stimulus.
- **Key points**: They are the proximal body parts from which the pathological reflex activity and the tone in the rest of the body part can be influenced.
- **Reflex inhibiting pattern (RIP)**: Is the pattern which change or break up the abnormal patterns due to release of tonic reflex activity.
- **Facilitation**: Facilitation incorporates the positioning of the patient in preparation for the automatic or the specific voluntary movements as the movements are easier to perform in certain postural sets.
- **Tapping rationale**: These techniques of tactile kinesthetic stimulation are similar to 'Kabat and Knott'. Recruiting and summation of nervous impulses by careful applied "Reciprocal Stimulations" to the muscles.
  - Effects:
    - To produce tone, increase in tone without producing hypertonia.
    - Facilitate muscular activity.
    - The treatment of hemiplegia is not a series of set exercises but sequences of learning or re-learning of movements for functional activities and maintenance of balance.

Principles of Treatment

The problem of the treatment is not that of strengthening or relaxing individual muscle groups but that of:

- Obtaining a more near normal muscle tone.
- Improving the coordination of posture and movements.
- A normal *postural reflex mechanism* is the prerequisite for normal movement. It consists of the interaction of various postural reactions, especially the *righting and the equilibrium and balance reaction* (Bobath B 1954, Bobath K 1959). A normal background of muscle tone for movements should be sufficiently high to make weight bearing against gravity possible and to give fixation to the movement but it must not be so high as to interfere

with the movement. Constant changes of posture are necessary accompaniments to the movements and changes of posture take place automatically, before a movement is initiated. (We don't think how we want to take turn, sit, stand or walk; we accomplish it totally, at an automatic level.)

Thus, every movement requires adequate *postural sets* to perform movements with ease and grace. Normal postural reflex activity is a prerequisite for normal muscle tone. Abnormal postural reflex activity is associated with abnormal muscle tone and set postural sets. The prime aim of the treatment is to normalize the tone by inhibiting abnormal postural reflex activity (Bobath B, 1955; Bobath K, 1957). These patterns are called reflex inhibitory patterns (RIP). Only after normalizing the tone at their "key points" of control (i.e. the head and neck and trunk), can the required movement pattern be performed without effort. Any effort will increase the tone, which will lead to abnormal reflex activity and abnormal performance of movement.

Principle Aims

- To change the abnormal tone by incorporating reflex inhibitory patterns.
- Reeducation of the abnormal postural patterns rather than to aim at strengthening or training of the individual muscle.
- The patient has to "re-learn" the movement patterns for functional activities and maintenance of balance. The therapist teaches and guides the patient to learn the movement patterns.
- The technique of the treatment is to treat the patient's reactions and the therapist is constantly guided by the responses of the patient to handling. There is continuous feedback between the patient and the therapist as therapist assesses during the treatment, the result of the technique utilized.
- The treatment techniques should be goal-oriented.
- The patient should always be treated as a whole. He is just not the arm, hand or leg. He has his middle—the trunk.
- Aim always at body symmetry and midline.
- Perceptual deficits are trained mainly by guiding and not by commands.

The Fundamental Principle of Treatment

As CNS is constantly seeking input for output, Davies (1994) focuses her treatment approach on the Input of the CNS emphasizing:
- Quality of touch.
- Minimization of fear.

- Removal of painful stimuli.
- Maintaining the dignity of the patient in every situation.

When damage occurs in one part of the brain, entire brain suffers from the lack of communication.

Treatment Concept

In the treatment of the hemiplegia the progress, residual disability and adjustments to affliction will depend on:

- Available resources in acute care.
- Severity of damage.
- Therapeutic approach.

Bobath's and Davies' concepts, from its very inception, are founded and evolved on current neuro physiological, neurodevelopmental and neuropsychological basis. The concept is based after considering the patient's movement problems, neuropsychological deficits and emotional status.

The entire concept is based on:

- Inhibition of spasticity and abnormal movement patterns.
- Facilitation of the movement patterns to near normal patterns of postures, balance and performance of movement sequences without effort.
- Holistic approach, treating the patient as a whole and not just his arm or leg.

As the problem is not the weakness of the muscles but that of the hypertonicity and spasticity and abnormal movement patterns. According to the treatments, principle of inhibition of spasticity and facilitation of near normal movements:

Normal movements cannot be superimposed on abnormal movement patterns and tone.

The abnormal tone is suppressed throughout the body by incorporating RIPs, at the key point of control in cardinal order. Proximally, these areas are head and neck and trunk, shoulder and pelvic girdles and distally the wrist and hand, ankle and foot, the weight bearing body parts. To estimate the potential ability and to plan systematic treatment approach, qualitative motor and somatosensory assessment is the basis for initial and follow up treatments.

The treatment from the day one is an ongoing process: That of teaching and relearning. The therapist teaches and the patient relearns the different patterns of posture, movements and balance. The nervous system learns by performance and needs to get *"in to the act"*, so the patient has to be actively involved in this activity and go through the process of learning to lay down the memory engrams. Communication is mostly by tactokinesthetic channel as the aim is to make the patient feel his environment (to be in touch with it). He must perform maximally at his peak level to activate the reticular system for attention and alertness.

In the early acute stage, respiratory care, correct positioning in semi prone position on both sides and careful handling of the shoulder girdle and shoulder joint helps to prevent setting in of strong hyper tonus and strong spastic patterns of hemiplegic posturing and compensation from the sound side. Assist in avoiding shoulder pain and shoulder problems.

The therapy program concentrates on:

- Head-neck orientation
- Activation of trunkal muscles, weight bearing and weight shifts.
- Through trunk activation of limbs movements, supporting the limb in RIPs and working in small ranges without effort.
- Bilateral activities of the limbs to prepare the patient for midline awareness, body symmetry and control and weight shifts in lying, sitting and standing.

As the spasticity reduces, the synergic element is broken down and the patient is able to actively perform motor activity. Body tonus and movement coordination are indivisible, they depend on each other. Retraining head neck orientation with a freely mobile head with intact balance and equilibrium reactions is very important for the patient to walk and move about without the fear of fall. Fear means instability. Instability means lack of center of gravity and base of support.

Where possible the patient must be taught to walk without support so that his good arm is free for balance. Patients who show little recovery in arm or leg can relearn the balance reactions remarkably well and recover ability to take quick steps to regain their balance in standing and walking.

Constantly evaluate your treatment technique for feedback response. If the desired response is lacking, analyze your handling (have you given too little support, was the effort too much, was the patient held in good RIP) and change your handling technique. Always start with the activity that the patient can achieve and watch for the reactions throughout his body. Splinting provokes exaggerated stretch reflex response, and hence, it is advocated to use the splinting judiciously.

In case of hypotonia or flaccidity, tactokinesthetic stimulations are advocated through:

- Inhibitory tapping
- Joint compressions
- Pressure tapping
- Brush and sweep tapping.

All these tapping procedures are to be cautiously applied to initiate motor activity. The motor output will be in response to the sensory input. Following restorative therapy, maintenance of the therapeutic care is very essential to monitor any deterioration in movement quality.

Let us now consider one of the most used techniques of treatment, the proprioceptive neuromuscular facilitation technique.

Proprioceptive Neuromuscular Facilitation (PNF)

Proprioceptive neuromuscular facilitation (PNF) is a philosophy and a method of treatment. It was started by Dr Herman Kabat in the 1940s. Dr Kabat and Margaret Knott continued to expand and develop the treatment techniques and procedures. At first PNF was used as a treatment for patients with poliomyelitis. With experience, it became clear that this treatment approach was effective for patients with a wide range of diagnosis. Today PNF techniques are widely used world over for the treatment of neurological and orthopedic cases.

Definition

- **Proprioception:** having to do with any of the sensory receptors that give information concerning movement and position of the body.
- **Neuromuscular:** involving the nerves and muscles.
- **Facilitation:** making easier.

PNF is a concept of treatment. Its underlying philosophy is that all human beings, including those with disabilities, have untapped existing potential (Kabat 1950). PNF is an integrated approach. Each treatment is directed at a total human being, not at a specific problem or body segment. The treatment approach is always positive, reinforcing and using that, which the patient can do, on a physical and psychological level. The primary goal of all treatment is to help patients achieve their highest level of function.

Basic Neurophysiological Principles

The work of Sir Charles Sherrington was important in the development of the procedures and techniques of PNF. The following useful definitions will provide an exact insight on the neurophysiologic aspect of the technique.

- **After discharge:** The effect of a stimulus continues after the stimulus stops. If the strength and the duration of the stimulus increase, the after discharge increases also. The feeling of increased power that comes after a maintained static contraction, is the result of after discharge.

- **Temporal summation:** A succession of weak stimuli (subliminal) occurring within a certain period of time combined (summate) to cause excitation.
- **Spatial summation:** Weak stimuli applied simultaneously to different areas of the body reinforce each other (summate) to cause excitation. Temporal and spatial summation can combine for greater activity.
- **Irradiation:** This is a spreading and increased strength of a response. It occurs when either the number of stimuli or the strength of the stimuli is increased. The response may be either excitation or inhibition.
- **Successive induction:** An increased excitation of the agonist muscles follows stimulation (contraction) of their antagonists. Techniques involving reversal of antagonists make use of this property.
- **Reciprocal innervation:** Contraction of muscles is accompanied by simultaneous inhibition of their antagonists. Reciprocal innervation is a necessary part of coordinated movement. Relaxation techniques make use of this property.

"The nervous system is continuous throughout its extent- there are no isolated parts."

Basic Procedures for Facilitation

The basic procedures for facilitation are:

- **Resistance**: To aid muscle contraction and motor control, to increase strength, aid motor learning.
- **Irradiation and reinforcement:** Use of the spread of the response to stimulation.
- **Manual contact:** To increase power and guide motion with grip and pressure.
- **Body position and body mechanics:** Guidance and control of motion or stability.
- **Verbal commands:** Use of words and the appropriate vocal volume to direct the patient.
- **Vision:** Use of vision to guide motion and increase force.
- **Traction and approximation:** The elongation or compression of the limbs and trunk to facilitate motion and stability.
- **Stretch:** The use of muscle elongation and the stretch reflex to facilitate contraction and decrease muscle fatigue.
- **Timing:** Promote normal timing and increase muscle contraction through timing for emphasis.
- **Patterns:** Synergistic mass patterns, components of functional normal motion.

A combination of these basic procedures is done to get a maximal response from the patient.

Techniques

The goal of the PNF techniques is to promote functional movement through facilitation, inhibition, strengthening and relaxation of muscle groups. The techniques use concentric, eccentric and static muscle contractions. These muscle contractions with properly graded resistance and suitable facilitatory procedures are combined and adjusted to fit the needs of each patient.

The techniques are,
- Rhythmic initiation
- Combination of isotonics
- Reversal of antagonists
    - Dynamic reversal of antagonists and slow reversal
    - Stabilizing reversal
    - Rhythmic stabilization
- Repeated stretch or repeated contraction
    - Repeated stretch from beginning of range
    - Repeated stretch through range
- Contract-relax
- Hold-relax
- Replication

Rhythmic initiation: Rhythmic motions of the limb or body through the desired range, starting with passive motion and progression to active resisted movement. It aids in initiation of movement, improves coordination and sense of motion, normalizes the rate of motion by either increasing or decreasing it, teaches the motion and helps the patient relax.

Combination of isotonics: Combined concentric, eccentric and stabilizing contractions of one group of muscles, i.e. agonists without relaxation. For treatment, start with the range where the patient has the most strength or best coordination. This technique activates control of motion, improves coordination, increases the active range of motion, strengthens the muscles and is effective in functional training in eccentric control of movement.

Reversal of antagonists: These techniques are based on Sherrington's principle of successive induction.
- **Dynamic reversals:** Active motion changing from one direction to the opposite without pause or relaxation is the characteristic of this motion. In normal life, we often see this kind of muscle activity, throwing a ball, bicycling, walking etc. It helps in gaining active range of motion, increase strength, develop coordination, i.e. smooth reversal of motion, prevent or reduce fatigue and increase endurance.

- **Stabilizing reversals:** Alternating isotonic contractions opposed by enough resistance to prevent motion. The command is a dynamic "push against my hands or don't let me push you", and the therapist allows only a very small movement. It increases stability and balance, increases muscle strength and increases coordination between agonists and antagonists.
- **Rhythmic stabilization:** It is characterized by alternating isometric contraction against resistance, no motion intended. It increases active and passive range of motion, increases strength, increases stability and balance and decreases pain.

Repeated stretch or repeated contractions:
- **Repeated stretch from beginning of range:** The stretch reflex elicited from muscles under the tension of elongation is the main characteristic of this technique. They facilitate initiation of motion, increase active range of motion, increase strength, prevent or reduce fatigue and guide motion in the direction desired.
- **Repeated stretch through range:** The stretch reflex elicited from muscles under the tension of contractions is the rationale of this technique. It helps to increase active range of motion, increase strength, prevent or reduce fatigue and guide motion in desired direction.

Contract-relax:
- **Contract-relax direct treatment:** It is resisted isotonic contraction of the restricting muscles i.e., antagonists, followed by relaxation and movement into the increased range. It increases passive range of motion.
- **Contract-relax indirect treatment:** The technique uses contraction of the agonistic muscles instead of the shortened muscles. "Don't let me push your arm down, keep pushing up."

Hold-relax:
- **Hold-relax direct treatment:** Resisted isometric contraction of the antagonistic muscles- shortened muscles, followed by relaxation. It increases passive range of motion and decreases pain.
- **Hold-relax indirect treatment:** In the indirect treatment with hold-relax, you resist the synergists of the shortened or painful muscles and not the painful muscles or painful motion. If that still causes pain, resist the synergistic muscles of the opposite pattern instead. It is indicated when the contraction of the restricted muscles is too painful.

Replication:
This is a technique to facilitate motor learning of functional activities. Teaching the patient, the outcome of a movement or activity is important for functional work, e.g. sports and self-care activities. It is helpful in teaching the patient

the end position or outcome of the movement and assesses the patient's ability to sustain a contraction when the agonist muscles are shortened.

Goals of PNF Techniques

- Initiate motion
  - Rhythmic initiation
  - Repeated stretch from beginning of range.
- Learn a motion
  - Rhythmic initiation
  - Combination of isotonics
  - Repeated stretch from beginning of range
  - Repeated stretch through range
  - Replication
- Change rate of motion
  - Rhythmic initiation
  - Dynamic reversals
  - Repeated stretch from beginning of range
  - Repeated stretch through range
- Increase range
  - Combination of isotonics
  - Dynamic reversals
  - Rhythmic stabilization
  - Stabilizing reversals
  - Repeated stretch from beginning of range
  - Repeated stretch through range
- Increase stability
  - Combination of isotonics
  - Stabilizing reversals
  - Rhythmic stabilization
- Increase coordination and control
  - Combination of isotonics
  - Rhythmic initiation
  - Dynamic reversals
  - Stabilizing reversals
  - Rhythmic stabilization
  - Repeated stretch from beginning of range
  - Replication
- Increase endurance
  - Dynamic reversals

  – Stabilizing reversals
  – Rhythmic stabilization
  – Repeated stretch from beginning of range
  – Repeated stretch through range
■ Increase range of motion
  – Dynamic reversals
  – Stabilizing reversals
  – Rhythmic stabilization
  – Repeated stretch from beginning of range
  – Contract-relax
  – Hold-relax
■ Relaxation
  – Rhythmic initiation
  – Rhythmic stabilization
  – Hold-relax
■ Decrease pain
  – Rhythmic stabilization or stabilizing reversals
  – Hold-relax

After discussing the rationale of the Bobath and the PNF techniques, let us now consider the Rood's technique, which focuses on the facilitation of neuromuscular system using various techniques.

The Rood Approach

The rood approach is based on the known physiological fact that the skeletomotor units with different enzyme profiles play a distinct role in control of movement and posture and how afferent input can influence different controls on these in the central nervous system. The techniques are many times used for all the neurological patients, majority being the hemiplegics. These techniques are also used effectively in conditions like rheumatoid arthritis, osteoarthritis, soft tissue injury and post-fractures. The techniques take the name after Margaret Rood, an American Physical Therapist who in 1956, stated that *'muscles have different duties. Most of them are a combination, but some predominate, in light work and others in heavy work* (Tables 8.1 and 8.2). The essential features of these techniques are:
■ Identification of goals
■ Identification of factors contributing to poor function
■ Following a sequence of positions and activities of normal motor development and selecting those most relevant to individual needs.

- Selection of appropriate afferent stimuli to exploit potentiality of tissues to change at molecular level. This facilitates attainment of motor goals and helps to prevent perpetuation of abnormal influences imposed by pathological needs
- Pertinent timing of stimuli.

Ensuring repetition in association with environs, and thus, managed without therapy, so that a lasting effect is obtained.

TABLE 8.1 Muscle work patterns

Light work	Heavy work
Phasic movement	Tonic co-contraction
Fast glycolytic motor units	Slow oxidative motor units
Superficial, usually multiarthrodial	Deep one joint
Fusiform or strap, small area of attachment	Pinnate, large area of attachment
Great increase in blood supply if active	Rich blood supply at all times
High metabolic cost, rapidly fatigue	Low metabolic cost, slow to fatigue
Flexors and adductors	Extensors and abductors

TABLE 8.2 Muscle work patterns

Light work patterns: Facilitated by	Heavy work patterns: Facilitated by
Quick stretch	Quick stretch
Unpleasant stimuli	Joint compression in correct alignment
Potentially harmful stimuli, pain (nociceptors)	Pressure on weight bearing surfaces, distal end fixed
Specific receptor sites on lips	Resistance distally to extension or abduction of proximal limb joint
Input from semicircular canals, e.g. movement of head in space	Input from utricle and saccule, static position of head in space
Inhibited by:	**Inhibited by:**
All stimuli for heavy work, e.g. compression of long axis of the body segments	All stimuli for light work, e.g. pain and movement of head

Total movement is facilitated in the normal early patterns of curl up, stretch out and rolling, omitting undesirable ones, e.g., total extension if extensor spasticity predominates. This will secure any component, muscle activity or movement, if necessary muscles are innervated and appropriate stimuli are used. Postural stability is facilitated by using positions with the distal segment fixed, and compression is given through correctly aligned head, trunk or limbs. Movement, active or passive, over the fixed distal segments prepares for dynamic stability. Lastly, movement is facilitated with the distal end of the part free. Objective and functional activities are used. In all these, head control is obtained before that of arms and upper trunk and lastly control of lower trunk and legs, thus, the principle of cephalocaudal development is observed. Movement control follows the sequence of flexion, extension, adduction, abduction and lastly, rotation as in ontogenetic development (Table 8.3).

Receptors

Receptors are divided into six types depending upon the area where they are found: cutaneous, muscle spindles, golgi tendon organs, mechanoreceptors in dermis and joints, labyrinthine system and receptors in special sense organs.

- **Cutaneous**
  - *Cutaneous stimulation by quick light brushing:* This is used as a preparatory facilitation to increase excitability of motor neurons which supply inhibited muscles. The area to be brushed is specific in terms of the nerve root supply to skin and muscle; these must be the same and the skin must lie on the same aspect of the part as does the muscle. In most cases, the skin overlying the muscle shares its root supply. A changing stimulus is needed and is continued only for a short time in one place. A soft artist's brush is used, or electronic brush may also be used. For skin supplied by anterior primary rami, the excitatory effect is local and mainly to superficial muscles, whereas, for the skin supplied by the posterior primary rami, the effect is excitatory to deep muscles. On the face, the effect is to the muscles of mastication and probably to the muscles of expression through the intersegmental connections of cranial nerves 5th and 7th. A delay of up to 20 minutes occurs before the maximal effect if the nerve pathways to the inhibited muscles have not been used recently. Rapid skin stimulation to the entire palm or sole of feet will increase the blood circulation of the entire part.
  - *Brief application of the cold:* In form of quick icing, this technique is used for excitatory facilitation. This is most effective when the part

TABLE 8.3 Sequences in gross motor development

A. Total Movement Patterns	Descriptions	Remarks
A1	Supine Withdrawal pattern, total flexion, tonic posture pattern, heavy work, trunk, neck and proximal extremity joints. Reciprocal innervations. Bilateral. Centered at 10th thoracic vertebra	Miss out in very young except those with extensor spasticity
A2	Roll over. Flexion top arm and leg. Phasic movement pattern	Use first for young child. CVA Hemiplegics
A3	Pivot patterns. Total extension. Reciprocal innervations. Bilateral. Centered at 10th vertebra	Avoid if extensor spasticity predominates
B. Fixed Distal Segments		
B1	Co-contraction neck, vertebral extension	Use for hyperkinesias of head and neck. Use to stabilize eyes if nystagmus
B2	Forearm support. Alignment must be correct to avoid trauma to glenohumeral joint	
B3	All fours	
B4	Sitting. Auto facilitation by pressure on knees through heels	
C. Movements over fixed distal segments to gain mobile stability	Examples: Rock side to side, backward and forward, turning movements	
D. Skilled movements Distal end of limbs free	Objective activities, e.g. reaching, crawling, walking	

to be treated is warm and almost immediate effect is observed when applied to the skin overlying the muscle.

– *Slow stroking:* If carried out from neck to sacrum, this can reduce choreoathetosis or excessive muscle tone. It should be applied rhythmically for three minutes.

– *Precautions:*
  • Use brushing for only three seconds in one place at one time, as, a longer duration of application will inhibit rather than facilitate.
  • In case of flaccidity, especially, in infant or young child with no mechanism for response, brushing may cause a seizure.
  • Avoid brushing to the external ears and outer thirds of forehead, as this has a central inhibiting effect.
  • Icing done behind the ear can reduce the blood pressure immediately.
  • Ice applied to special receptor areas in the sole of foot or palm of hand is potentially nociceptive so its usage should be avoided in very young children and sensitive individuals.
  • Ice can safely be applied over the lips and tongue as this is pleasant but teeth can be avoided as it is painful.
  • Ice applied over the skin supplied by the posterior primary rami may set up a chain of effects on viscera over which one has no control.
  • Ice used in the region of the left shoulder may be dangerous if there is known cardiac disease.

■ Muscle Spindles

– *Quick unexpected stretch:* On any muscle, this has a facilitatory effect via the spindle afferents from a primary ending (1a) and must therefore be avoided in spasticity.

– *Slow full stretch:* If this is applied to deep muscle components passing over one joint only it will be inhibitory to the muscle stretched and excitatory to the antagonists. Full length is gradually obtained and should be held for five minutes. Other stimuli than follow to elicit correct postural use of the part. The inhibitory effect is mediated via secondary spindle endings (2). The therapist should avoid synergic muscles which are multi jointed for the stretch as it would produce reflex inhibition in extensors and excitation in flexors. A chain reaction can be gained—if slow stretch is applied to soleus muscle, with the knee flexed, reciprocal activation of dorsiflexion is obtained which in turn inhibits the gastrocnemius muscle; the extensor thrust is prevented and a normal stance is facilitated. Other groups of deep muscles which respond well are vastus medialis and lateralis, the hip abductors, the lumbar and cervical deep extensors, the posterior muscles of the glenohumeral joint and the shoulder girdle retractors.

– *Vibration:* Muscle spindle can be stimulated by vibrations applied by a mechanical device at the musculotendinous junction with the muscle on stretch. The facilitation gained increases the strength of contraction and may overcome inhibition in a muscle. This reflex is known as Tonic vibratory reflex (TVR). Burke et al have shown that some fusimotor drive to a muscle is essential for production of the TVR. Cutaneous brushing prior to the use of vibrator should enhance its effect.

■ **Golgi Tendon Organs (1b)**

– These receptors lie in series with contractile muscle fibers at the musculotendinous junction and are also known as contraction receptors and are auto inhibitory to a non-resisted repeated contraction of a muscle. Their inhibitory effect can be cancelled by concurrent facilitatory influences, so to exploit the inhibition no resistance is given even by the force of gravity and a small range repeated contraction is requested.

– The patient is taught to produce repeatedly, very small range contraction of the spastic muscle and its antagonist. There must be no resistance even from gravity, the part should be supported, effort avoided and no facilitation given. After many repetitions, stimuli can be given to elicit strong isotonic contraction of the antagonistic extensor or abductor groups. The spastic group of muscles is thus lengthened and the process can be repeated using a starting position in which the spastic muscles are longer than previously. Gradually, by several series of repetitions, considerable relaxation can be gained.

– This technique is particularly useful for the adductors of hip and shoulder joints.

■ **Mechanoreceptors in Dermis and Joints**

– Receptors found in the ligaments and capsules of joints are known to play a vital role in the control of posture and movement. A classification of these receptors is given by Wyke (1972).

– Pressure on normal weight bearing areas increases activity in slow acting motor units which are stabilizers of the posture. For example, pressure under the medial side of the heel activates the dorsiflexor muscles which evert the foot, facilitates dorsiflexion in eversion and corrects the tendency to plantarflex and inversion in a spastic leg.

– If in the upper limb, the pressure is given to the heel of hand, spasticity and protective muscle spasm are reduced and deep postural tone is increased.

– Firm rubbing along the posterior border of the ulna and compression through the long axis of the upper or whole arm, with the head of humerus in its correct contact position with the scapula, will aid in decreasing the spasticity. No pain should be elicited.

– When pressure from the top of the skull to the ischial tuberosities is given through a correctly aligned and trunk, the deep postural muscles are activated and the head and trunk stabilizes. A weighted cap or weight cuff on shoulder can be used for this purpose.

– Prone positions, with the head or trunk unsupported, facilitate stability by increase in postural tone.

– Pressure on the distal attachment of the superficial muscles and on the palmar surfaces of the metacarpals allows the long flexor muscles to be released.

■ Labyrinthine System

– The position or movement of the head in space stimulates the receptors in the utricle and saccule and in the semicircular canals. Static positions will stimulate the utricle and saccule and influence postural tone; the tonic labyrinthine reflexes of the neonate are modified as righting and equilibrium reactions develop. The influence of retained or released tonic reflexes must be observed and positions must be selected to reduce these.

– Movement of the head stimulates the semicircular canals and elicits movement, reducing excessive postural tone and aiding the initiation of movement in cases of bradykinesia. This is most effective with the head in a vertical position and is easy to achieve by seating the patient in a revolving chair.

– To elicit total extension of head, trunk and extension and abduction of the limbs the patient is placed prone on a tilting plinth with the pivot pattern.

■ Receptors in Special Sense Organs

– Use should be made of stimulation of receptors in the nose and mouth to mobilize the face or to elicit tongue movements. Examples include using a drop of a dilute solution of quinine placed on the back of the tongue to overcome tongue thrust and solutions of ammonia held under the nose to release a Parkinsonian mask. Diluted unsweetened lemon juice stimulates secretions from the throat.

– Optical righting reactions can be elicited and motivation is gained either by looking at objects or following their movement. Rood techniques have been used to facilitate the respiratory muscles in unconscious patients.

Timing

A selection of body positions and activities can be made so that the sequences followed are timed for maximum facilitation. For example; skin brushing precedes all other stimuli to allow for the delay in its facilitatory effect. Verbal commands should coincide with the application of stimuli which gain an immediate effect.

Repetition

Axoplasmic flow along nerve processes produces changes in the molecules of nerve and muscle tissue. Repetition of regimes of activity over sufficient periods of time is needed to effect changes in muscle unit so that they are more suited to the demands made upon them. Regimes are planned for sufficient periods regularly and over a long enough span to ensure lasting beneficial effects.

Treatment Planning

- Hypokinesia
  - Skin brushing
  - Total movement will facilitate any weak component
  - Bone taps, quick ice, vibration
  - Deep muscles—distal end of segments fixed, then applying compression and resistance distally to gain co-contraction
  - Rocking movements.
- Bradykinesia
  - Semicircular canals—revolving chair, passive or active head and shoulder rotation, alternate punching a suspended target
  - Preparation for walking—use of poles held by patient and by therapist from behind
  - Auditory stimulation during each step.
- Hyperkinesia
  - Ontogenetic sequences are used
  - Stimulation of mechanoreceptors until deep muscles contract and hold the position
  - Weight bearing on prone is used.
- Spasticity
  - Spasticity with some voluntary movement control:
    a. Light brushing
    b. Slow stretch
    c. Non-resistant repeated contractions

d. Weight-bearing to facilitate mechanoreceptors. Compression pressure on weight-bearing areas
   e. To teach movement over fixed distal segments, finally eliciting selective motor function
   f. Specific position such as molding a hand around the cone.

■ Released grasp reflex

Firm slow massage using the heel of the hand applied to the nonweight bearing areas of the patients palm or the medial side of the sole of the foot will inhibit grasp in an adult.

■ Facilitation of swallowing and speech

– Light brushing to the upper lip, face and throat is used.
– Application of ice to lips and tongue gives facilitation.
– Resisted sucking is used as facilitation as well as it increases muscle strength.
– Application of a wipe of ice to the lower neck anteriorly.
– Sucking or sipping a drink of diluted unsweetened lemon juice helps to clear secretion in the throat by stimulating flow of thin saliva.

The following is an overview of a generalized protocol in the treatment of hemiplegic patients.

Motor Control Training

General Considerations

Training should focus on improving motor control by stressing selective movement patterns. Movement combinations that allow success in functional tasks should be emphasized. Patients frequently respond to movement commands with gross or mass patterns of movement and excessive effort. The linking together of the proper components and the refinement of isolated control requires a great deal of mental concentration and volitional control. Inhibition of unwanted activity and excessive effort is crucial to the patient's success. Movements that are performed too quickly or too strongly will be ineffective in producing the control needed. Initially, the therapist should select postures that assist the desired motion and/or reduce tone and reflex interference. As control develops, postures can be changed to more difficult ones that challenge developing control. Resistance to movement should be minimal. Often the resistance of gravity acting on the body, or slight manual resistance, is enough to initiate or facilitate the correct muscular responses. Normal function implies a tremendous variability in movement performance. Muscles need to be activated in a variety of patterns and contexts. Eccentric contractions are generally easier to perform than concentric. Isometric contractions are also important since increased recruitment of static gamma motoneurons occurs, thus providing additional facilitation for weak or hypotonic muscles. The clinician should stress slow reciprocal movements. This emphasis on balanced interaction of both agonists and antagonists is crucial for normal coordination and effective function.

If the patient is hypotonic and/or unable to initiate movement, effective strategies may include direct facilitation of movement using a variety of different stimuli. Exteroceptive, proprioceptive and reflex stimulation techniques can be utilized. Some disagreement exists, however, over the type of movements that ought to be stimulated. Brunnstrom advocated the use of synergistic patterns in early recovery for those patients unable to move at all. These patterns are viewed as part of recovery and used to bridge the gap between flaccidity and early movement. Once voluntary movement is achieved, synergistic patterns are then modified to selective patterns. The use of synergistic patterns is therefore limited to a small number of patients who demonstrate no voluntary return of movement. Patients who have voluntary control would be inappropriate candidates for this type of training.

Still others, adhering to the neurodevelopmental treatment (NDT) philosophy developed by Bobath believed that emphasis on synergistic movements can lead to an increase in spasticity, poor control of selective movement patterns and widespread abnormal reflex activity. In NDT, the patient learns to control tone and movement through the use of reflex inhibiting patterns that promote "normal" selective movements during functional activities. Automatic reactions are facilitated through the use of postural and sensory stimulation.

Coordination movement can also be promoted using PNF movement patterns. For example, the therapist might select extension with the knee flexing if the patient were experiencing incomplete knee flexion with hip extension at toe-off. Appropriate PNF techniques might include slow reversals, timing for emphasis with repeated contractions if components are deficient, or hold relax active movement, if initiation of movement is difficult. The technique of agonistic reversals is effective in developing the eccentric control necessary for normal function. Thus, activities of bridging, stand to sit, or kneeling to heel-sitting might be practiced.

Since patients with Hemiplegia present with variable symptoms, rigid adherence to any one approach may yield unsatisfactory results. Most therapists take an eclectic approach, selecting procedures from the different approaches that have the greatest chance of success. Choice of therapeutic techniques may also be dependent on other factors, including ease of delivering care, cost-effectiveness and length of treatment. The success of a particular technique also depends upon the physiotherapist who is delivering the therapeutic technique and the response of the patient towards the same. There are multiple variables in the patient care and hence, control of all is highly improbable. Thus, it becomes next to impossible to actually quantify the research comparing any two of the treatment approaches in the patients suffering from hemiplegia.

Tone Reduction

Patients who demonstrate the strong spasticity typically seen during the middle phases of recovery may benefit from a number of techniques designed to modify or reduce tone. These include positioning out of reflex-dependent postures, reflex-inhibiting patterns that encourage movement of the weak and hypotonic antagonists and avoiding excess effort and heavy resistance. Rhythmic rotation of limbs with slow, steady passive movement out of the spastic pattern may also serve to decrease tone, while providing ROM to the spastic limb. A reduction in truncal tone can be promoted through techniques of rhythmic initiation or slow reversals combined with upper and lower trunk rotation. Postures of sidelying, sitting, or hook lying are frequently used. Proprioceptive neuromuscular facilitation extremity or trunk patterns (chopping or lifting) that emphasize diagonal and rotational movements combined with techniques designed to reduce tone (e.g. rhythmic initiation) may also be helpful. Local facilitation techniques may prove successful in stimulating weak antagonists and reducing spasticity in some patients. However, as Bobath points out, reciprocal relationships are not always normal, particularly in the presence of strong spasticity, so that these techniques may be ineffective, serving to increase rather than decrease tone in the spastic muscles. Exercise procedures that take advantage of prolonged pressure on long tendons and the resultant inhibition are also effective in reducing tone. A common exercise for hemiplegics involves weight bearing on an extended, abducted and externally rotated arm with the wrist and finger extended. Slow rocking movements add to the inhibitory effect on the spastic wrist and finger flexors. Spasticity in the quadriceps can be similarly inhibited through weight bearing in kneeling or quadruped positions. Orally inflatable pressure splints have also been used effectively, to assist in the maintenance of inhibiting patterns by providing prolonged stretch and inhibition to spastic muscles. They also aid in providing stability and allow early weight bearing on a limb during training activities.

Techniques that promote a generalized reduction in tone by decreasing CNS arousal mechanisms, include slow stroking down the posterior primary rami, and soothing verbal commands. Gentle rocking works through the vestibular system to also produce a generalized reduction in tone.

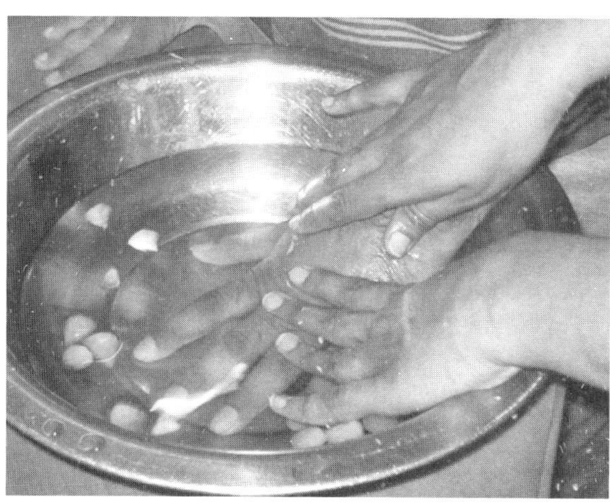

FIGURE 8.1: Quick ice dipping for activating finger extension, left hemiplegia

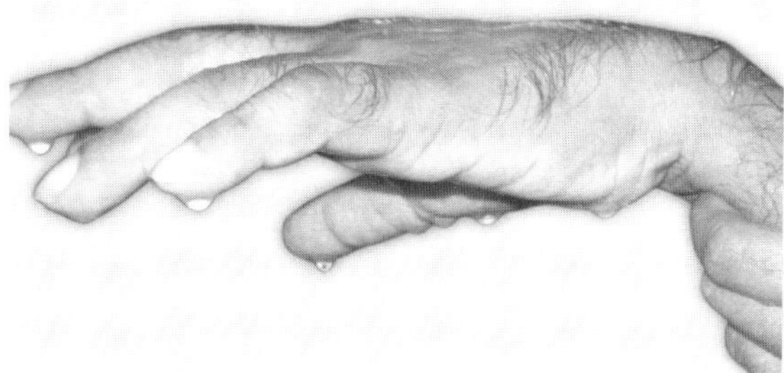

FIGURE 8.2: Active finger extension after icing, left hemiplegia

Myofascial release techniques, better known as MFR, can reduce the tone of the spastic muscles, significantly. During the process itself, when the therapist's fingers are moving on the patient's spastic muscles, relaxation of the muscles and soft feel of the relaxed muscles can be perceived. All the other techniques of treatment usually follow MFR and prolonged icing in a spastic case (Figure 8.1). The ease of the other exercises increases with this method.

Prolonged icing using ice wraps, ice packs, or ice massage may decrease spasticity by slowing conduction in nerves and muscles and decreasing muscle spindle activity (Figure 8.2). Once tone is reduced, the therapist should emphasize active movement out of the positions of spasticity. This can prolong the inhibitory effects and produce restrictive movements.

Compensation for Sensation Loss

Patients who have significant sensory loss may demonstrate impaired or absent spontaneous movement because of the lack of feedback signals before and during movement. The more the patient can be made to use the affected side, the greater the chance of increased sensory awareness and function. Conversely, the patient who refuses to use the hemiplegic side contributes to the problem of persistent lack of sensorimotor experience. Without attention during treatment, this 'learned nonuse' phenomenon can contribute to further deterioration. Treatment should, therefore, involve the patient using the hemiplegic side in volitional motor tasks.

The presentation of repeated sensory stimuli will maximize use of residual sensory function and CNS reorganization. Stretch, stroking, superficial and deep pressure and weight bearing with approximation can all be used during therapy to increase sensory input (Figure 8.3). Training should also focus on localization of touch. Electrical stimulation has been used to assist in activation and localization of sensorimotor responses. The selection of inputs should be directly related to the functional task at hand and provided to those surfaces directly used in the task (Figure 8.4). Stimulation should be of sufficient intensity to engage the system but not to produce adverse effects (Figure 8.5).

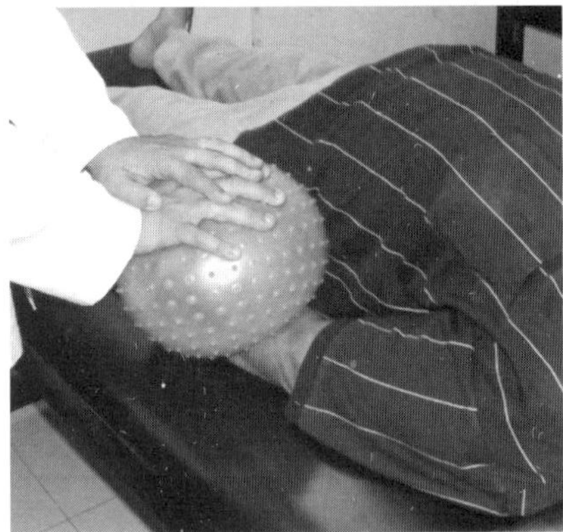

FIGURE 8.3: Sensory stimulation using deep pressure by texture ball, left hemiplegia

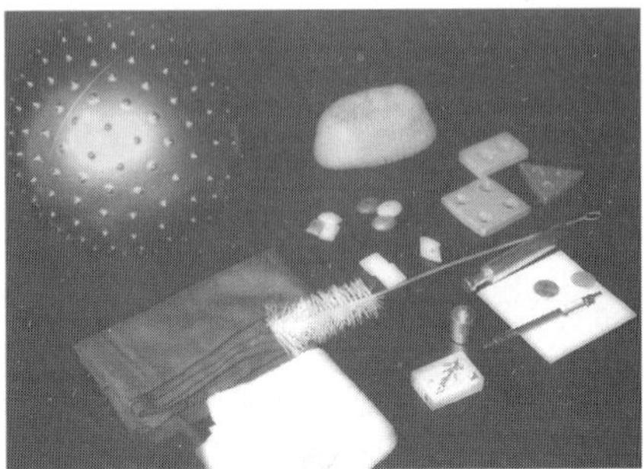

FIGURE 8.4: Various articles used for sensory stimulation and stereognosis

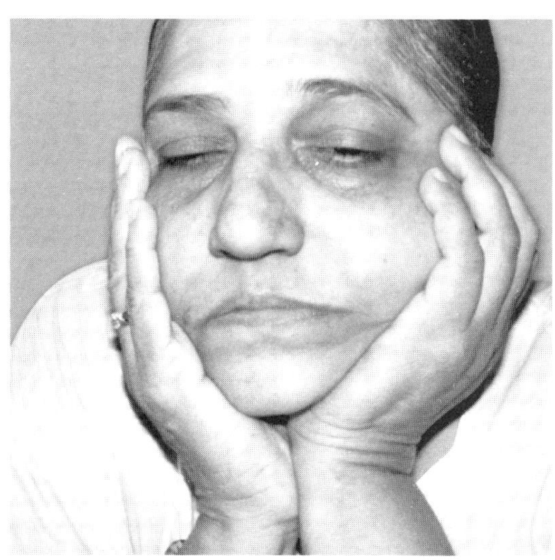

FIGURE 8.5: Self sensory activation by using palmar surface on face, left hemiplegia

Johnstone suggests that inflatable pressure splints can be used during treatment to provide additional sensory stimulation to deep pressure, muscle and joint senses. In more severe cases, she suggests a program of intermittent pressure therapy to stimulate movement within the tissues and overcome problems of sensory accommodation.

A safety education program for awareness of sensory deficits and care of anesthetic limbs should also be instituted. This is particularly important for preventing upper limb trauma during transfer and wheelchair activities. Training for those patients with hemianopsia and unilateral neglect traditionally includes emphasis on scanning the visual environment on the affected side.

Motor Learning Strategies

Recovery from hemiplegia is based on the brain's capacity for reorganization and adaptation. An effective rehabilitation plan capitalizes on this potential and encourages movement patterns closely linked to normal performance. Function should be stressed at all times and the function should be meaningful and important to the patient. Optimal motor learning can be ensured through attention to a number of factors. Demonstrate the desired task at the ideal performance speed. Manually, guide the patient through the desired movement to assist in his or her understanding of the task and its components. Encourage early active participation of the affected side. Practicing the movements on the unaffected side first (Figures 8.6 to 8.8) can yield important transfer effects to the affected side.

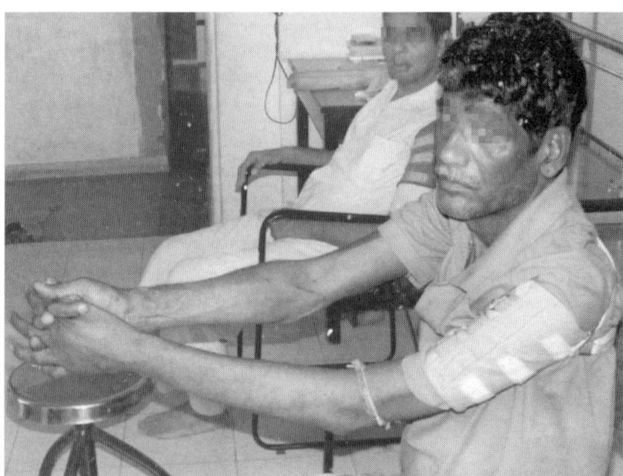

FIGURE 8.6: Bilateral upper limb usage, note the use of subluxation strap, Bobath type, left hemiplegia

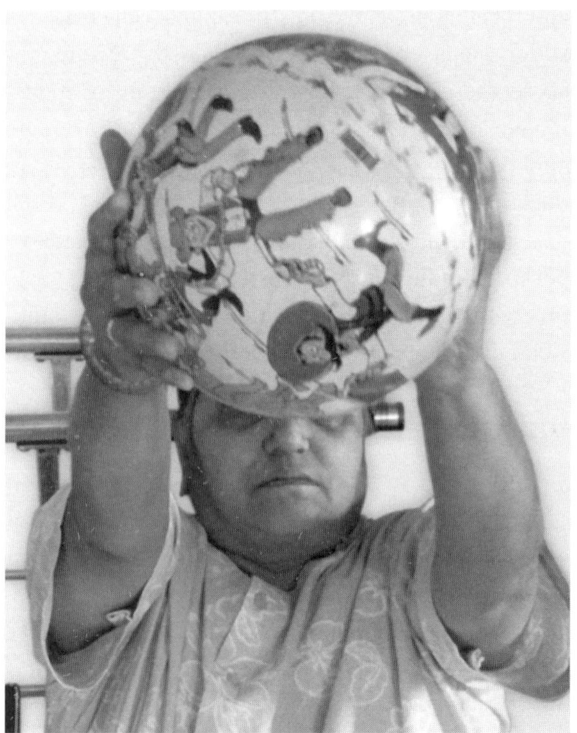

FIGURE 8.7: Bilateral upper limb usage using a dynamic object like a ball, left hemiplegia

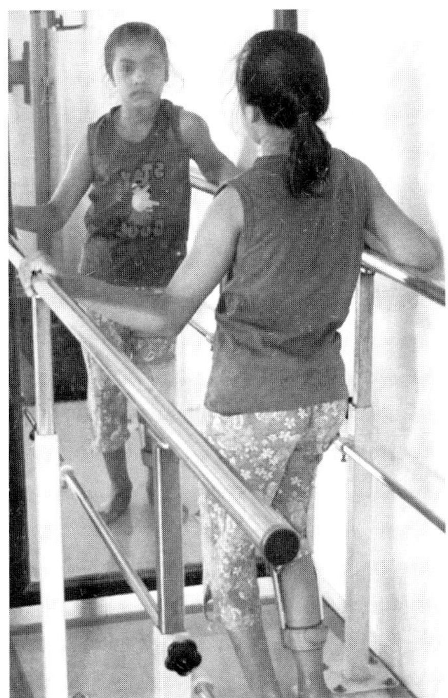

FIGURE 8.8: Weight-bearing in parallel bar

Simultaneous practice of similar movements on both sides can also improve learning, while promoting integration of both sides of the body. Visualization of the movement components can help some patients in initially organizing the movement. During early learning visual guidance is extremely important. This can be facilitated by having the patient watch the movement. If the patient needs glasses, make sure they are worn during therapy. Use of mirror can be an effective technique for some patients to improve visual feedback, especially during postural activities.

During later learning, proprioception becomes important for movement refinement. This can be encouraged by early and carefully reinforced weight bearing on the affected side in upright activities. Additional proprioceptive inputs (manual contacts, tapping, stretch, tracking resistance, antigravity postures, or vibration) can be used to improve movement feedback and stimulate the necessary components. The patient should be encouraged to "feel the movement" and learn to recognize correct movement responses from incorrect ones. Assist the patient in learning to eliminate the unnecessary movement components. Exteroceptive inputs (light rubbing, brushing, and ice application) may provide additional sources of information, particularly where distortions of proprioception exist. However, great care must be taken to avoid sensory bombardment or feedback dependence. To do this, requires careful assessment during each treatment session. Pain and fatigue (either mental or physical) should be avoided, since each will be associated with a decrease in motor performance. Careful attention to the learning environment will also yield important therapeutic gains. Reduce distractions and provide a consistent and comfortable place in which the patient can exercise. Provide clear, simple verbal instructions; do not overload the patient with excessive or wordy commands. Monitor performance carefully and give accurate feedback. Reinforce correct performance and intervene when movement errors become consistent. Organize the patient's schedule so that practice sessions are relatively short and the patient has adequate rest. Coordinate staff efforts to ensure that the patient is being asked to perform the task consistently with the same performance expectations. Progress and challenge the patient with a new task as soon as the previous one has been mastered. Encourage the patient to be self-sufficient and to develop self-assessment skills, goals, and problem-solving skills. Begin and end treatment sessions on a positive note, ensuring the patient has success in treatment and continuing motivation. Finally, communicate, support, and encourage the patient; recovery from stroke is an externally stressful experience and will challenge the abilities of both patient and therapist.

Treatment Program in Acute Stage

INTRODUCTION

The entire treatment program given in the following sections is integrated and designed so that all the important aspects of effective techniques are incorporated. The practicing therapist can modify the program as per the requirement of the patient.

Initially, when the patient is diagnosed with hemiplegia due to any of the causes, the effect on the patient as well as the close relatives is that of a catastrophe. The word *'paralysis'* itself has a huge weight attached to it. Thus, in the initial stages, it is important that the primary caretakers as well as all the members of the rehabilitation team educate the near and dear ones of the patient regarding the realistic prognosis. Many a times, it is not possible to give an exact picture of the prognosis, but nevertheless, the negative effect of the word *'paralysis'* should be counteracted by the positive approach.

Physiotherapy for the hemiplegic patient can be grossly divided into 5 stages which are as follows:

1. Neurointensive care unit (NICU).
2. Transient care unit (TCU).
3. Wards.
4. At patient's residence.
5. Outpatient-based department of the physiotherapy clinic.

Let us discuss the mode of physiotherapy treatment in all these stages.

DURING NICU AND TCU STAY

Initial stages of the treatment at the intensive care units are of utmost importance in saving the valuable life of the patient. From first few hours to a few days

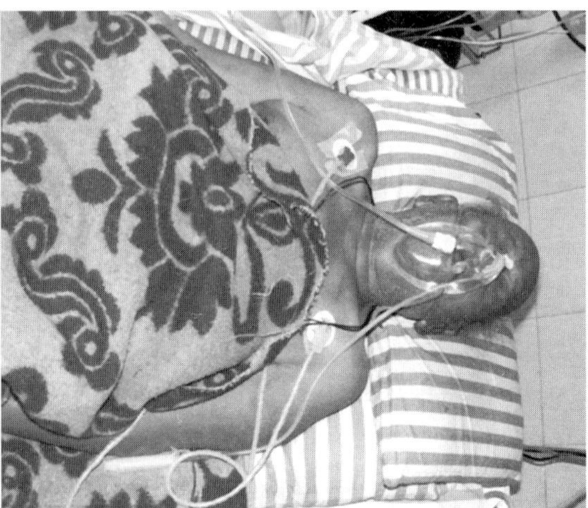

FIGURE 9.1: Patient in NICU

are very critical for the patient as well as the caretakers. For a physiotherapist, apart from being prompt and technically correct in therapy, being polite, caring, dedicated and remaining positive and using a positive and affirmative language will make wonders for the patient, as well as, for the near and dear ones. Usually, the patient may have a number of lines like: the Ryle's tube for feeding, parenteral line for fluid balance and medicines, endotracheal tube, indwelling urinary catheter or external catheter, etc. (Figure 9.1). Managing physiotherapy with these lines will be a challenge. Virtue of patience will pay off during this time.

Rehabilitation during the acute stage can begin as soon as the patient is medically stabilized, typically within 72 hours. Goals of physical therapy during the early rehabilitation will include:

■ Maintain ROM (range of motion) and prevent deformity
■ Promote awareness, active movement and use of the hemiplegic side
■ Improve trunk control, symmetry and balance
■ Improve functional mobility
■ Initiate self-care activities
■ Improve respiratory and oromotor function
■ Prevent secondary complications
■ Monitor changes associated with recovery
■ Minimize the feeling of fear of 'paralysis' for the patients and immediate relatives.

Treatment must commence immediately after the onset of hemiplegia. Progress will be more rapid if the patient is treated two or three times a day in the early stages, even if only 10 minutes at a time. The patient's ability and tolerance are directly related to the site and severity of the lesion and his physical condition prior to the illness rather than to the length of time since the incident. Treatment must progress accordingly. Most patients are able to sit out of bed within a few days and it is important for them to move from the ward or bedroom so that they are stimulated by the changes of surroundings. Shaving, wearing make-up and dressing in everyday clothes, all help to overcome the feeling of being an invalid.

Rehabilitation in a hospital department has the advantage of invaluable contact with other people and patients with similar problems as well as the stimulation of leaving home and dealing interdependently with new situations. Adequately instructed relatives and friends can provide a very effective learning environment and are often able to give more reinforcement to the concept of rehabilitation.

PULMONARY OR CHEST PHYSIOTHERAPY

In the initial stages, if the patient is unconscious, pulmonary physiotherapy in form of airway clearance and minimizing and treating lung complications is vital. Following methods are usually employed for the same.

- **Segmental Breathing Exercises:** The segmental breathing exercises are carried out by placing the hands on the chest wall of the corresponding part of the lung i.e., apical, middle and basal. Basal lobes are more likely to be involved during the long term stay in bed. Just by placing the hands on the part, expansion can be maintained as the air fills up that part of the lungs. Adding gentle pressure will provide sensory input to the part which is being treated. At the end of expiratory phase, gentle overpressure can be given to aid in increased inspiratory phase in the next breathing cycle.
- **Abdominal Breathing and Activation of Diaphragm:** Place the hands on the diaphragm and the lower costal margins. Gentle overpressure will aid in abdominal breathing. A palm placed directly over the upper abdominal region with gentle overpressure will also aid in abdominal breathing. For a right handed therapist, the right elbow flexed can be placed on the right side of the iliac crest and the forearm should cross the abdomen and the palm should rest on the left lower costal margin. With the thumb of the extended right palm resting on and palpating the diaphragm, gentle breathing by the patient is allowed to continue. This technique is beneficial for the patients who do not possess adequate strength of the diaphragm.
- **Vibrations and Percussions:** Vibrations given during the expiration phase will allow secretions to mobilize and get collected near principle bronchus

from where, they can be suctioned out. Vigorous percussions like shaking and clapping can be avoided in the initial stages but can be used judiciously. However, in case of complications like pneumonitis (which is fairly common), or lung consolidation and collapse, vigorous chest Physiotherapy three to four times a day and two to three times in the night time is strongly indicated.

■ **Suction:** Nebulizers are used prior to and after the treatment to expand the airways and aid in draining out the secretions. Suction is always done immediately after the therapy and again after a time period of about 15 minutes. This suction which we are talking about is in addition to the suction which is regularly carried out by the nursing staff round the clock. Suction catheter should be kept in the cavity for not more than 3 seconds at a time, as more time will create negative pressure within the airways of lungs. This procedure can be repeated as many times as required, till majority of the secretions are drained. The suction catheter should be introduced very slowly and gently with circular motion around its axis to avoid any injury inside the pharynx, the larynx or the bronchus. If by oral suction the secretions are not properly drained, an oral airway can be used to avoid the biting of the suction catheter. Many a times, a nasal airway has to be used to clear out the pharyngeal secretions. A laryngoscope has to be used to reach deeper into the larynx for more effective suction. During suctioning, a fall in the saturation of patient's oxygen level or fluctuations in heart rate are taken care of and any change if seen, suctioning is immediately discontinued till the patient stabilizes. It should be a matter of common sense to take all the necessary aseptic precaution while dealing with the patient in ICU or elsewhere. It is beneficial for both the patient as well as the therapist. Physiotherapy for the patient on artificial respirator or ventilator should be referred to additional reading recommended as it is a specialized subject in itself.

■ For chest physiotherapy, a compromise on the patient's positioning can be made as it may not be possible to give a head low position to majority of the patients with hemiplegia due to brain dysfunctions. Also, due to various lines and drains, it may be difficult to maintain side lying position and hence, whatever available position is used to deal with the lungs. Head up position of 30 to 40 degrees is strongly recommended, as this position avoids falling back of tongue which may be a cause of asphyxia. This position will drain the apical lobes automatically. The pressure of the abdominal organs on the lungs will be avoided by this position.

■ **Proprioceptive neuromuscular facilitation (PNF):** Proprioceptive patterns can be used to increase the chest expansion. Intercostal stretch is a useful tool to gain chest expansion. Mobilization of thorax in side lying will ensure maintenance of thoracic cage mobility. Overpressures to entire thoracic cage during expiration will facilitate draining of secretions as well as inspiration. Mild resistance to inspiration will facilitate it furthermore.

If the patient during the ICU stay is conscious and obeying verbal commands, the therapy program can be:

- Deep breathing exercises with pursed lips
- Deep breathing exercises with elongated expiratory phase
- Segmental breathing exercises
- Segmental breathing exercises with gentle vibrations
- PNF
- Active positioning
- Huffing and coughing
- Inspiratory incentive spirometry with calibrations for records of the daily progress of vital capacity
- Balloon spirometry for expiration and fun
- Chest expansion active and assisted
- Abdominal breathing exercises.

Usually a program of 5 to 10 deep breaths per hour is excellent workout. Over the day, a program of spirometry can be done many a times. Remaining therapies can be coordinated at every 2 to 3 hours. Making the patient sit up in the bed as soon as possible, will enable the chest to remain healthy. All the therapies may be discussed with the consultant of the patient for smooth functioning.

POSITIONING

Within the first few days, the physiotherapist should meet the patient's relatives and explain patient's difficulties and how they can help to overcome them. They will appreciate being involved and having something concrete to do while visiting; they often have more time to spend with the patient than either tend to sit on his unaffected side as his head is usually looking that way and, it is easier to gain his attention. They should sit on his affected side and be shown how to turn his head towards them by placing a hand over his cheek and applying a firm prolonged pressure until the head stay round. They should then strive to attract his attention by encouraging him to look at them and talk to them. Their conversation presence will stimulate him and help to restore his state of awareness. Holding his affected hand will give sensory stimulation and bring awareness of the limb. Initially, interested relatives can encourage the patient to do his self-assisted arm exercises and later, they can encourage other appropriate activities such as correcting posture and assisting in the therapeutic performance of self-care activities.

Instruction for Nurses and Relatives

Careful instructions and involvement of nurses and relatives are of paramount importance and will eliminate or minimize many of the complications associated with hemiplegia.

Position of the Bed in the Ward

The patient benefits if the position of his bed in the ward or room makes him look across his affected side at general activity or items on his affected side; he has to reach across the midline for a glass of water, napkin, etc.

Nursing Procedures

Great therapeutic value can be incorporated in routine procedures by encouraging the patient's participation. While bathing him in bed, the nurse can focus his attention on each part of the body by naming it and, asking for his help to facilitate washing, e.g. rolling on to his side with her and holding up the affected arm with the sound hand; or rolling actively as she is making the bed. When a bedpan, medicine or food is brought to the patient, the approach should be from his affected side, thereby increasing his awareness of it.

Position the Patient in Bed

The bed must have a firm mattress on a solid base and the height should be adjustable. It will need to be lowered to enable easy and correct transfer of the patient into a chair. Five or six pillows will be required to maintain the correct alignment of the head, trunk and limbs. The patient's position should be changed frequently. Two to three-hourly turning is advisable in the early stages while the patient is confined to bed. Even when he is out of bed during the day and more active, correct positioning at night must continue.

Position Lying on the Affected Side

- The head is forward with the trunk straight and in line
- The underneath shoulder is protracted with the forearm supinated
- The underneath leg is extended at the hip and slightly flexed at the knee
- The upper leg is in front, on one pillow
- Nothing should be placed in the hand or under the sole of the foot because this would stimulate undesirable reflex activity, i.e. flexion in the hand and extensor thrust in the leg.

Position Lying on the Sound Side

- Patient is in full side lying, not just a quarter turn.
- The head is forward with the trunk straight and in line. If necessary, a pillow under the waist will elongate the affected side further.
- The affected shoulder is protracted with the arm forward on a pillow.
- The upper leg is in front, on one pillow. (The foot must be fully-supported by the pillow and not hang over the end in inversion).
- A pillow is behind the back.
- Nothing should be placed in the hand or under the sole of the foot.

Position in Supine

- The head is rotated towards the affected side and flexed to the good side.
- The trunk is elongated on the affected side.
- The affected shoulder is protracted on a pillow with the arm elevated or straight by the side.
- A pillow is place under the hip to prevent retraction of the pelvis and lateral rotation of the leg.
- Nothing should be placed in the hand or under the sole of the foot.

In the supine position, there will be the greatest increase in abnormal tone because of the influence of reflex activity, and this position should be avoided whenever possible.

Positioning of the patient is one of the first considerations during early rehabilitation. The room should be arranged to maximize patient awareness of the hemiplegic side. A bed positioned with the hemiplegic side towards the main part of room, door and source of interaction will stimulate the patient to turn toward and engage the affected side. The resulting sensory stimulation to the stroke side promotes integration and symmetry of the two sides of the body. However, this may be contraindicated in cases of unilateral neglect or anosognosia, since the arrangement may contribute to sensory deprivation and withdrawal.

Early on, the patient is likely to spend significant time in bed and effective positioning program seeks to prevent undesirable postures, which can lead to contractures or decubitus ulcers. Since, most stroke patients will become spastic, a positioning program also aims to position the patient out of tone-dependent and reflex-dependent postures. Patients are generally placed on a positioning schedule, with turning every 2 to 3 hours. Assumption of upright postures is promoted as soon as possible.

The following postures should be 'totally avoided':

- Lateral side flexion of the head and trunk toward the affected side with head rotation toward the unaffected side.
- Depression and retraction of the scapula, internal rotation and adduction of the arm, elbow flexion and forearm pronation, wrist and finger flexion.
- Retraction and elevation of the hip, with hip and knee extension and hip adduction; or hip and knee flexion with hip abduction. Ankle plantar flexion is common to both.

The supine position should be balanced with other positions since there is a high risk of pressure sore development in the sacral area, heel and lateral malleolus, if the leg is externally rotated. It also maximizes reflex effects. Thus, extensor tone associated with the tonic labyrinth reflex and tonal responses associated with head positions of the tonic neck reflexes may be promoted. A footboard should be avoided since abnormal extensor responses of the foot and leg may be stimulated with a contact stimulus to the ball of the foot. Similarly, objects should not be placed in the hand, since the grasp reflex may be stimulated, increasing flexor spasticity. Attention should also be directed to the hemiplegic shoulder. Correct positioning protects the shoulder from downward displacement by controlling the scapula position in slight protraction and upward rotation. Gentle approximation forces through the shoulder joint can also assist in preventing shoulder subluxation.

Due to presence of various indwelling lines for the intravenous fluids, Ryle's tube, indwelling catheter, nasal or oxygen with mask and/or endotracheal tube, it is difficult for the nurses and the therapist to give a proper positioning to the patient. Care should be taken so as to avoid the disturbance to the lines which are life-saving. Nevertheless, the importance of the proper positioning should not be compromised at any cost. Initially, the Medical staffs as well as the patient's relatives are anxious about the lifesaving measures for the patient. Thus, it is the duty of the therapist to make sure about the avoidance of the faulty postures and promotion of good positioning.

Common positions that should be promoted include:

- **Lying in the supine position:** As explained above, the head and trunk should be positioned in midline or flexed slightly toward the sound side to elongate muscles on the hemiplegic side. A small pillow or towel under the scapula wall assists in scapula protraction. The arm can rest on a supporting pillow, extended and in abduction, with wrist and finger extension. The pelvis is protracted with the leg in a neutral position relative to rotation. The affected knee is positioned with a small towel roll to prevent hyperextension.

■ **Lying on the sound side:** When the patient is lying on the unaffected side, the trunk should be straight. A small pillow under the cage can be used to elongate the hemiplegic side. The affected shoulder is protracted with the elbow extended and the forearm is neutral or supinated. The pelvis is protracted and the affected leg flexed at the knee with hip extended, in neutral rotation and supported by a pillow (Figures 9.2 and 9.3).

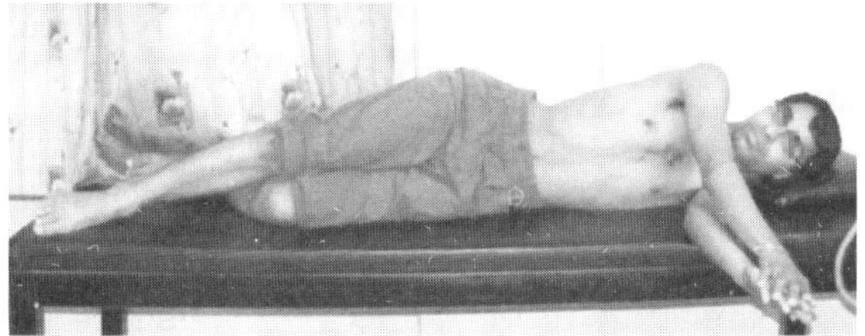

FIGURE 9.2: Lying on the sound side, right hemiplegia

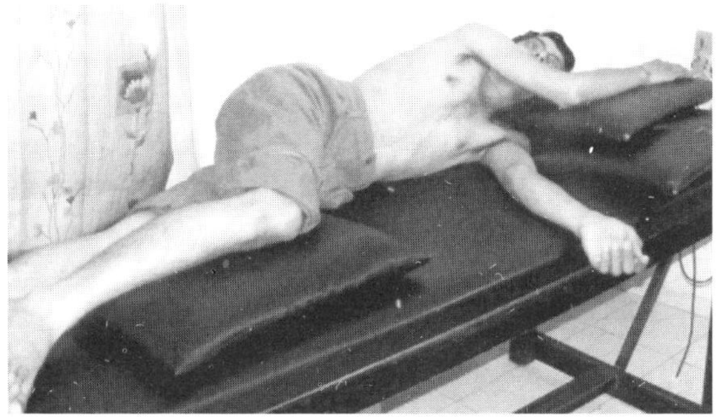

FIGURE 9.3: Lying on unaffected side with pillow support, right hemiplegia

■ **Lying on affected side**: When the patient is lying on the affected side, the trunk should be straight. The affected shoulder underneath is positioned well forward with the elbow extended and forearm supinated. The affected leg is positioned in hip extension with knee flexion. An alternate position has slight hip and knee flexion with pelvic protraction. The unaffected leg is positioned in flexion on a supporting pillow.

■ **Sitting:** The patient should sit upright with trunk and head in midline alignment. Symmetrical weight bearing on both buttocks should be encouraged. The legs should be in neutral with respect to rotation. When sitting in bed, pillows may be needed to bring the trunk to the upright position. When sitting in a chair, the hips and knees should be positioned in 90 degrees of flexion, with weight bearing on the posterior thighs and with the feet flat. In bed, the arm can be supported on a pillow or adjustable

table, while in a wheelchair, an arm board or lap board can be used. The scapula should again be slightly protracted with wrist and fingers extended in a functional open position.

PASSIVE RANGE OF MOTION EXERCISES

Passive ranges of motion exercises are most vital during initial stage. They create an imprint on the brain, aid in peripheral blood circulation, prevent tightness, contractures and deformities, and prevent bedsores and deep venous thrombosis (DVT). Passive movements can be carried out in full range of motion wherever applicable, 10 to 15 repetitions for each joint, 4 to 5 times a day. Therapist can start from periphery (fingers and toes) to head or from head to periphery. Usually, head righting and trunk righting is recommended, prior to any limb mobilization for increased effectiveness. Positioning for head and trunk, as discussed earlier is important for a sequential rehabilitation. For a patient who is unable to maintain the position, frequent change in position has to be organized by the caretakers. For ease in application, a sequence is described below:

- **Head and neck:** Flexion, extension, side flexion to right, side flexion to left, rotation to right and rotation to left.
- **Trunk:** Upper trunk rotation to right and left, lower trunk rotation to right and left, assisted pelvic tilts, flexion of trunk, extension using pillows in supine-lying, or another easier method is stretching in side-lying position, side stretches on both the sides when the patient is in side-lying position. One hand can be kept on the anterior-superior iliac spine and other hand crosses and is held beneath the scapula at its inferior angle. Stretch is applied by taking the two points apart.
- **Scapulae:** All the mobilization of scapula is done along the thoracic cage only. If viewed from sides, the thoracic cage is convex from top to bottom and from side to side, hence, the scapula moves in the similar fashion on the thoracic cage. Scapular mobilization, passively, can be carried out either in supine or side-lying. Side-lying position is a better position as moving scapula can be viewed easily. Care should be taken as to not suspend the flail hemiplegic limb to protect the glenohumeral joint, which is suspended only by the muscular support.

  Sequence of the movements may be: Elevation, depression, protraction, retraction, upward rotation, downward rotation, and combination of these movements. Tipping of scapula is avoided due to chances of injury to the rotator cuff musculature.

- **Shoulder (glenohumeral) joint:** The entire upper extremity should be well supported while performing movements. One hand of the therapist holds the palm with abducted thumb and other hand is kept at the elbow joint to stabilize it. The sequence of the movement can be: Flexion, extension, abduction, adduction, internal rotation, external rotation in full range of motion. Passive movements can be also performed in a PNF pattern, e.g. scapula: Elevation, retraction; shoulder: Flexion, abduction, external rotation; elbow: Extension; radioulnar: Supination; wrist: Extension, radial deviation; fingers: Extended and abducted; thumb: Extended and abducted.
- **Elbow joint:** Flexion and extension is carried out in a gentle manner. Risk of myositis ossificans is kept in mind.
- **Radioulnar joint:** Pronation and Supination. In this mobilization, grip is of importance. One hand is kept on the elbow at the cubital fossa and other hand grips the lower end of radius and ulna, just before the wrist joint and the pivot force is applied. The therapist's hand should not cross the wrist joint while mobilization because, if done so, a shearing force (twisting) is diverted towards the wrist joint, in case of a stiff radioulnar joint which will produce pain in the wrist.
- **Wrist joint:** Flexion, extension, radial deviation, ulnar deviation.
- **Fingers:** Flexion, extension at metacarpophalangeal (MCP), distal interphalangeal (DIP), and proximal interphalangeal (PIP) joints individually as well as together for all fingers, abduction (fanning) and adduction of fingers, intermetacarpal glides.
- **Thumb:** Flexion and extension at carpometacarpal (CMC) and interphalangeal (IP) joints, abduction, adduction, opponens and circumduction.
- **Hip joint:** Flexion, extension (up to neutral in supine, can be extended further in side-lying), abduction, adduction, external rotation, internal rotation.
- **Knee joint:** Flexion, extension. Proper care is taken while carrying our passive or assisted knee mobilization. One palm of the therapist is kept beneath the knee joint on the popliteal fossa to prevent the knee from snapping during extension. As during the initial stages, the muscles are flail, ligaments of the knee may get damaged due to improper handling.
- **Ankle and subtalar joints:** Dorsiflexion, plantar flexion, inversion and eversion.
- **Foot and toes:** Intermetatarsal glides, toes flexion and extension.

All the above mentioned movements are carried out gently without much application of force. The speed of movement is kept slow and rhythmic. Undue stimulation of sensitive structures is avoided, e.g. sole of feet, ball of great toe, palmer area, as it may produce exaggerated response due to sensory loading.

These movements can be carried out in the sets of 10 to 15 repetitions, 4 to 5 times in a day or as the need be.

If the patient has regained lost consciousness and is in a position to obey verbal commands, assessment of the volitional activities is carried out and accordingly, active exercise treatment protocol is designed and planned. General contraindications of movements and mobilizations are kept in mind. Jerky movements and gross movement patterns using momentum are not allowed as it leads to development of abnormal reflex pattern activity. E.g., clenching fists prior to the development of wrist and fingers extensors will inhibit opening of fingers. Straight leg raisings will promote extensor thrust in lower limbs which is decremental for patient's gait.

RANGE OF MOTION AND PREVENTION OF LIMB TRAUMA

Range of motion exercises during early recovery maintains normal range in flaccid, non-functional limbs and maintains mobility of the joint capsule. In the upper extremity, correct ROM techniques should include careful attention to external rotation of the arm with scapular mobilization and upward rotation during shoulder elevation activities (Figures 9.4 and 9.5). If the motions are not performed, the patient is likely to experience shoulder impingement, rotator cuff injury and pain. The use of overhead pulleys for self-ROM is generally contraindicated for the above reasons. Full ROM should be performed in all shoulder motions. Inadequate ranging can lead to the development of adhesive capsulitis and/or shoulder hand syndrome. Tightness and swelling of the wrist and finger flexors may develop. Daily range of motion, elevation, massage, icing, or compression wrapping may improve the status of the hand. Splinting in a functional position can also be considered. Either dorsal or volar resting pan splints that incorporate the forearm, wrist, and hand are commonly used.

During position changes, care must be taken not to pull onto the arm or let it hang unsupported, since the risk of traction injury would be increased. A hemi sling with pads beneath the elbow and wrist and/or hand may be used to support the arm and prevent subluxation. While such slings are effective in mechanically supporting the shoulder during activity, they have the negative feature of positioning the arm close to the body in adduction and internal rotation. With prolonged use, contracture and increased flexor tone may develop. Slings may also impair trunk mobility, balance reactions, and positive body image. An alternate approach to the tradition sling is a humeral cuff maintained by a figure-eight harness (Bobath sling). This device supports the upper arm and shoulder with a cuff while avoiding the internal rotated, flexed arm. Careful monitoring of

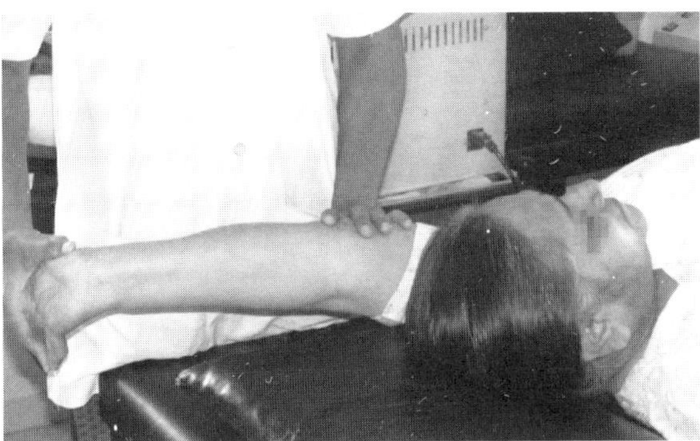

FIGURE 9.4: Range of motion exercise, left hemiplegia

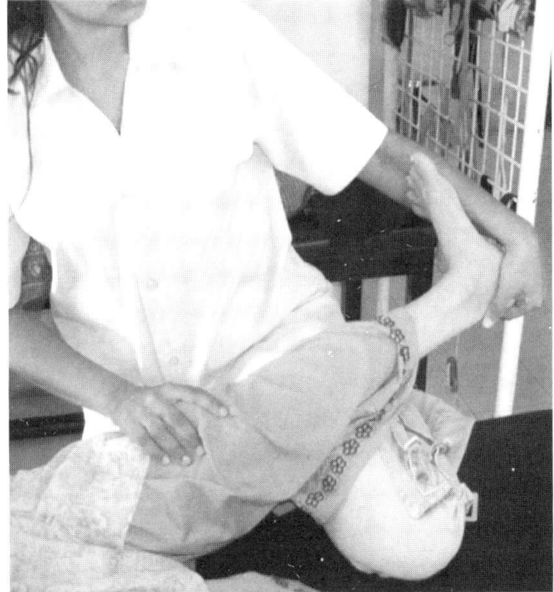

FIGURE 9.5: Range of motion exercise for lower extremity, left hemiplegia

circulation is necessary when using this type of sling. A padded arm through attached to the arm of a wheel chair is a third type of device commonly used. The support height and arm position are adjusted to control subluxation. In a study comparing the effectiveness of three different devices, the hemi sling and arm though proved more effective than the Bobath sling in controlling subluxation.

As spasticity emerges, the use of a sling is generally contraindicated. Care must be taken to mobilize the arm and prevent prolonged posturing, especially in internal rotation and adduction with pronation, wrist and finger flexion. Full range of motion in shoulder elevation activities (stressing elongation of the pectoralis major and latissimus dorsi with scapular rotation) should be maintained. Exercise procedures should concentrate on the action of the serratus anterior, emphasizing scapula upward rotation. This can be accomplished in a number of postures (supine, side-lying, or sitting) using the techniques of placing and holding, or modified hold-relax active movement with the arm externally rotated and extended, and an open hand.

START WITH THE MIDLINE

As soon as the patient is able to comprehend the instructions given, midline orientation in a more active form is started. All the reactions are practiced in midline so as to improve the memory of normal truncal movement in the brain. After the head and neck righting as described earlier, abdominal activation is started. It can be done by various methods. Initial protocol is described below.

- In supine-lying, gradual stroking is done on the abdominal muscles in an oval route with three fingers (index, middle and ring) of the therapist by applying gentle pressure. Both the sides are stroked starting from end of the sternum to the area below the umbilicus in the line of anterosuperior iliac spines. This is done in an oval route covering also the obliques. In the Figures 9.6 and 9.7, rib cage elevation is seen which is due to insufficient abdominal muscles.
- If during the respiration, lower rib cage is elevated as seen in the Figure 9.7, then, during the activation of abdominals, gentle compression of the rib cage is carried out for facilitation of the muscles.
- Head raises will contract the abdominals as they act as stabilizers.
- Bridging which is a common exercise with all therapists is not practiced unless the abdominal activation is present.
- Turning to both the sides with total flexion pattern is taught to the patient.

Many goals and treatment activities, begun during early recovery, are continued throughout the course of the patient's rehabilitation. Some are modified to appropriately challenge the patient and propel him or her to optimal recovery. During the middle and late stages of recovery, the patient is out of bed and involved in a variety of activities and therapies. It is important to monitor cardiorespiratory endurance carefully and avoid overtiring the patient. Physical therapy goals typically include:

- Prevent or minimize secondary complications.
- Compensate for sensory and perceptual loss.
- Promote selective movement control and normalized postural tone.
- Improve postural control and balance.
- Develop independent functional mobility skills.

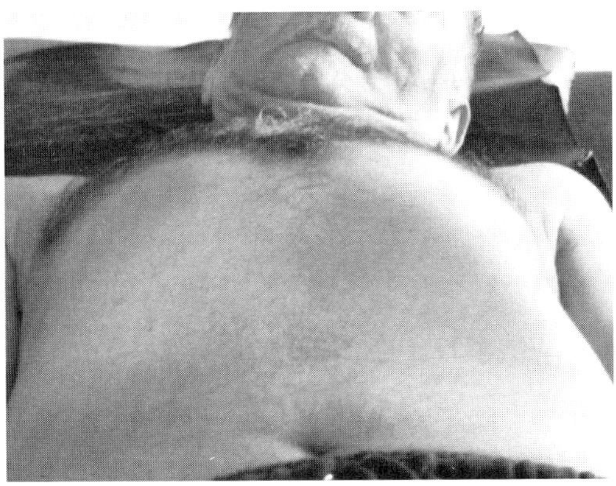

FIGURE 9.6: Rib cage elevation

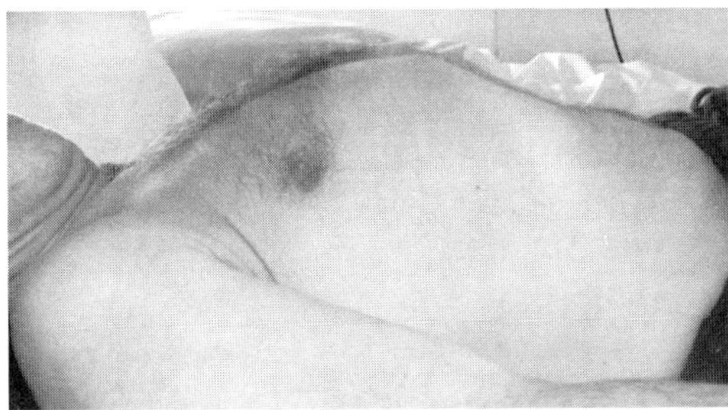

FIGURE 9.7: Lower rib cage elevation

- Develop independent activities of daily living.
- Develop functional cardiorespiratory endurance.
- Encourage socialization and motivation.

Let us now consider the general mistakes the people make while carrying out rehabilitation of a hemiplegic patient.

DO'S AND DON'TS

- Squeeze a ball: "NO"
  - Exception: Molding the hand round the cone or a ball (in lumbrical position), can benefit in shoulder hand syndrome, where there is hyperextension at MCP joints and reduced web space which results in useless hand but should evaluate for grasp reflex.
- Monkey poles: "NO"
- Overhand pulley exercises: "NO"
- If hand hurts, it's doing you good: "NO"
- Parallel bar for walking: "NO"

- Springs, weights help to regain muscle power: "NO"
- Testing of muscle strength: "NO"
- If recovery does not occur in 3–4 months, it is unlikely: "NO"
- Work or try harder: "NO"
  - Exception: Only use it carefully to boost the morale.
- Paddling a cycle. "With Caution"
  - Exception: Patient who have regained good functional movements.
- Forced passive stretching should be strictly avoided.
- Do not compare two stroke patients.
- Hot water fomentation and diathermy should not be used in patients with impaired sensations.
- Do not label the patient unmotivated, confused, demented unless properly assessed.
- Never walk a hemiplegic hanging his sound arm or hemiplegic arm around assistant's neck.

10

Activities in Lying

INTRODUCTION

For ease in carrying out the treatment practically, let us now divide the treatment protocol as per the position in which they are carried out: Lying position, sitting position and standing position in subsequent chapters.

In the acute stage, all the movements are carried out in lying down position, as tone of antigravity muscles is not sufficient enough to keep the body in upright position. Many a times, new activity is taught in lying position as many of the patients feel unsafe in unsupported position. All the transition activities from supine to side-lying, side-lying to prone and from lying to sitting are carried out in lying position. As soon as the patient is able to sit upright, activities in sitting are started as sitting is a more functional position of the two.

After moving the patient passively, a more active movement protocol is employed. Treatment is always started by explaining the patient about the nature of the movement and its functional outcome. Before the movements are started, there are a few techniques which inhibit spastic patterns and facilitate the normal movement patterns, which are explained below.

BRUSHING

Techniques of Rood approach are used at the start of the treatment. Slow or rapid brushing or stroking can be used for reducing the spasticity or for excitatory purpose early on as there is a latent period of about few minutes before the effect starts. That is why Rood's approach can be used at the beginning so that the tissues become receptive to the session in which active control is expected out of it.

Brushing by a small horse hair brush on the desired part is carried out. Brushing is carried out slowly but firmly, directly on the skin of the corresponding muscle which is to be stimulated. The sequence can be:

- Extensor aspect of the forearm—from lateral epicondyle of humerus to distal aspect of wrist joint. It stimulates activity of long extensors of forearm and wrist and fingers
- From distal aspect of dorsal aspect of the wrist to dorsal tip of all fingers—stimulates area of the tendons of extensors of fingers and thumb and dorsal interossie muscles
- On the triceps muscle
- On the abdominal
- From ischial tuberosity to popliteal fossa for knee flexors
- On the lateral aspect of the leg for ankle eversion with dorsiflexion
- Any other group of muscles as and when required.

ICING

Quick icing can immediately stimulate the contraction. There is a controversy regarding the direction of the stroke of ice whether from distal to proximal or vice versa, here, the judgment of the practitioner is advocated. Slow icing is used to decrease the tone of the muscles. Quick icing can be done by using the ice cube directly on the skin with vary fast strokes. For slow icing on spastic muscles, usually ice bags are more useful for practical purposes. Quick icing can be carried out on the parts which were enumerated for brushing also.

Slow icing can be carried out on:
- Flexor aspect of forearm
- Flexor aspect of arm
- Pectoral region, distally
- Anterior thigh for quadriceps overactivity
- Calf area for gastrocnemius overactivity
- Other area, if needed.

Careful assessment of present movement pattern and expected development of synergistic patterns is expected to be carried out by the therapist before attempting to use facilitatory or inhibitory techniques.

CONNECTIVE TISSUE RELEASE

Connective tissue release or myofascial release MFR is of valuable help as an adjunct to the therapy. A general procedure used in patients suffering from hemiplegia is described here.

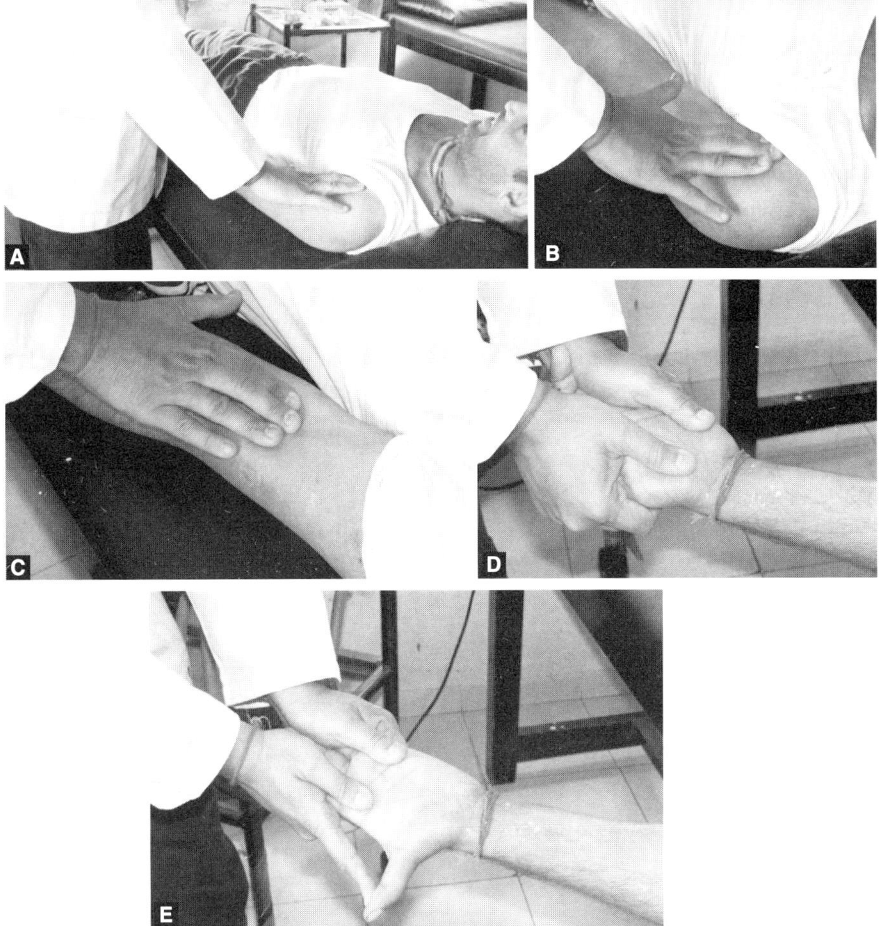

FIGURES 10.1A to E: MFR to upper extremity, left hemiplegia

Technique

- Patient lies supine in a comfortable position
- The part to be treated is exposed
- Talcum powder can be used to reduce friction
- Take your 3 fingerbreadths to perform this technique on the patient as shown in the Figure 10.1A and the pressure is evenly applied by the pulp of the fingers
- Pressure is adjusted so that the patient should not feel the pain as well as should also not feel ticklish (Figure 10.1B)
- With continuous application of pressure, fingers are slided on the surface of the patient's body from proximal attachment of the muscle to the distal attachment (Figures 10.1C to E).

- This procedure is repeated 3 to 4 times gradually, or as per requirement
- The therapist would 'feel' the 'melting away' of spasticity as the treatment is administered
- The patient is made aware of this feeling of relaxation.

Spastic muscles feel 'hard' on touch as compared to the muscles having normal tone. Softening of the muscles on touch, occurs if the tone of the muscle normalizes. In chronic spastic cases, the superficial and the deep fascia become adherent to the other structures and it becomes difficult for the patient to move actively. Connective tissue techniques also helps in such cases. Nevertheless, few sittings of this technique are required to produce sustainable results.

Sites of Application (Figures 10.1 to 10.4)

- Sternocleidomastoid, pectoralis major, biceps, brachialis, coracobrachialis, forearm flexors, and palm with opening of thumb and fingers.
- Quadriceps for extensor thrust, gastrocnemius, plantar aspect of sole of foot with opening up of great toe and other toes (extension and abduction)
- For patellar tendon and entire quadriceps mechanism, following technique is useful (Figure 10.2)
  - Therapist stands on the affected side (e.g., right) of the patient
  - Therapist places the right hand on the patient's right anteriosuperior iliac spine (ASIS), and left hand just above the patella, both the hands crossing each other
  - The patella rests between the 1st web space of the therapist
  - Thereafter, a gentle force by both the hands is applied in opposite direction to take away the *slack*. The hand on the ASIS gives force on the cephalic direction while the hand on patella gives force in caudal direction
  - This force is sustained for 90 seconds, and then gradually released. Usually 3 to 4 repetitions are sufficient.

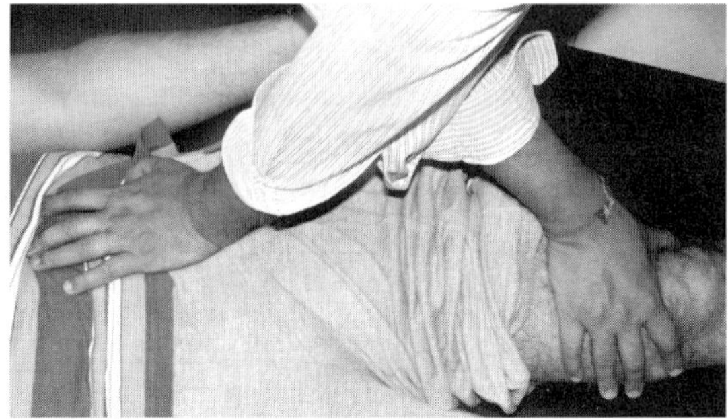

FIGURE 10.2: MFR to quadriceps, crossed hand technique, left hemiplegia

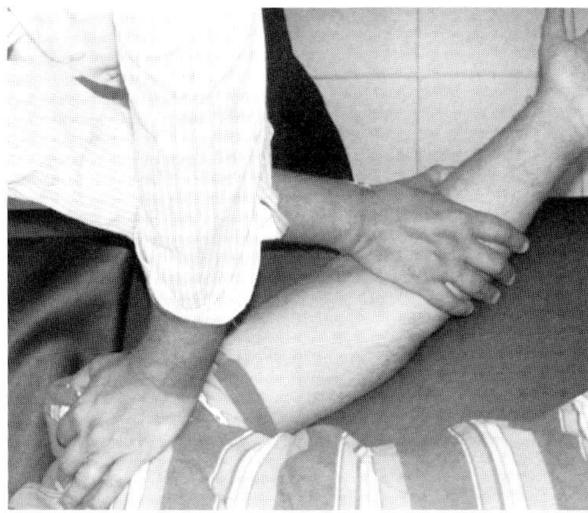

FIGURE 10.3: MFR to biceps, crossed hand technique, left hemiplegia

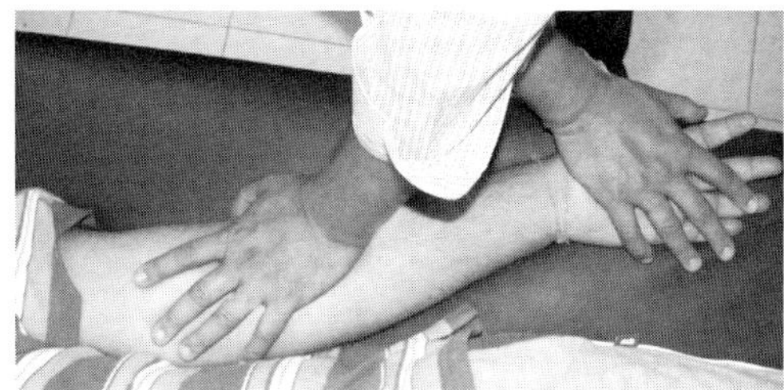

FIGURE 10.4: MFR to long flexors, crossed hand technique, left hemiplegia

This technique is also beneficial in releasing the tone in any part of the body. Apart from quadriceps, it can be easily and effectively applied in the muscles of arm and forearm as shown in the Figures 10.3 and 10.4. The force which is applied is just to take up the 'slack' in the system and it should not be more than that otherwise there is a risk of skin of the part to be stretched, which is not desired.

Benefits

- Body contact imparts tactile stimulation
- The muscle tone normalizes 'on table', thus improving its flexibility, stretchability, contractility immediately
- Decreases the chances of tissue contractures
- As this technique loosens up the fascia, it helps in the entire kinematic chain function
- Improves the circulation of the part and normalizes the part temperature.

NEURAL TISSUE STRETCH

Prior to exercise program, neural tissue stretch can be beneficial for the ease of the movement. It decreases the pain and improves active and passive range of motion. For the upper quadrant, the sequence of movement is:

Median Nerve

- Neck side-flexed and rotated to opposite direction
- Scapula downwards
- Humerus externally rotated and abducted at 90 degrees
- Elbow extended
- Forearm supinated
- Wrist extended
- Fingers extended and opened up and thumb extended and abducted.

Ulnar Nerve

- Neck side-flexed and rotated to opposite direction
- Scapula downwards
- Shoulder externally rotated, abducted at 90 degrees
- Elbow completely flexed
- Forearm pronated
- Wrist extended and radially deviated
- Fingers extended and thumb extended and abducted.

Radial Nerve

- Neck side-flexed and rotated towards opposite direction
- Scapula downwards
- Shoulder internally rotated, and abducted
- Elbow extended
- Wrist flexed
- Fingers and thumb flexed and placed in palm.

The sequence for lower quadrant is:

Sciatic Nerve

- Trunk side-flexed to opposite direction
- Hip medially rotated, flexed and adducted
- Knee extended

For further reading, refer to Butler and Shaklock.

- Ankle dorsiflexed and subtalar joint may be inverted or everted
- Toes extended.

Femoral Nerve

- Trunk side-flexed
- Hip medial rotation, adducted and extended; For hip is externally rotated, abducted and extended
- Knee flexed
- Ankle plantar flexed
- Toes flexed.

Obturator Nerve

- Trunk side-flexed
- Hip is externally rotated, abducted and extended
- Knee flexed.

For upper quadrant, either lying or sitting position is chosen for the treatment. For lower quadrant, lying position is the position of choice for ease of application. The above described positions are used to assess the tension in the neural mechanism. The patient complains of pain and sometimes paresthesia in any region along the course of the nerve which is affected. After the assessment is done and the nerve tissue localized, mobilization in a gentle manner is carried out step by step. First, proximal parts are mobilized and gradually, other parts can be added to it. For the purpose of treatment, either proximal part is kept fixed and distal part is moved or vice versa. The mobilization which is carried out is of oscillatory in nature. Oscillations are quick and can be done at a frequency of 1 to 2 per second. If pain is more, the frequency can be decreased and gradual, sustained mobility is done. Neural tissue mobilization is also valuable in preventing and breaking the synergistic patterns of movement.

SUSTAINED STRETCH

After carrying out connective tissue release, sustained stretch technique can be used if spasticity is still present. Spasticity is velocity dependent, if the speed of stretch is high, spasticity increases due to stretch reflex. Thus, for decreasing spasticity and for maintaining stretchability of the muscles, slow and sustained stretching is advised. In the Figure 10.5 sustained stretch of the upper extremity is demonstrated. Similarly, sustained stretch of any

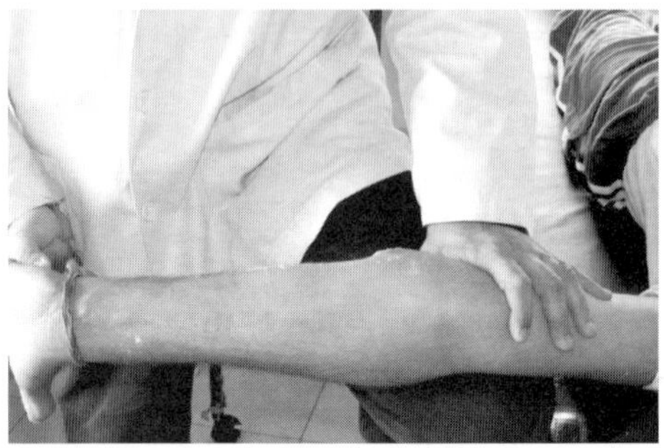

FIGURE 10.5: Sustained stretch of upper extremity, left hemiplegia

of the desired part of the body can be done. The end range position is held for at least 90 seconds for relaxation. It can also be held for 3 to 5 minutes if need be. This technique inhibits the spastic muscles and hence, antagonistic muscles are facilitated. The new length of the tissue is registered in the brain and the base line is shifted. In this manner, the new length of the tissue gets maintained and after a time, the tissue gets used to the new length and hence, even after the synergistic pattern is activated due to some reason, the relaxation time taken for the treated tissue is less than the tissue which is not treated by sustained stretch. The therapist should take care about the pain during the stretch, if any. Initially, the stretching pain is common which decreases during the 90 seconds of hold. Sometimes, the pain may not subside, and in such a case, the sustained stretch is discontinued till the cause of pain is found out and treated. Pain elicits the hypertonicity and hence, it is not advisable to elicit any form of pain during any of the treatment session. Therapy sessions should be enjoyable to the patient and not stressful or painful. Sustained stretch used in the synergistic patterns prior to active control exercises will be tremendously beneficial in providing the quality of the movement. These techniques can be taught to the patient and patient's relatives so that, it can be carried out several times a day. Uses of weight bearing on limbs, standing, wall stretches, auto-assisted stretches, etc. are different forms of sustained stretches.

PRESSURE OVER BODY PARTS

Application of pressure by the use of a heavy medicine ball can be used for decrease in spasticity, activation of the proprioception and tactile stimulation. It is a useful tool at the start of the therapy session. In the Figures 10.6A and B, a medicine ball of 2 pounds weight is used for the pressure.

Pressure can be applied by any of the technique but in practical purposes,

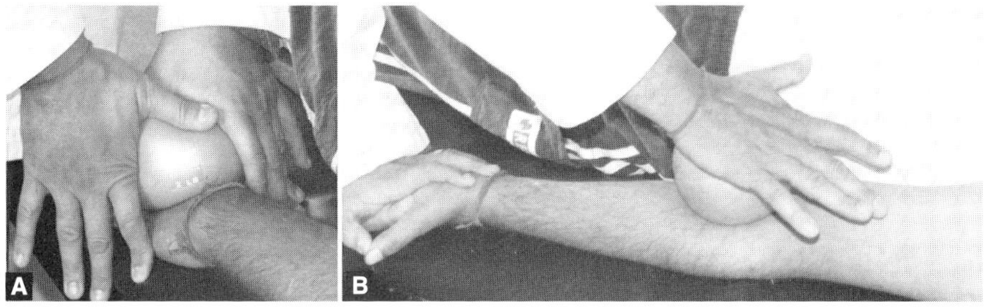

FIGURES 10.6A and B: Applying pressure over upper extremity by medicine ball, left hemiplegia

ball is most user-friendly as it can roll freely on the body surface. Application of the pressure can be done by the therapist all over the body (including trunk and chest) on the affected side. In patients with sensory problems, pressure is applied first on the unaffected side to get the 'feel' of the procedure. Patients can also be taught to apply pressure with a ball themselves using their normal upper extremity to improve sensory perception.

SELECTIVE TRUNK ACTIVITY

By studying the pathological manifestation in the periphery, we can realize the significance of sound middle or center part of the body, that the functional movements must have a healthy center and the key is the trunk for the performance of various functional movements and skillful activities economically, with ease and speed and for normal head and neck orientation in space. Bobath concept has stressed the importance of the trunk and its rotation as a key to reducing spasticity in the proximal areas and progressing to inhibit in distal parts. Selective truncal activity is a prerequisite to standing, walking, to turn in bed, in moving between lying and sitting, and sitting to standing. All these movements involve muscle activity in relation to the pull of gravity. Sitting to standing activity that is performed numerous times a day, is the most challenging, requiring shifting the body mass against the pull of gravity over to the feet for the maintenance of balance. This activity recruits extensor muscles in the trunk and the lower extremities.

Our upright posture, narrow base and freedom of upper extremity movements demand a stable and yet a mobile trunk. The pelvic girdle forms a stable base for the long moving lever of the vertebral column in upright postures against gravity. The connection between the trunk and the upper extremities is quite different. The scapula floats in a muscular suspension to permit great ranges of movements at the glenohumeral joints. It provides stability for the grasping and prehensile hand functions. The shoulder girdles have no direct articulation with the vertebral column, arms are freely mobile to explore and experience the environment from early childhood. The vertebral column must have a very finely coordinated muscle activity for the stability and mobility against gravity. The body moves forwards, backwards and sideways and the precise muscles must be activated to prevent falling in the direction of the gravity. All movements of the spine require muscle activity to oppose the pull of gravity. The therapist must have a thorough knowledge of the truncal mechanics to selectively activate the desired muscles in relation to the pull of gravity. The ideas of the bridge and the tentacle (Kleinvogelback, 1990) will help to clarify the analysis of muscle activity.

Bridge is formed when two parts of the body hold the arch; the muscles on the underside of the arch maintain the bridge.

Tentacle moves against the gravity, distal part is free, as in open chain lower limb movements.

Problems associated with loss of selective trunk activity are:
- Breathing
- Inability to come to sitting from lying
- Difficulty associated with maintenance of balance in sitting, standing and walking
- Loss of shoulder girdle activity.

CORRECTION OF ANTERIOR CHEST POSITION IN LYING

Before the actual active movement pattern activities are started, position of the patient is aligned in midline. Any excess tone in the neck and scapular muscles is reduced. The neck is kept neutral in relation to the thorax. As the Figure 10.7 suggests, the tip of the shoulders are held in the position by applying adequate pressure. The palm of the therapist's hand should push the distal end of clavicle and acromioclavicular joint downwards. The hands should not push the head of the humerus as this may result into subluxation of the glenohumeral joint. This procedure is carried out on both sides for symmetry of the body parts. Gentle oscillatory motion in downwards direction may be necessary for a few times before obtaining a substantial symmetry. This procedure stretches sternocleidomastoid muscle to some extent and is helpful in stretching of upper trapezius muscle on both the sides. The thorax thus is ready for further activation.

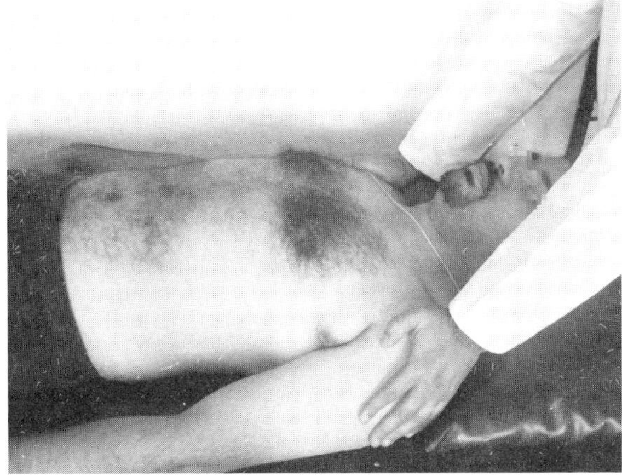

FIGURE 10.7: Aligning tips of shoulder, left hemiplegia

RIB CAGE ALIGNMENT

As earlier explained, the rib cage may be elevated and flared outwardly due to the loss of tone on the affected side. As shown in the Figures 10.8A and B, the rib cage alignment is first assessed on both the sides and correction is made on both the sides by pushing the rib cage down and inwards. This position is held for a few seconds and is repeated for several times. This procedure facilitates the contraction of intercostal muscles and abdominal muscles, stretches the fascia on the anterior aspect of neck and thorax and help to stretch the anterior muscles. It improves conduciveness of the anterior structures for stretching and hence, active activation. The scapular alignment is facilitated due to alignment of the thorax and thus indirectly, the shoulder functions are facilitated.

If during any of the active movements, the rib cage gets elevated, it can be held down by the unilateral pressure on the affected side till the active control is achieved by the patient. During this procedure, patient is constantly asked to keep the attention on the direction of the movement for faster learning.

MOBILIZATION OF THORAX

The position for mobilization of the thorax in lying is as shown in the Figure 10.9A. The therapist cradles the patient's hemiplegic upper limb as shown. The therapist then assists the patient to flex and rotate while the patient keeps the head off the couch. This is important because if the patient is keeping the head down, extensor tone may take over rendering the activity useless as we are working towards the activation of the flexion pattern which is

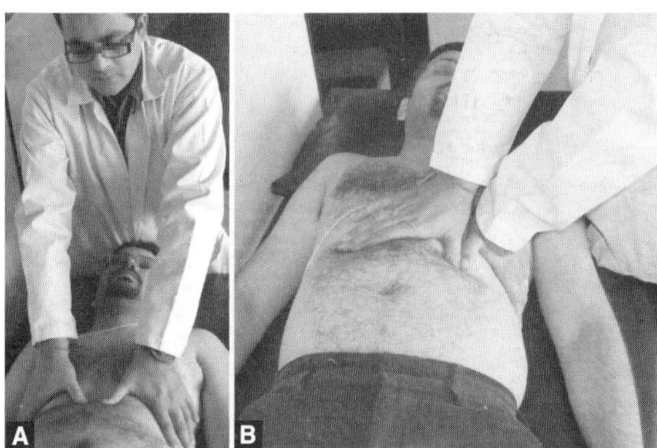

FIGURES 10.8A and B: Pushing the ribcage down and inward, left hemiplegia

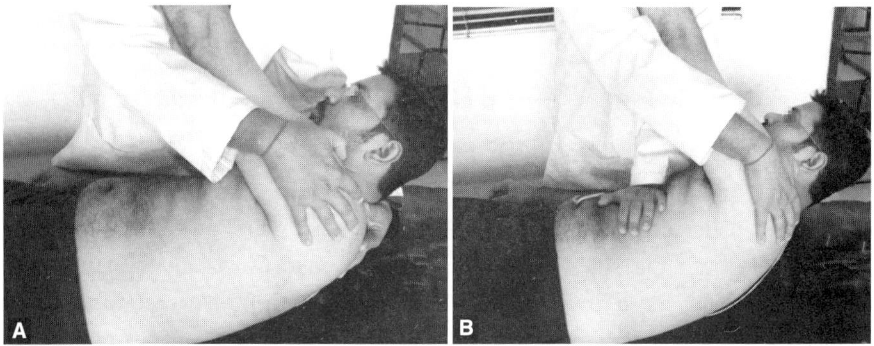

FIGURES 10.9A and B: Mobilization of thorax, left hemiplegia

antagonistic to the abnormal total extensor pattern. Gradually, the assistance by the therapist is reduced till the patient is able to carry out the movement. The therapist may have to stabilize the thorax with one hand if the rib cage gets elevated or if the lumbar spine starts flexing due to stiff thorax, as shown in the Figure 10.9B.

The Figure 10.10 shows the active progression with the flexion of thorax along with the activation of lumbar flexion, recruiting the abdominal muscles. Notice the position of the head and neck flexion. Notice the position of the scapular forward rotation and protraction recruiting serratus anterior and pectoralis major and minor. The upper limb may be assisted by the therapist from the wrist and fingers, till the active upper limb holding is possible.

MOBILIZING THE ARM

A stiff painful arm impedes balance and movement of the whole body, limits treatment and interferes with daily living. If full passive elevation of the arm

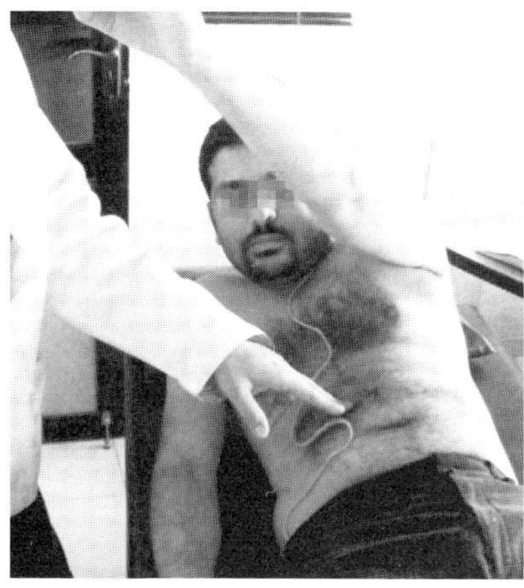

FIGURE 10.10: Active mobilization of thorax with upper limb and abdominal activation, left hemiplegia

is performed everyday, the complications may never arise. The movement should be performed in such a way that no pain is elicited. Pain around the shoulder would indicate that sensitive structures around the joint were being compromised (Davies, 1985).

Elevation of the Arm

Maintaining lateral rotation at the shoulder, the elbow is extended, and the arm lifted into full elevation with supination of the forearm, extension of the wrist and fingers and wide abduction of the thumb (Figures 10.11 and 10.12).

Mobilization of upper limb is begun in an active fashion by a technique of placing. Initially, an appropriate position is selected and assistance is given to achieve that position. Then after, assistance is reduced and patient is asked to actively hold the position. As shown in the Figures 10.13A to C, a position of shoulder flexion and external rotation is selected and elbow is kept extended. Wrist and fingers are kept extended. The patient is asked to actively hold the position. This way, functions of upper limb can be achieved in varieties of ways. Different angles of motions are selected and desired results can be achieved.

The arm is moved until it will stay in elevation without pulling down into flexion. Care must be taken not to drop the arm before any of the active control is developed. Arm should never be allowed to go into abduction as it will elicit abduction of the arm along with the internal rotation of the shoulder which is not desirable.

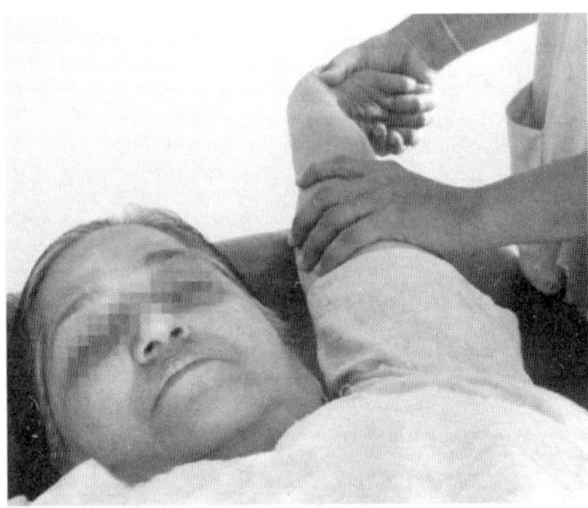

FIGURE 10.11: Mobilization of upper limb in RIP, left hemiplegia

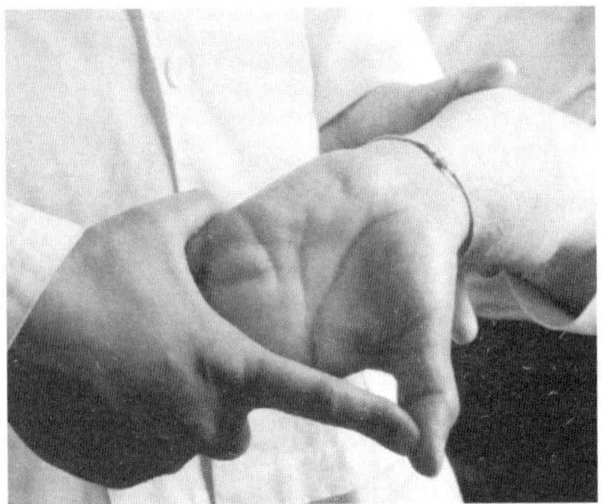

FIGURE 10.12: Grip for mobilization, left hemiplegia

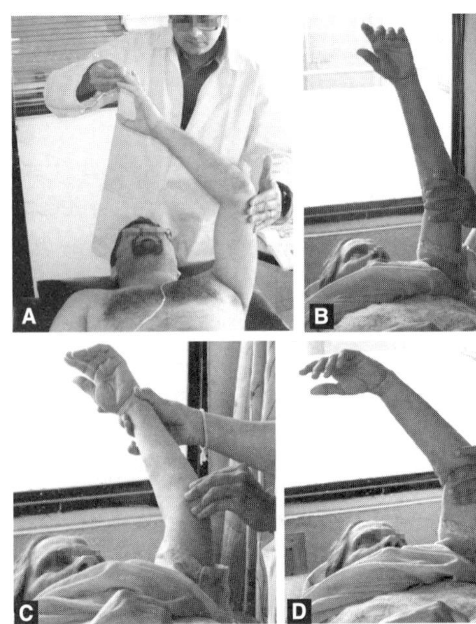

FIGURES 10.13A to D: Active assisted mobilization of upper limb, left hemiplegia

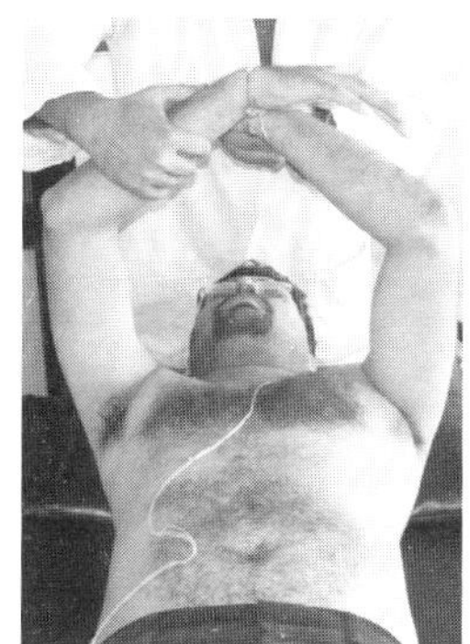

FIGURE 10.14: Bilateral symmetrical pattern of movement in upper limbs, left hemiplegia

From full elevation, the arm is taken out to the side in abduction and up again maintaining the external rotation of shoulder, extension at the elbow, fingers and wrist with supination of the forearm.

After achieving the active control of upper limb in lying, bilateral symmetrical movements are started as shown in the Figure 10.14. The elbows are actively extended on both the sides and assistance is given as and when required. The bilateral symmetrical movements facilitate the adequate control in the affected limb. During this procedure, the thorax is actively stabilized and contraction of abdominals is achieved by active posterior pelvic tilt by keeping the lumbar spine touched to the couch. Lower limbs can assume a position of flexion at knee and hip (crook lying) initially progressing to lower limbs extension.

PROPRIOCEPTIVE NEUROMUSCULAR FACILITATION (PNF) PATTERN ACTIVITIES

Movements can be carried out in proprioceptive neuromuscular facilitation (PNF) patterns. Facilitation is carried out in entire pattern of activity or the patterns can be broken up into segments and hence, concentration on individual movement can be gained. Example of the pattern of activities can be:

Starting position:
- Shoulder: Extension, adduction, internal rotation
- Elbow: Flexion
- Radioulnar: Pronation
- Wrist: Ulnar deviation, flexion
- Fingers: Flexion
- Thumb: Flexion, adduction

End position:
- Shoulder: Flexion, abduction, external rotation
- Elbow: Extension
- Radioulnar: Supination
- Wrist: Radial deviation, extension
- Fingers: Extension
- Thumb: Extension, abduction

Other patterns which can be used are:

Shoulder flexion, adduction, internal rotation, with elbow flexion and supination, wrist and fingers flexion, thumb flexion and adduction, as a starting position to the end position of shoulder extension, abduction, external rotation, with elbow extension and pronation wrist and fingers extension and thumb extension and abduction.

Any of the PNF patterns can be used with a variety of combinations. The ultimate goal of achieving normal functional movement patterns is always kept in mind while choosing the activity pattern. For an example, if tone in elbow extensor is higher than that of the flexors, then a pattern with elbow flexion can be selected. Many such combinations can be made by judicious use of the patterns. Initially, assistance from the therapist may be needed for completion of the task. Techniques like stretch reflex, quick stretch, and irradiation may be used as and when required. In later stages, according to strength of individual muscle and comparative strength of the muscle in a movement pattern, resistance to the individual part or entire pattern can be given. After the session, the tone of the muscles is checked for and if hypertonia occurs, the effort on the part of the patient is decreased in the subsequent sessions.

SIDE-LYING ACTIVITIES

Activities in side-lying can be started as soon as possible. As explained earlier, total flexion pattern is used while turning to any side. While turning to hemiplegic side, the use of normal lower limb extension as in 'pushing' as well as normal side upper limb pushing is not allowed. Also, while turning to normal side, pushing with extensor thrust of hemiplegic lower limb or 'pulling' from normal upper limb is not allowed (Figures 10.15A and B). Instead, a total flexion pattern is used for turning by activation of trunk flexors and counteracting extensor thrust.

Correct rolling brings awareness of the affected side, release of spasticity by rotation between the shoulder girdle and pelvis and facilitates active movement in the trunk and limbs.

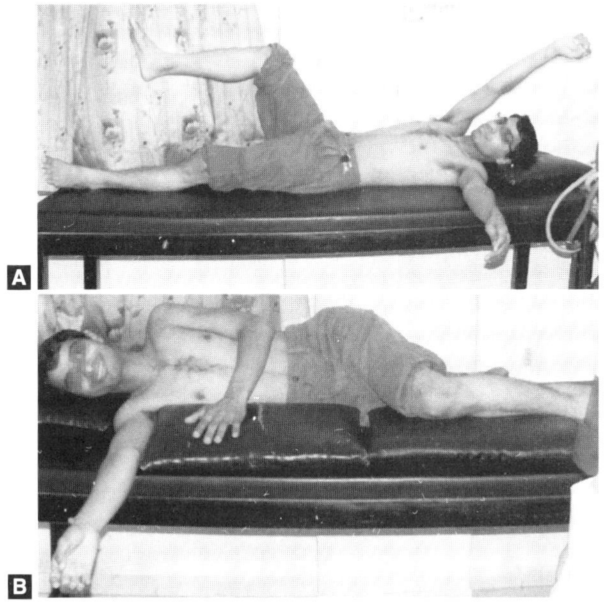

FIGURES 10.15A and B: (A) Turning to sound side using total flexion pattern, right hemiplegia; (B) Turning to affected side, right hemiplegia

To the Affected Side

With the affected arm in abduction, the patient is asked to lift the head and bring the sound arm across to touch the other hand, pushing off the bed.

To the Sound Side

The patient's affected leg is guided over his other leg with less and less assistance until the patient can perform the action himself. The patient can clasp both hands together and rotates the upper trunk by moving both arms to the sound side. Rolling should be encouraged in both directions, onto the sound side to promote early independence and onto the affected side to encourage functional reintegration of the hemiplegic side. Extremity movement patterns can facilitate improved rolling through momentum and the fostering of segmental trunk rotation patterns. With both hands clasped together in a prayer position, the patient can actively assist flexion and upper trunk rotation onto a side lying on elbow posture.

During early transfers, the patient may be more or less a passive participant. Adjusting the hospital bed to the height of the chair or wheelchair will help to ease the transfer. Staffs often emphasizes the sound side by placing the chair to that side and having the patient stand and pivot a quarter turn on the unaffected leg before sitting down. While this technique promotes early and safe independence in transfers, it neglects the affected side and may make subsequent training more difficult. The patient should be taught to transfer to both sides early on.

Transferring to the hemiplegic side may be more difficult at first but will assist in overall re-education and reintegration of the two sides of the body. When transferring, the patient's affected arm can be stabilized in extension and external rotation against the therapist's body. Alternately, the patient's arms (hands in prayer position) can be placed to one side on the forward weight shift by using manual contacts, either at the upper trunk or pelvis. The affected leg may be stabilized by the therapist's knee exerting a counterforce on the patient's as needed.

As shown in the Figures 10.16 and 10.17, the side-lying to affected side with the arm at 90 degrees will facilitate external rotation at shoulder and eventually supination of forearm, extension of elbow and hence, will facilitate the movement of wrist and fingers extension.

The side-lying position is also useful for the selective elbow flexion and extension (Figure 10.18). In this position, the shoulder is in a fixed position of external rotation and abduction. The force of the contraction is concentrated upon the elbow and the radioulnar joints. Firstly, supination is tried and keeping the forearm supinated, elbow flexion is gradually carried out. Then, it is gradually lowered towards extension. Care must be taken not to allow the jerky movements to take place. The eccentric lowering of the forearm in extension will promote a good facilitation to active extension of elbow joint in more functional position of sitting and standing. The patient can visualize their own upper limb moving which will provide with a visual biofeedback.

SCAPULAR MOBILIZATION

Scapular control is extremely valuable in rehabilitation and functional recovery of hemiplegic upper extremity. Initially, the scapula is kept mobile passively. Gradually, as the tone of the muscle starts developing, more active protocol is incorporated. As with all the activities, the addition of adequate and optimum resistance will further more improve the function. The position of glenoid

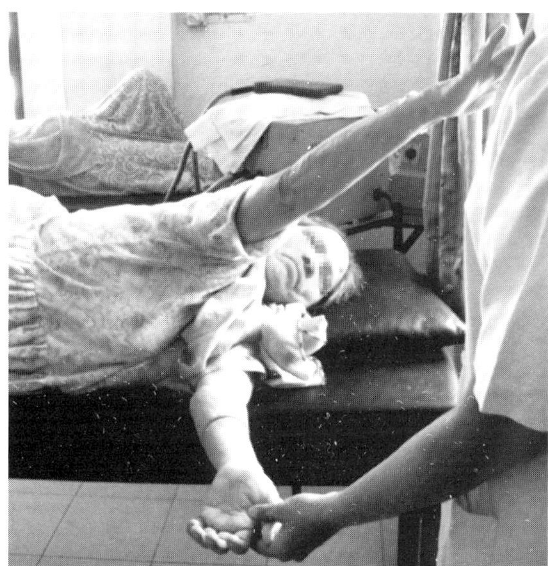

FIGURE 10.16: Weight bearing on affected side with reach outs using sound arm, left hemiplegia

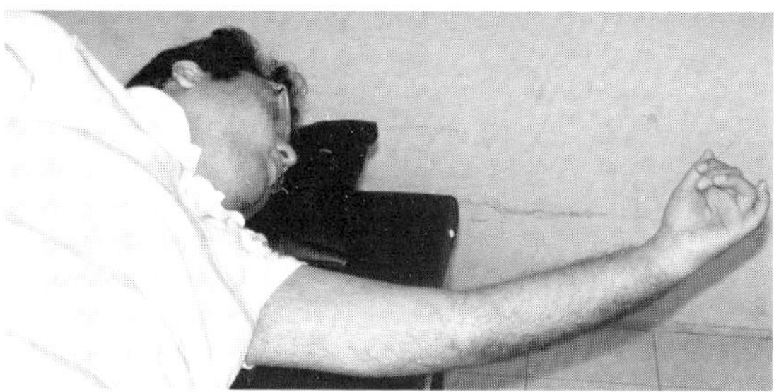

FIGURE 10.17: Shoulder external rotation with forearm supination in side-lying, left hemiplegia

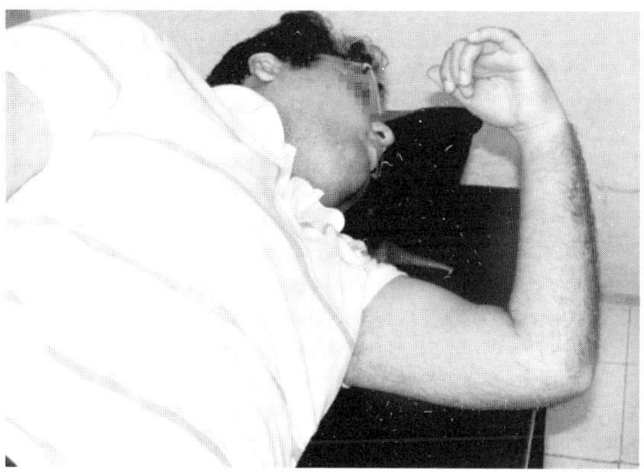

FIGURE 10.18: Selective elbow flexion, extension in side-lying, left hemiplegia

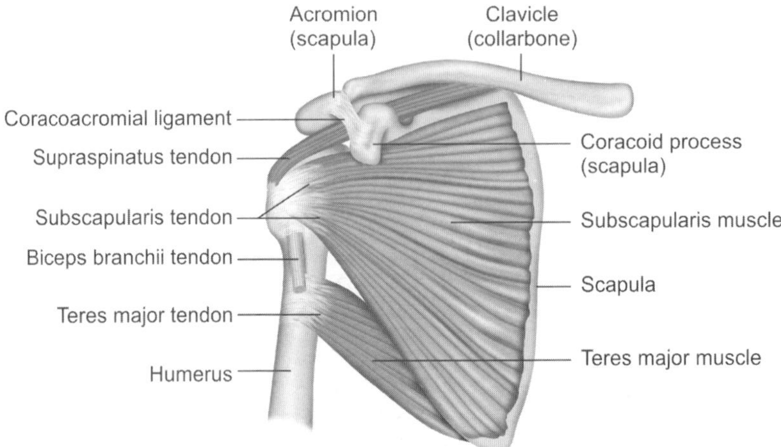

FIGURE 10.19: Scapular muscles from front

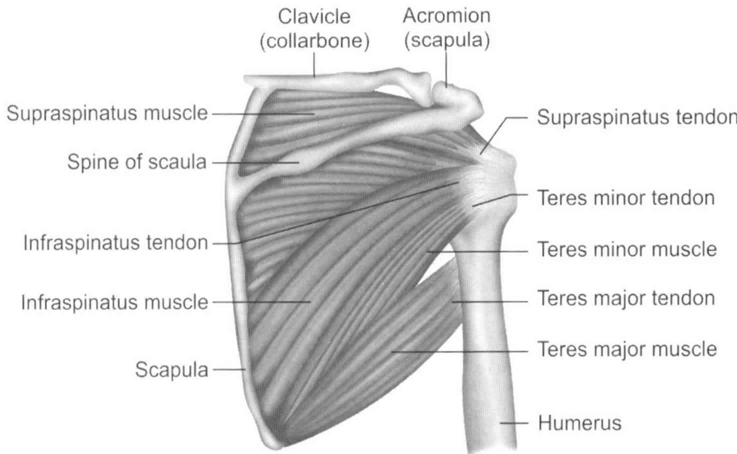

FIGURE 10.20: Scapular muscles from behind

cavity in relation to the head of humerus is vital for the functioning of the shoulder movements and hence the functioning of the entire upper extremity. As it is well known that the shoulder complex is dependent on the muscle activity only and the glenohumeral joint has compromised stability in gaining mobility. This stability is provided by the rotator cuff muscles and other joint structures. Thus, strengthening of rotator cuff muscles and the muscles of entire shoulder complex is vital in upper extremity rehabilitation (Figures 10.19 and 10.20). The muscles which need special attention are:

- Upper trapezius
- Middle trapezius
- Lower trapezius

- Serratus anterior
- Rhomboids major
- Rhomboids minor
- Teres major
- Teres minor
- Latissimus dorsi
- Subscapularis
- Supraspinatus
- Infraspinatus
- Pectoralis major
- Pectoralis minor
- Deltoid—all fibers

To start with, 'scapular clock exercises' can be given to the patient.

Posterior Depression

These activities are done initially passively or with optimum assistance and gradually progressed to active contractions in the specified direction or resisted at a later stage. The position of the therapist is behind the patient initially to get a full view of the moving scapula. As such, any part which is moved is to be exposed for proper visualization of the part, but in case of scapular activities, it becomes more important as scapular movements are difficult to exercise with the clothes on. Right hand of the therapist is placed on the tip of the shoulder as shown in the Figure 10.21 and the scapula is moved posteriorly and downwards. Other hand of the therapist stabilizes the thoracic cage and trunk for avoiding trick movements. End position is shown in the Figure 10.21. Figure 10.22 shows the scapular activity during upper extremity movement.

- Muscles activated:
   Serratus anterior—lower portion
   Rhomboids major and minor
   Latirsimus dorsi

Anterior Elevation

Scapula is moved anteriorly and in elevation. The position of the hands is similar, but the direction of the movement and resistance is adjusted according to the end movement. The Figure 10.23 shows the end movement. Figure 10.24 shows the scapular activity during upper extremity movement.

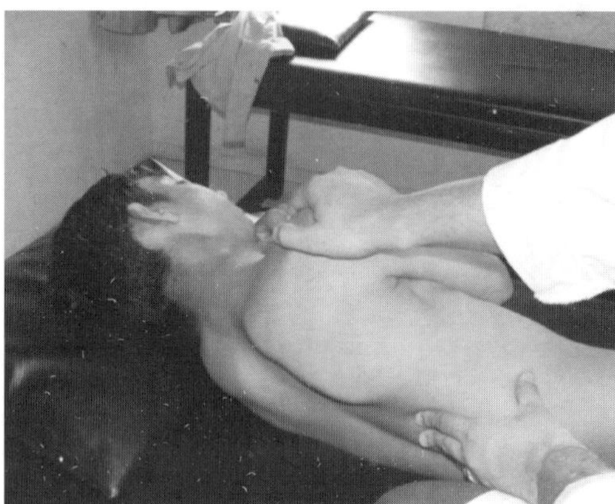

FIGURE 10.21: Scapula—posterior depression

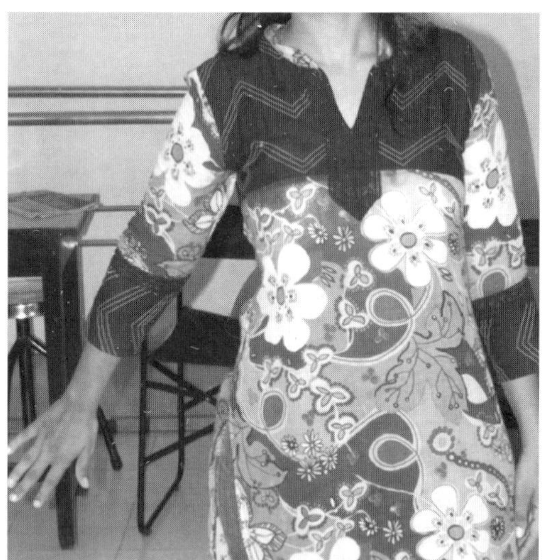

FIGURE 10.22: Scapula—posterior depression, entire upper limb PNF

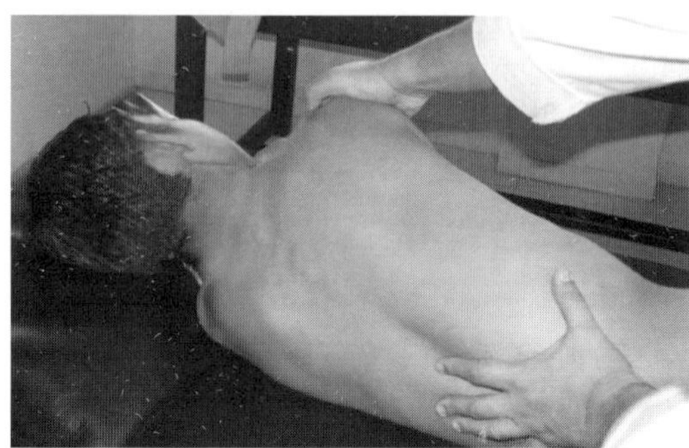

FIGURE 10.23: Scapula—anterior elevation

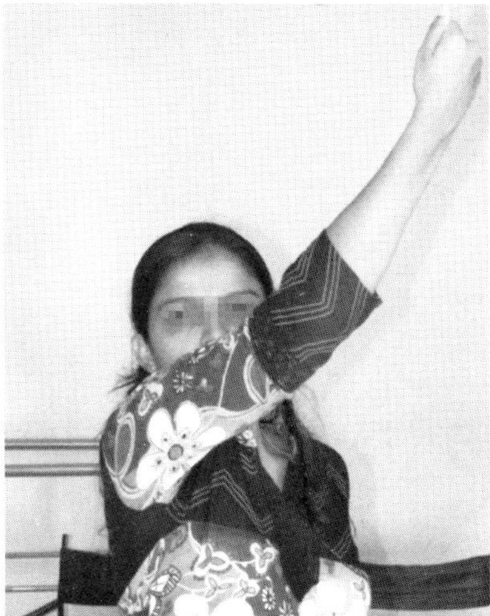

FIGURE 10.24: Scapula-anterior elevation, entire upper limb PNF

Anterior Depression

- Muscles activated:
  - Rhomboids
  - Serratus anterior—upper portion
  - Levator scapulae
  - Pectoralis minor

The scapula is moved anteriorly and downwards. For the ease of application, the therapist may stand on front of the patient but care should be taken to visualize the movement for accuracy of treatment.

The Figure 10.25A shows the end position. Figure 10.25B shows the scapular activity during upper extremity movement.

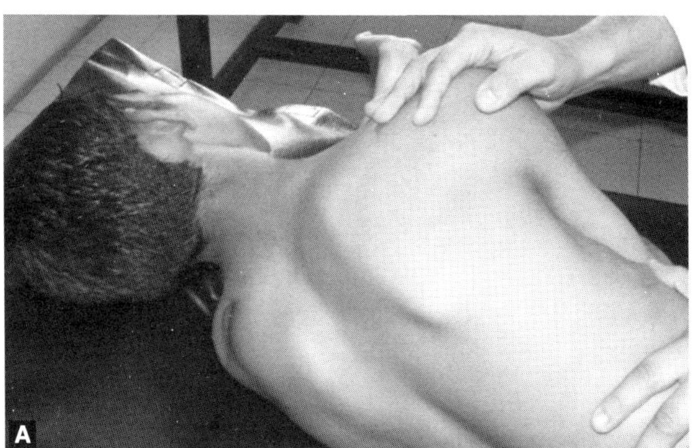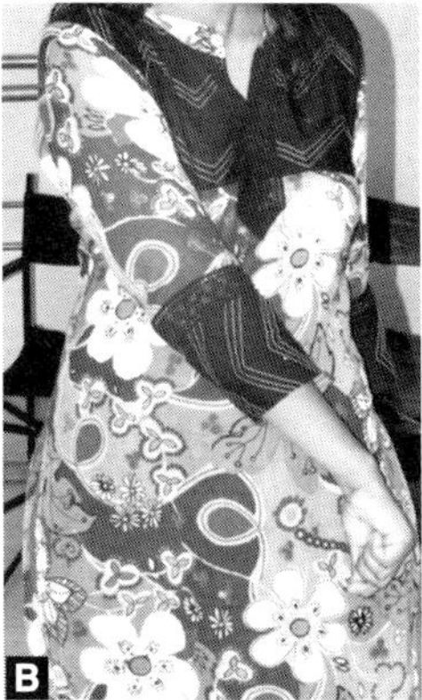

FIGURES 10.25A and B: (A) Scapula—anterior depression, (B) scapula—anterior depression, entire upper limb PNF

■ Muscles activated:
  Serratus anterior
  Pectoralis major
  Pectoralis minor
  Rhomboids

Posterior Elevation

The scapula is moved posteriorly and upwards. Figure 10.26A show the end position and Figure 10.26B shows the scapular activity during upper extremity movement.

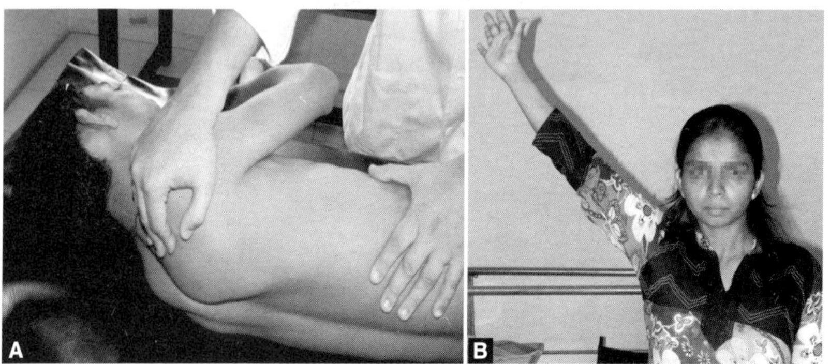

FIGURES 10.26A and B: (A) Scapula-posterior elevation, (B) scapula-posterior elevation, entire upper limb PNF

■ Muscles activated:
  Trapezius
  Levator scapulae.

Workout for Serratus Anterior

Important muscles like serratus anterior is rehabilitated specifically from the initial stages itself. The protocol of progressing from assisted to active and then to resisted workout is followed throughout. The position which is shown in the Figures 10.27A and B can be used both for assisted as well as resisted workout.

Note the position of left hand of the therapist which is palpating the lateral aspect of scapula. The serratus anterior can also be rehabilitated in side-lying position.

Workout for Middle Trapezius

Note the position of external rotation of the shoulder during trapezius workout in the Figure 10.28. The upper limb is horizontally abducted at 90 degrees.

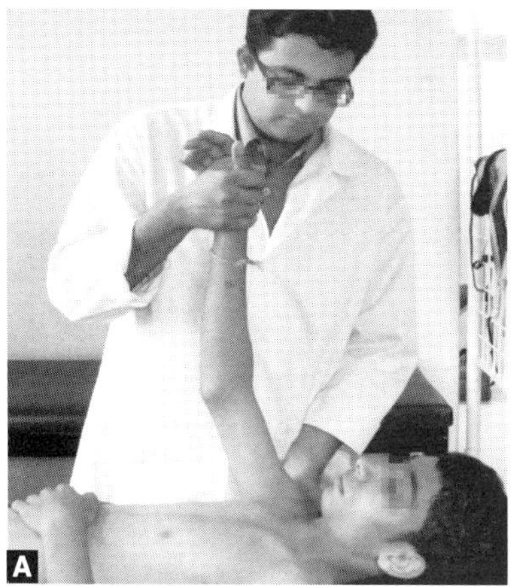
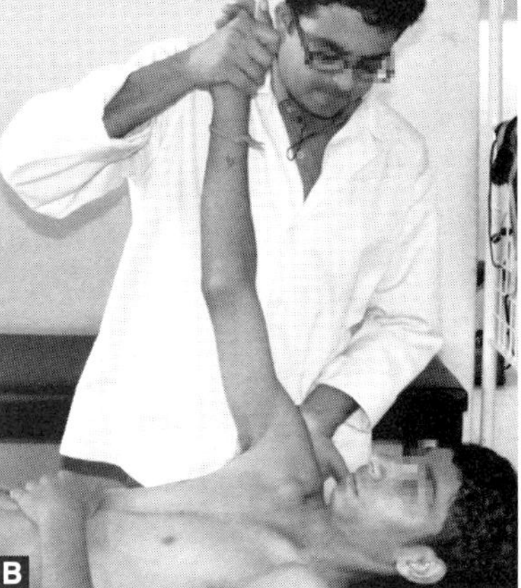

FIGURES 10.27A and B: Workout for serratus anterior in lying

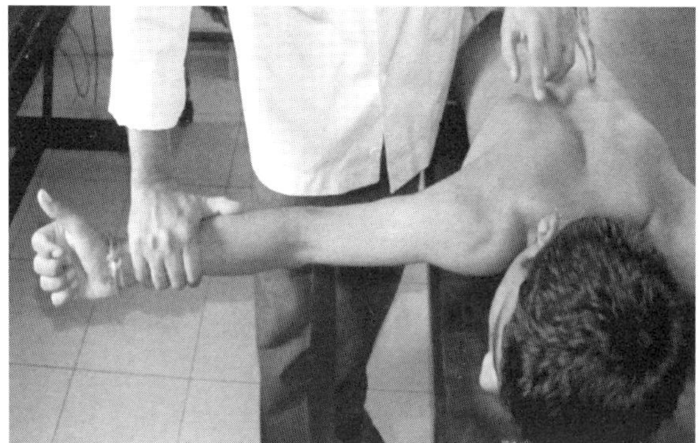

FIGURE 10.28: Workout for middle trapezius in prone-lying

Workout for lower trapezius

The upper limb is horizontally abducted and flexed in scaption (Figure 10.29).

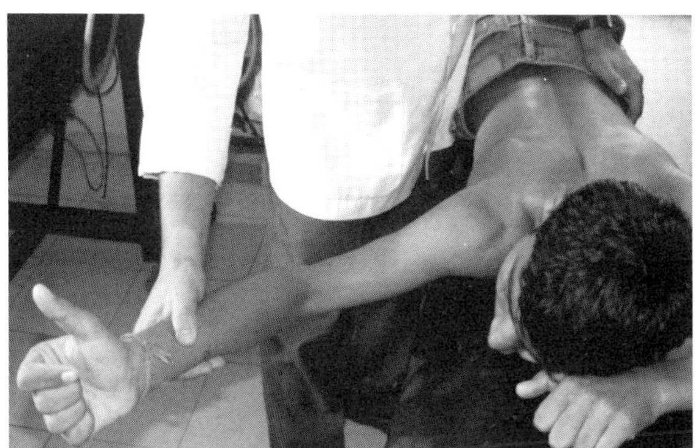

FIGURE 10.29: Workout for lower trapezius in prone-lying

Workout for Subscapularis

In the position of extension and internal rotation of shoulder, the elbow is taken in the direction of the roof. Resistance can be added in the later stage (Figure 10.30).

The workout of the muscles like trapezius and subscapularis in the open kinematic chain is difficult for the patient in the initial stages due to either hypotonia, or in the later stages by hypertonia. Thus, it is advised to carry out the scapular muscle activation from the earlier stages itself, in close chain and then moving towards open chain activities. This would ensure a smooth rehabilitation of the upper extremity.

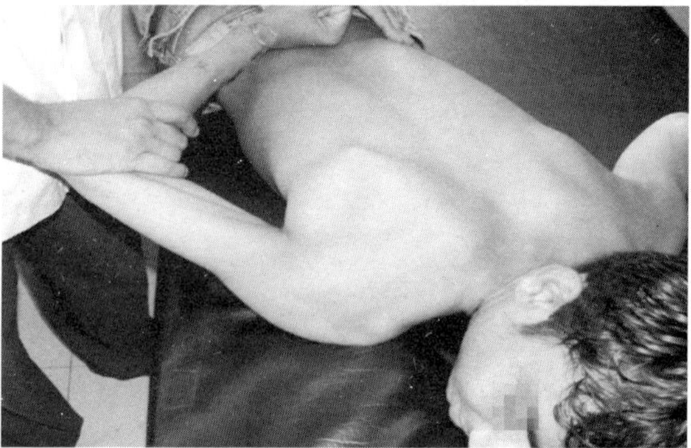

FIGURE 10.30: Workout for subscapularis in prone-lying

ACTIVATION OF LOWER TRUNK

For activation of lower abdominals, obliques, and stabilizers like transverse abdominis, lying position is useful in the initial stages. In the same position, resistance can be used to strengthen the muscles. As in the Figure 10.31A, both legs of patient are flexed at the hip and the knee and ankles are kept neutral. The trunk is flexed by asking the patient to take the buttocks off the couch. Patient is asked to keep the head stable. Assisted/resisted rotation on either side is carried out to rehabilitate obliques. This technique counteracts the extensor thrust of the spine.

Figure 10.31B shows the extreme position of flexion and rotation of the lower abdominal region.

Hemiplegic leg of the patient is crossed on the sound leg which is in crook position. As in the Figure 10.32, the hemiplegic side is left. The patient is asked to maintain the position. The pelvis is kept posteriorly tilted by keeping lumbar spine flat on the couch (lumbar lordosis obliterated). Next step is to rotate the trunk to left and then to the right by moving the leg. Note the position of the therapist's right hand which is on patient's left knee. This

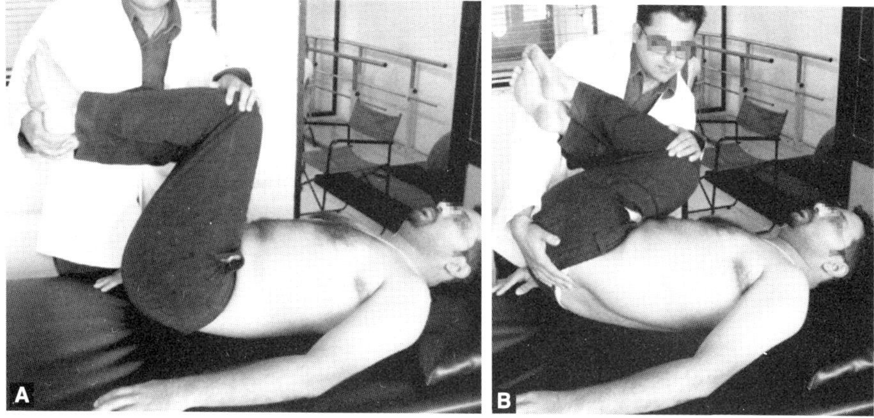

FIGURES 10.31A and B: (A) Activation of lower abdominals, left hemiplegia; (B) Flexion and rotation of trunk with lower limbs flexed, left hemiplegia

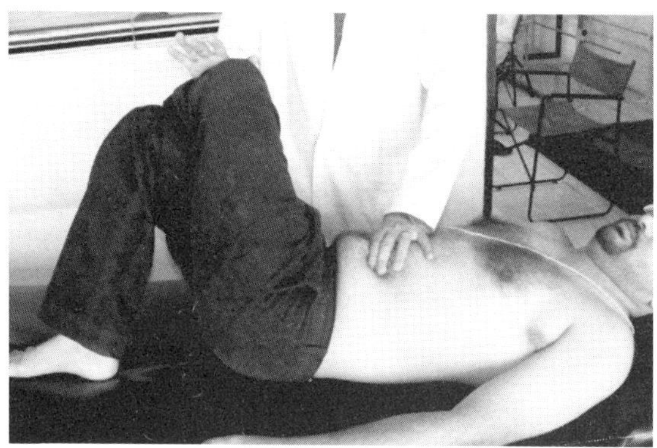

FIGURE 10.32: Abdominal activation, left hemiplegia

hand assists, controls as well as resists the motion of rotation while the left hand palpates the quality of the abdominal muscle contraction.

Figure 10.33 shows rotation towards right. Note the increase in lumbar lordosis which should be prevented.

Figure 10.34 shows rotation towards left. Note the position change of therapist's right hand. The left hand of the therapist constantly palpates the contracting muscles.

Extreme position of rotation will force the therapist to stabilize the upper trunk on the right side to ensure only the lower trunk rotation. All the above mentioned activities can be resisted to strengthen the muscles. Slight modification in the position may be required for practical purposes (Figures 10.35).

Furthermore, the sound upper limb is held in 90 degrees flexion as shown in the Figure 10.36. The active holds of the sound limb will elicit the contraction of thoracic area. By this activity, active stabilization of thorax is achieved along with the contraction of upper abdominal muscles which work as stabilizers.

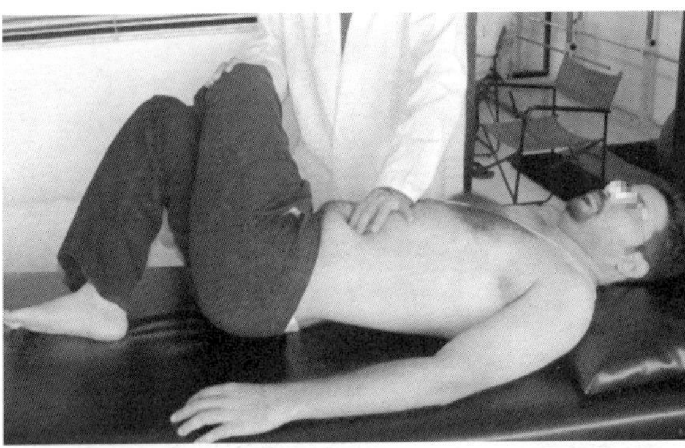

FIGURE 10.33: Abdominal activation with crossed legs with trunk rotation to right, left hemiplegia

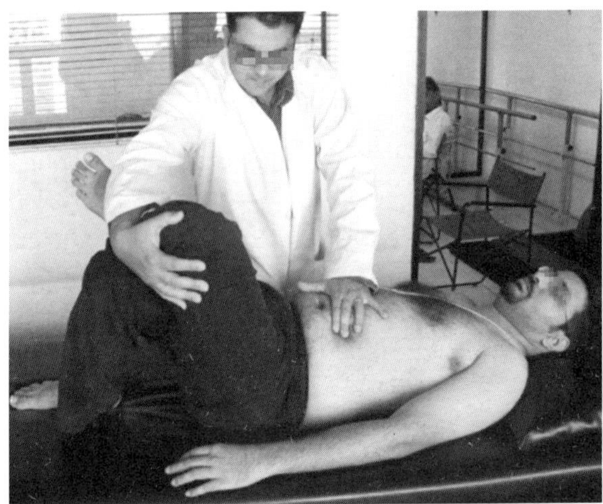

FIGURE 10.34: Abdominal activation with crossed legs with trunk rotation to left, left hemiplegia

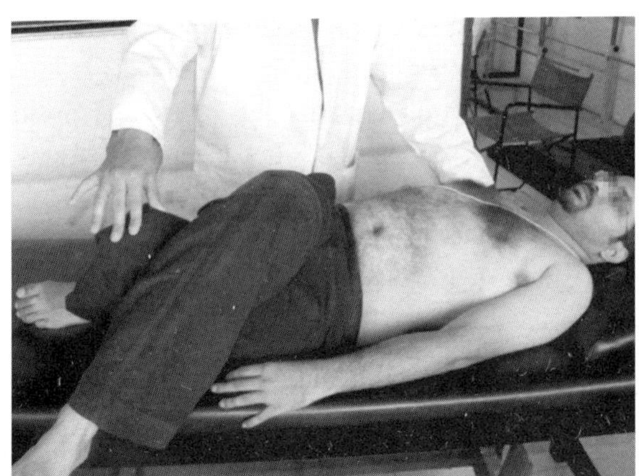

FIGURE 10.35: Extreme position of rotation, left hemiplegia

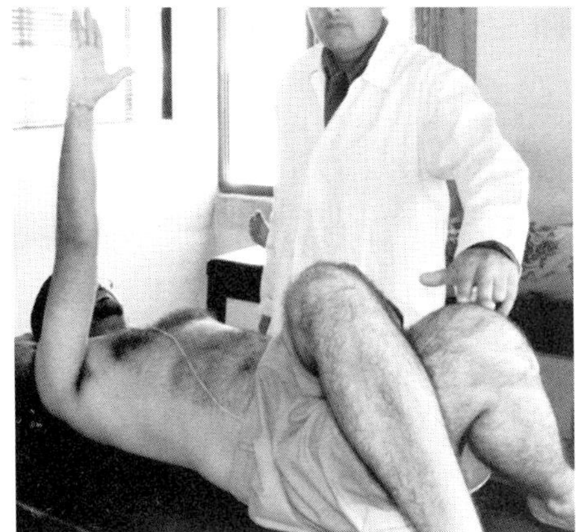

FIGURE 10.36: Abdominal activation with stabilization of thorax using sound upper limb, left hemiplegia

Figure 10.37 shows the incorrect method of bridging. The patient uses the force of hip extensors rather than abdominals for lifting the pelvis off the couch. This can be noticed by increase in the amount of lumbar lordosis. The correct position of bridging with posterior pelvic tilt by using the muscle force of abdominals is shown in Figure 10.38. This is the correct position of bridging activity and should be always encouraged from the initial stages.

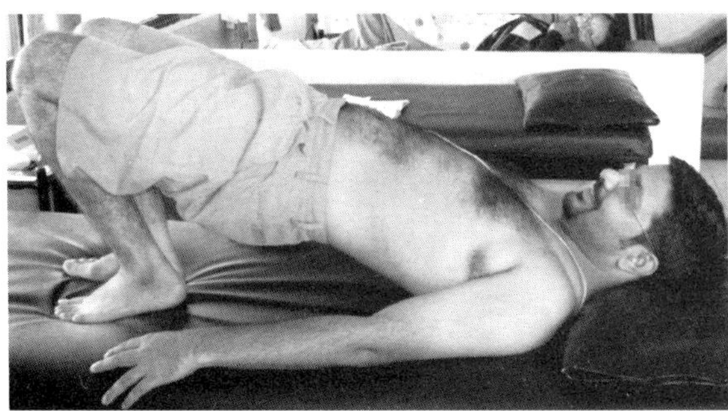

FIGURE 10.37: Incorrect method of bridging, left hemiplegia

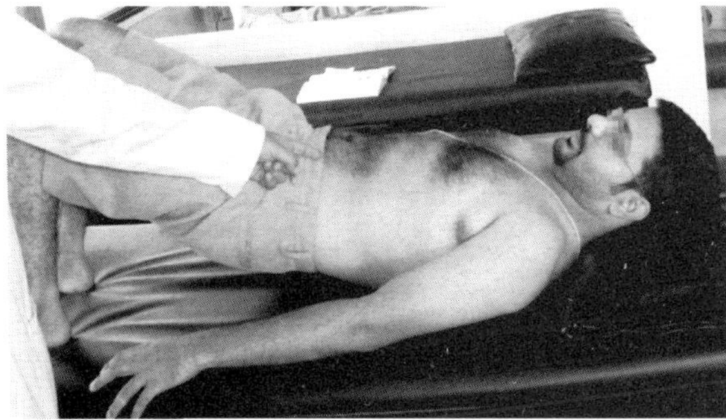

FIGURE 10.38: Correct method of bridging, left hemiplegia

Notice the contraction of abdominals in the Figure 10.38. The patient is left sided hemiplegic.

Progression in bridging is made by elevation of sound upper limb and sound lower limb, simultaneously. This will provide strong contractions of trunk muscles (Figure 10.39). Note the active maintenance of posterior pelvic tilt throughout the movement. Extra undue effort on the part of the patient will increase the spasticity on the affected side and hence, care is taken to check affected limbs while carrying out this activity. If the tone on the affected side increases, either limbs are kept in reflex-inhibiting postures or the grade of effort is reduced.

Rhythmic knee flexion and extension with hip and pelvis fixed is practiced for the total weight bearing on the affected limbs and this is useful functionally in activities like moving, sitting and stance phase of walking (Figures 10.40 to 10.42).

Bridging activities develop pelvic control, advanced limb control (hip extension with knee flexion, foot eversion), and early lower extremity weight bearing. Bridging activities should include assisted and independent assumption of the posture. If the affected lower extremity is unable to hold in a hook-lying position, the therapist will need to assist by stabilizing the foot during

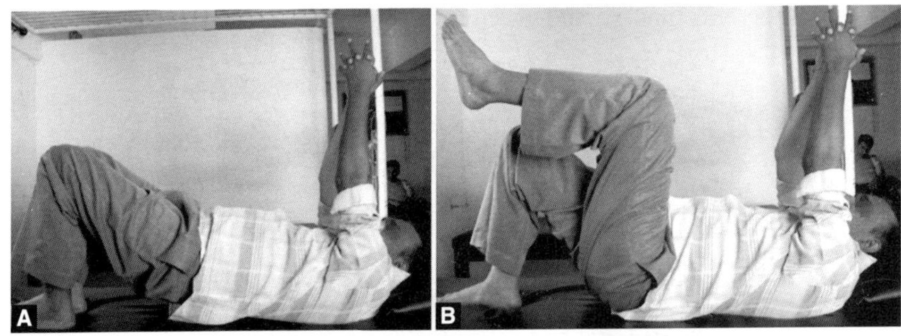

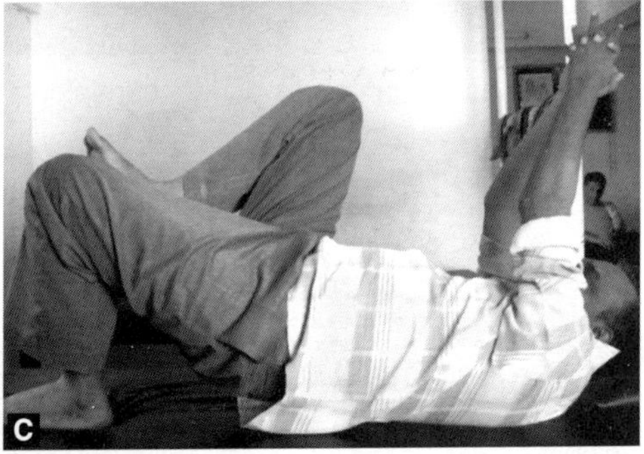

FIGURES 10.39A to C: (A) Bridging with both upper limbs held in flexion, right hemiplegia, (B) unilateral bridging with weight bearing on hemiplegic side, right hemiplegia and (C) unilateral bridging with weight bearing on sound side, right hemiplegia

the bridge activity. Care should be taken as bridging activates the trunk extensors, if there is a lack of abdominal control for posterior pelvic tilts. Assistance for the posterior tilt maintenance for bridging should be given by the therapist till the active control develops.

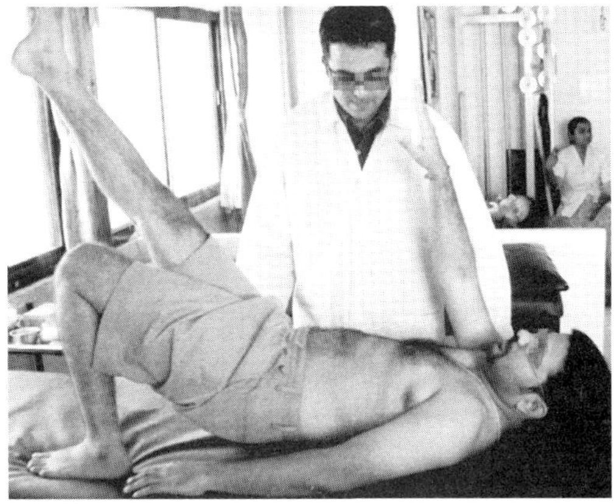

FIGURE 10.40: Unilateral bridging with thoracic stability, left hemiplegia

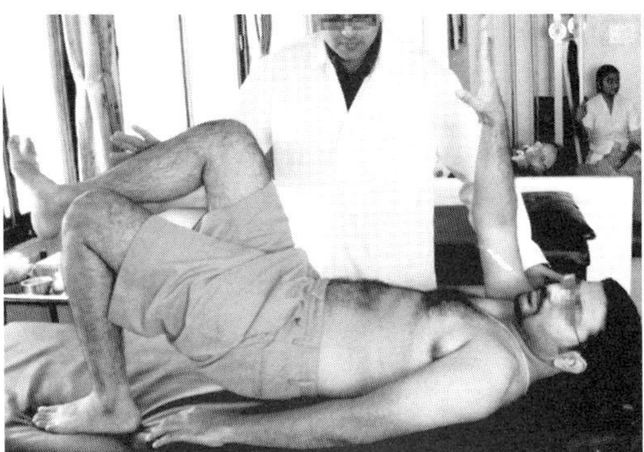

FIGURE 10.41: Unilateral bridging with dynamic activities, left hemiplegia

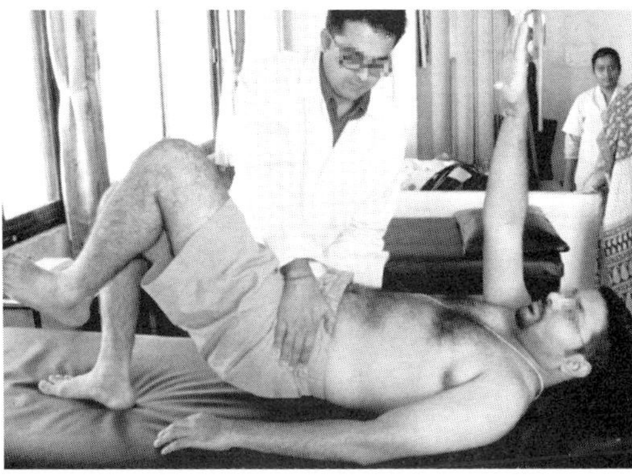

FIGURE 10.42: Unilateral bridging with resistance, left hemiplegia

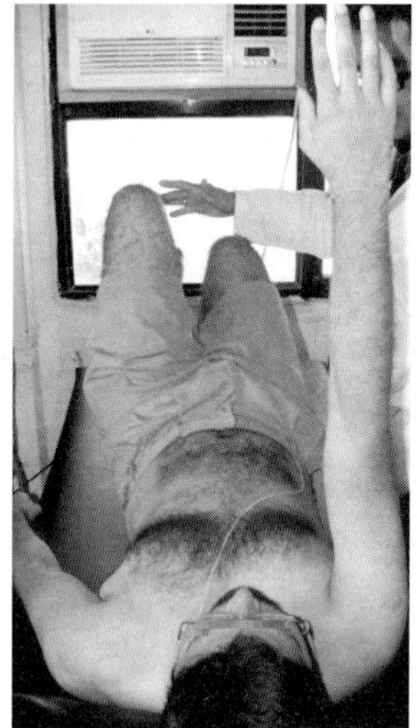

FIGURE 10.43: Unilateral bridging with the control of lower extremities, left hemiplegia

Affected lower limb is raised with knee in flexion while the sound upper limb is lifted up (Figures 10.42 and 10.43). The contralateral action is useful in reactions of pelvis during activities of turning and walking. Initially, the therapist may have to assist the pelvis in upward direction and prevent it from falling off. Later on, the same grip can be changed to resist the upward movement of pelvis.

Elongation of the Trunk

The patient lies in half crook-lying with his affected leg flexed and adducted. Place one hand on his pelvis, the other hand over his shoulder and elongate his trunk until the hip remains forward off the bed (Figure 10.44).

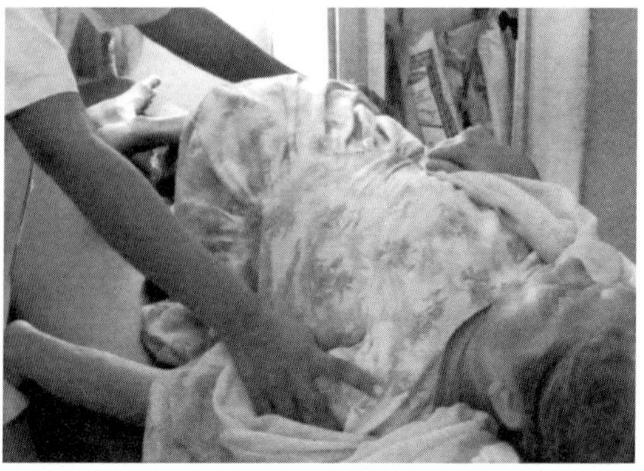

FIGURE 10.44: Elongation of the trunk, left hemiplegia

Movement of the Scapula

One hand is placed over the scapula, the other supporting his arm (Figure 10.45). With the shoulder protracted, the scapula is elevated and depressed until spasticity is released and it moves freely. While the scapula is being moved, the arm is eased into lateral rotation.

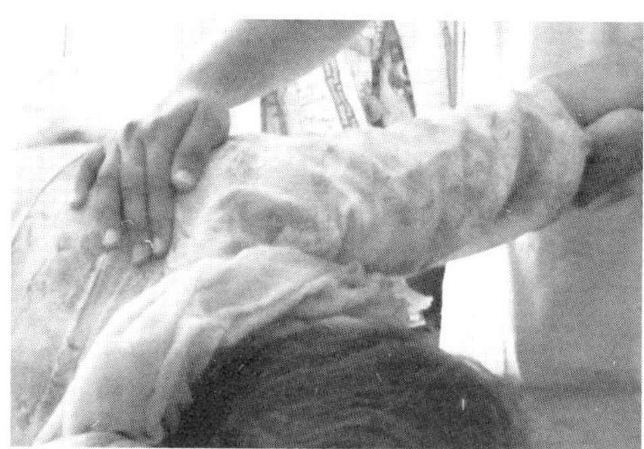

FIGURE 10.45: Mobilization of scapula in side-lying, left hemiplegia

LOWER EXTREMITY CONTROL

Training of the lower extremity essentially prepares the patient for ambulation. Pre-gait mat activities should concentrate on working muscles in the appropriate combinations needed for the gait. For example, hip and knee extensors need to be activated with abductors and dorsiflexors for early stance. Strong synergy combinations also need to be broken up. A variety of activities can be used, including bridging, supine knee flexion with hip extension over the side of the mat, or standing modified plantigrade with knee flexion. Hip adduction should be stressed during flexion movements of the hip and knee, while abduction should be stressed during extension movements (e.g. supine, PNF D1 lower extremity diagonal; sitting, crossing and uncrossing the hemiplegic leg). Pelvic control is important and can be promoted through lower trunk rotation in a number of postures (e.g. side-lying; supine, modified hook-lying with the hemiplegic leg pushing off; kneeling; or standing).

An effective progression increases the challenge to the patient gradually by modifying postures until synergy influence is completely lacking (e.g. hip abduction can be performed first in hook-lying, then supine, side-lying, modified plantigrade and standing positions). Contraction patterns should also be varied. Thus, dorsiflexors can be first activated in a sitting posture by using first a holding contraction, then an eccentric letting go, and finally a shortening contraction. This stimulates the functional expectations of normal gait cycle as the foot goes in swing phase through stance.

Voluntary control of eversion is often difficult to achieve, since these muscles do not function in either synergy. The application of stretch and resistance to these muscles during a pattern that activates dorsiflexors may be effective in initiating a response. Postural challenges may also elicit these muscles automatically, even though voluntary control is lacking. Control of knee function is also problematic. Reciprocal action should be stressed early, beginning first in sitting, then in supine hook-lying, prone, modified plantigrade, or supported standing positions, and progressing to standing and walking. Dissociation of arm movements during lower extremity training is also an important consideration and may be achieved through the use of pre positioning and voluntary control (e.g. having the patient hold clasped hands together overhead in a "prayer position", during a lower extremity activity).

Since most patients regain some use of their lower extremities early in recovery, range of motion techniques should focus on specific areas of deficit. For many patients, the foot and ankle control remains limited and tone quickly progresses from initial flaccidity to spasticity, typically in the plantar flexors (Figure 10.46). Techniques are designed to elongate plantar flexors through slow, maintained stretch and to activate weak dorsiflexors, thereby reciprocally inhibiting plantar flexors, may prove more successful than straight passive ROM. Thus, weight bearing and rocking in modified plantigrade or prolonged static positioning using adaptive equipment (i.e. tilt table with toe wedges) can gain motion while inhibiting spastic plantar flexors. Johnstone suggests using orally inflated pressure splints to maintain limbs in antispasm positions and to promote sensory re-education. To prevent associated reactions, the hands can be clasped in elevation or, preferably, the patient can learn to inhibit the reaction by letting the arm remain relaxed at the side.

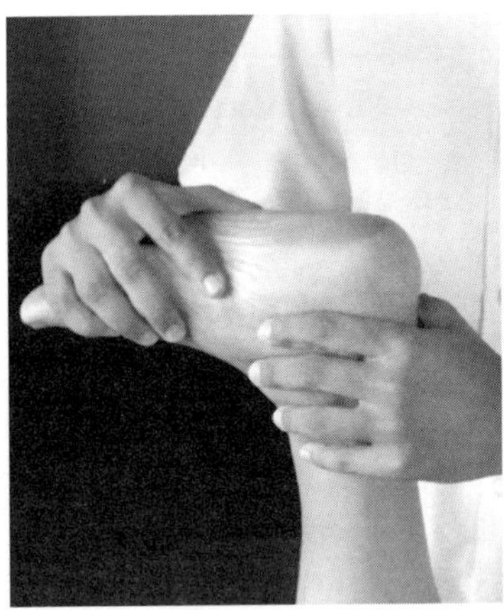

FIGURE 10.46: Plantar flexion in prone lying, left hemiplegia

Hip and Knee Flexion over the Side of the Bed

Place the leg of the patient over the side of the bed with the hip extended and hold the knee in flexion and the foot in full dorsiflexion until there is no resistance. Maintain the position of the foot and knee and guide the leg up on to the bed while the patient actively assists (Figures 10.47A to C). Repeat the movement preventing any abnormal pattern occurring, e.g. extension of the knee or lateral rotation of the hip. If the exercise is perfected, the patient will be able to bring the leg forward when walking and climb stairs in a normal manner, one foot after the other.

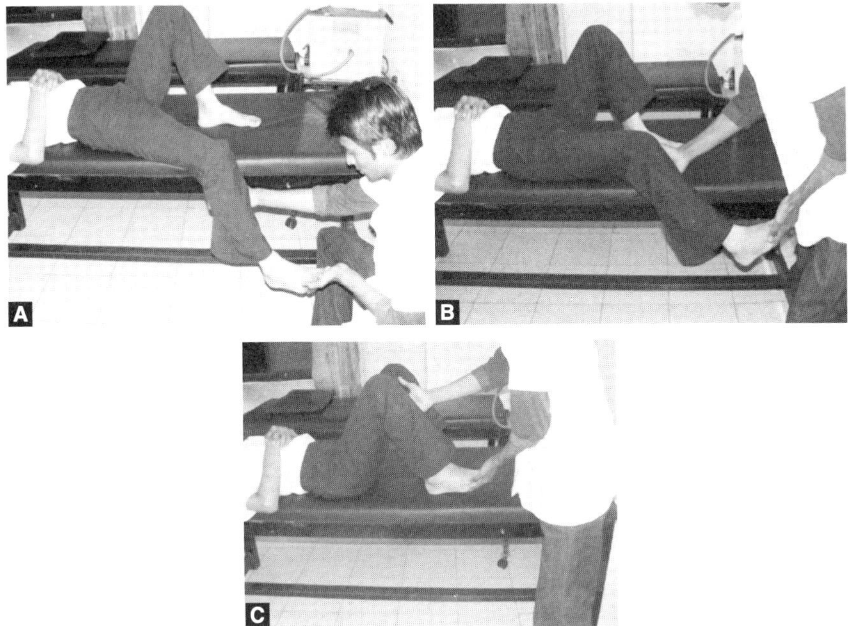

FIGURES 10.47A to C: Training for taking the hemiplegic leg up on the couch, right hemiplegia

Knee Extension with Dorsiflexion

The foot is held in dorsiflexion, and patient's leg is moved from full flexion into extension without the toes pushing down and without rotation at the hip. The patient takes the weight of his limb, making it feel light throughout. The similar activity can be carried out with the patient's affected heel resting on a ball as shown in the Figure 10.48. The patient tries to dorsiflex the ankle with moving the hip and knee in flexion and then gradually returns to a position of hip and knee extension keeping the ankle dorsiflexed throughout. If the ankle starts moving in plantar flexion, the patient immediately controls the movement actively.

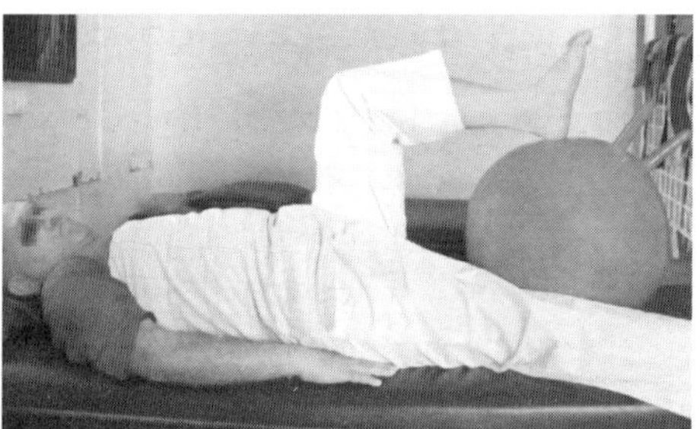

FIGURE 10.48: Counteracting extensor thrust dynamically, left hemiplegia

Hip Control with the Foot on the Bed

In crook-lying, the patient moves alternate knees smoothly into medial and lateral rotation without the other leg moving and without tilting the pelvis (Figures 10.49A to C).

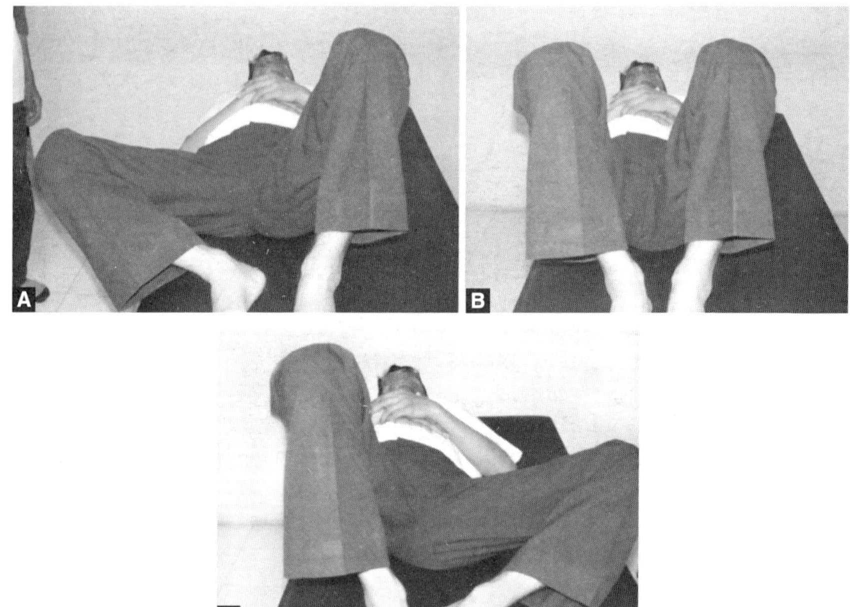

FIGURES 10.49A to C: (A and B) Selective training for hip rotation while the foot maintained on the couch, right hemiplegia (C) control maintained by affected side while the sound side is moving

Hip Control with the Hip in Extension

In half crook lying with affected leg flexed and adducted the patient lifts affected hip forward off the bed and, maintaining hip flexion, moves knee out and in.

Independent Movement of the Legs

To prepare for walking, teach the patient to move the legs without moving the trunk, one leg at a time, asking to make it feel light by taking the weight himself. They must maintain control while the leg is lowered on to the bed. The patient is asked to keep his trunk still and not to lean back throughout the activity. Controlled movements of the leg can be achieved by asking the patient to hold the limb in various positions in which the therapist puts (Figures 10.50A and B) where the therapist puts the patient's affected lower limb in a position of knee flexion with hip in flexion and asks the patient to hold the position. As a part of progression, the hip can be held actively in flexion while the movements of knee flexion and extension can be practiced for increase in motor control. Use of a ball can give a dynamic base for moving the leg. The patient can either use it for assistance as it can decrease friction of leg with the couch or can use as a means of achieving eccentric control as the ball has to be controlled when moving in gravity (Figure 10.51).

Contralateral movements with the sound lower limb and affected upper limb held steady in elevation. Note the quality of trunk muscles contractions.

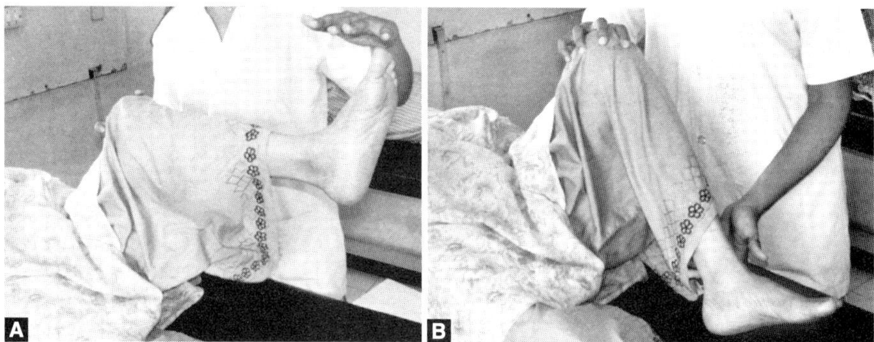

FIGURES 10.50A and B: Controlled movements of lower limb in lying, left hemiplegia

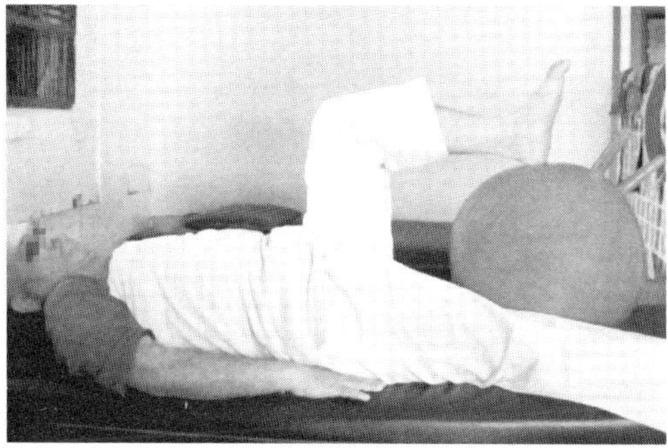

FIGURE 10.51: Control of lower extremities, left hemiplegia

The affected lower limb, left as in the Figure 10.52, is bearing full weight even as the pelvis is lifted off the couch and is posteriorly tilted.

Once there is some amount of active contractions in the lower limbs, usually, all the movements follow the synergistic patterns of extensor thrust, if the patient is left unattended to. To counteract the effect of strong extensor thrust, it is always better to start the proceedings initially as prevention is better than cure. Guidance from the sound lower limb as well as from the therapist is given. Therapist stands at the foot end of the patient in the middle. Both the lower limbs of patient are held in semiflexed position at hip and knee as shown in Figure 10.53. The therapist holds patient's foot which is maintained in dorsiflexion at ankles and extension at toes.

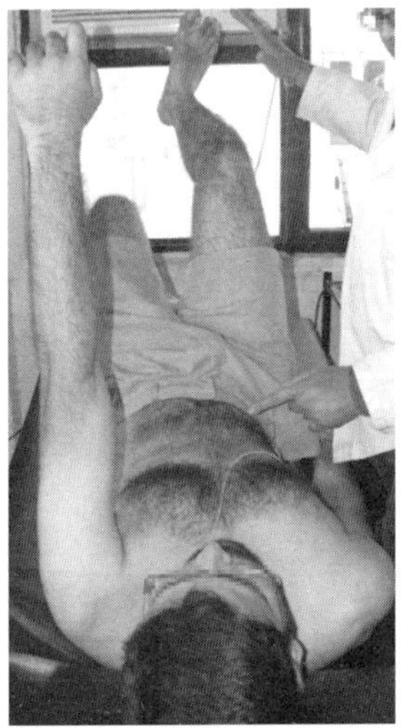

FIGURE 10.52: Activation of trunk muscles in bridging with contralateral extremity patterns, left hemiplegia

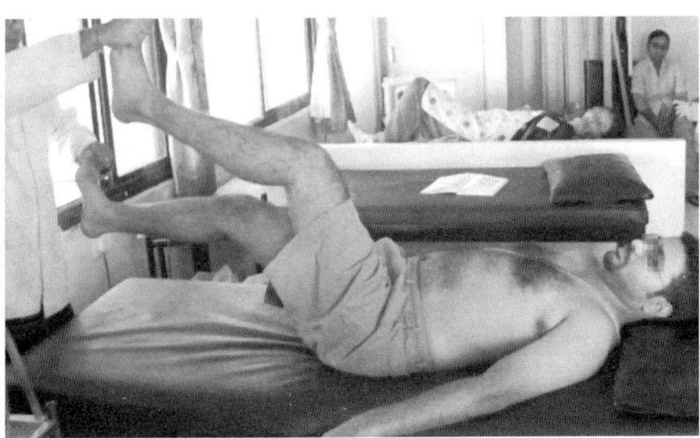

FIGURE 10.53: Controlled bilateral lower limb movements in lying, left hemiplegia

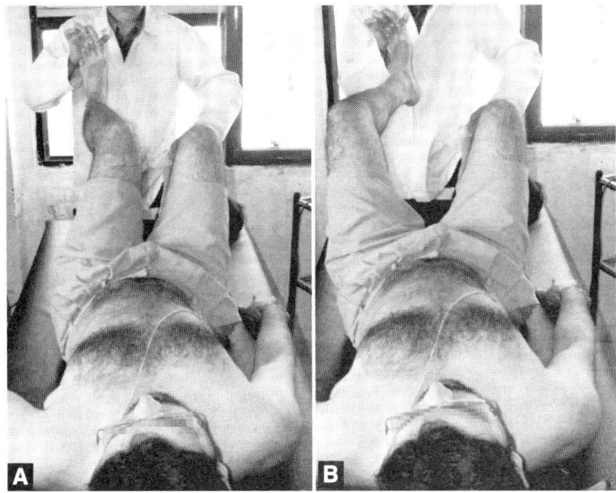

FIGURES 10.54A and B: Controlled bilateral lower limb movements in lying, left hemiplegia

Patient is instructed to keep lumbar spine flat on couch by contraction of abdominals. Both the lower limbs are moved in a cyclic fashion with the therapist assisting and guiding the movements on both the sides. Gradually, the patient actively moves the sound limb in a rhythmic fashion, while the therapist only guides. On the affected side, however, more assistance may be required to maintain the position. During the movement, both the limbs are not allowed to extend from the knee completely (Figures 10.54A and B). This elicits the contractions of quadriceps muscle eccentrically and gradual release of quadriceps as well as gluteus maximus muscles, is helpful in counteracting extensor thrust. Gradually, as the patient progresses, amount of assistance and henceforth, guidance can be decreased till the patient actively controls the limb in full range of motion. During this movement, the hip joint is held actively in neutral rotation. For this, the patient is instructed to keep the knee in center of the plane of movement and not allow the knee to drop either to right or to the left i.e., no amount of hip rotation. This elicits the control of hip rotators, abductors, adductors and extensors which will be of vital importance during every phase of the gait cycle. Patient should always watch the moving limbs throughout.

The Figures 10.55A and B show full weight bearing on the left side of the body which is affected side and actively lifting the pelvis off the couch. This activity may be difficult for most of the patients and hence, assistance to the pelvis may be used in upward direction. This movement strengthens side-flexors of trunk, latissimus dorsi, and lateral muscles of hip. Stabilizers of thorax, rotator cuff muscles and stabilizers of neck and head also get strengthened.

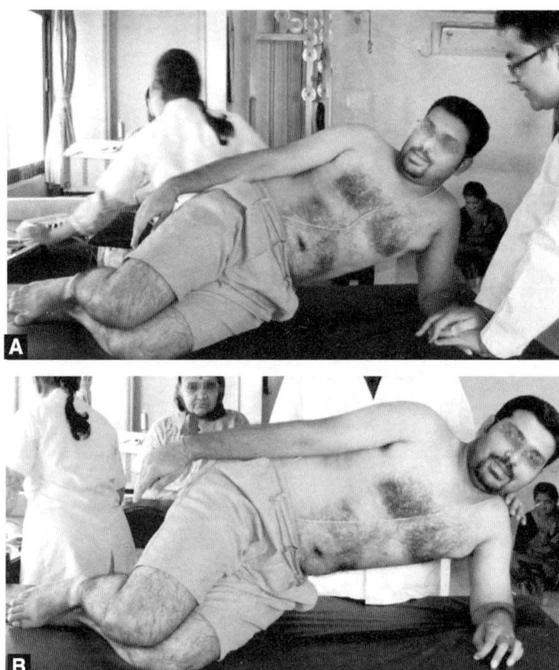

FIGURES 10.55A and B: Pelvic raising sideways with weight bearing on affected side, left hemiplegia

Trick motion of pelvis rotation to either direction and use of excess movement at hip is counteracted by the watchful therapist through proper holds. If any synergistic pattern is getting elicited in the limbs, the limbs are held in reflex inhibiting postures, and here, the judgment of the therapist is advocated.

ELONGATION OF TRUNK AND PELVIC CLOCK EXERCISES

Figure 10.56 shows the method of elongation of trunk on the hemiplegic side. Here in this case, the left side is the hemiplegic side. The patient turns to the sound side and thus the hemiplegic side is kept up. A small pillow is kept below the thoracolumbar region as shown in the Figure 10.56. Both the knees of the patient are kept slightly flexed to avoid the toppling off of the patient on either side. Right hand of the therapist is kept on the left iliac crest and left hand crosses the right and is kept either at lower border of scapula or at mid scapular region. 'Slack' in the system is taken up and a gradual force is applied so that side-flexors of the trunk are stretched. By using the same grip and position, rotation of the trunk can also be mobilized.

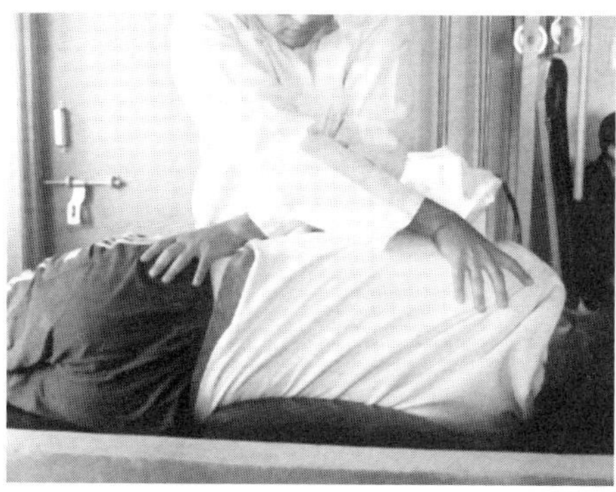

FIGURE 10.56: Elongation of trunk in side lying, left hemiplegia

Anterior Depression

As with the scapula, the pelvis can also be mobilized in the combination of movement patterns preferably in side-lying position. These patterns help in normalizing the gait faster and dynamic postural reflexes are trained. Figure 10.57 shows the anterior depression of pelvis. This is useful in stance phase. A logical progression of passive, assisted, guided, active and resisted workout is used. Grip of the therapist may vary accordingly. For assisted workout as shown in the Figure 10.57, the therapist may stand behind the patient diagonally. The therapist assists the patient's pelvis anteriorly and in downward direction. Other hand of the therapist stabilizes the trunk at lower costal margins as shown.

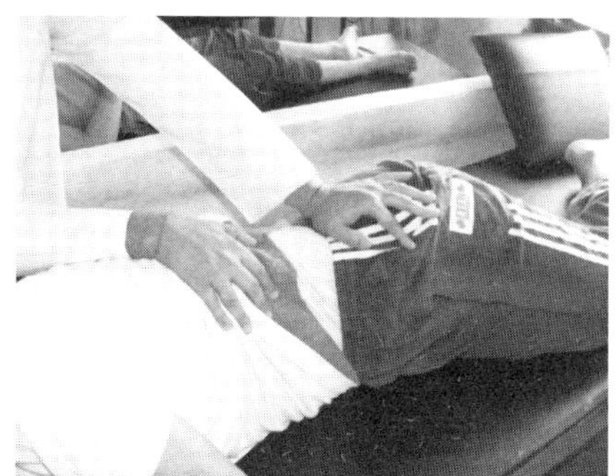

FIGURE 10.57: Anterior depression of pelvis, left hemiplegia

Posterior Elevation

Posterior elevation of pelvis is used in terminal stance and initial swing phase of the gait cycle. Here, the pelvis is moved posteriorly and in upward direction (Figure 10.58).

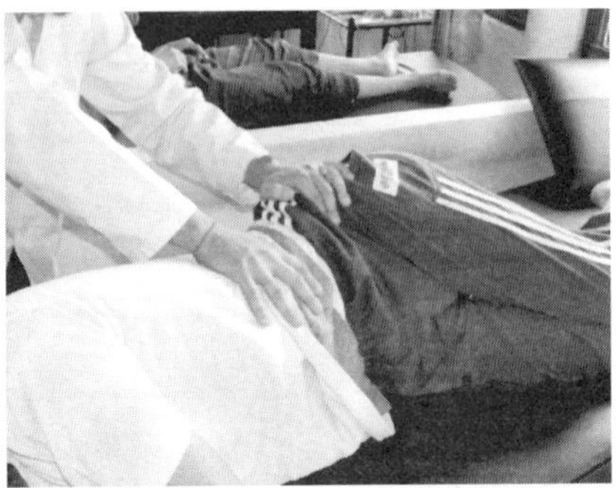

FIGURE 10.58: Posterior elevation of pelvis, left hemiplegia

Anterior Elevation

In anterior elevation of pelvis, the therapist guides and later resists the motion of pelvis anteriorly and upwards. Stability is carried out as already explained before (Figure 10.59).

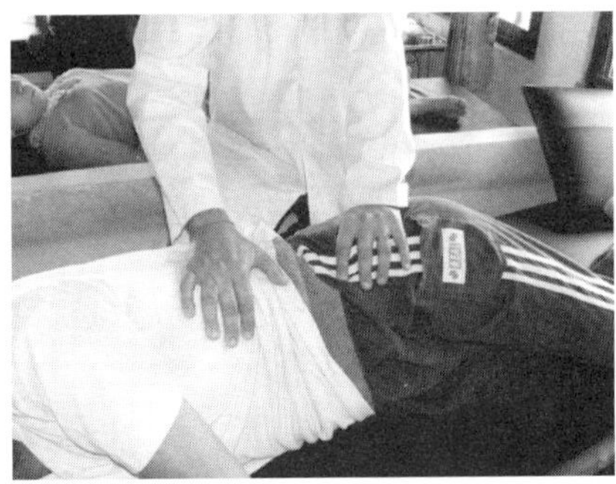

FIGURE 10.59: Anterior elevation of pelvis, left hemiplegia

Posterior Depression

In posterior depression, the therapist guides and later resists the motion of pelvis posteriorly and in downward direction (Figure 10.60).

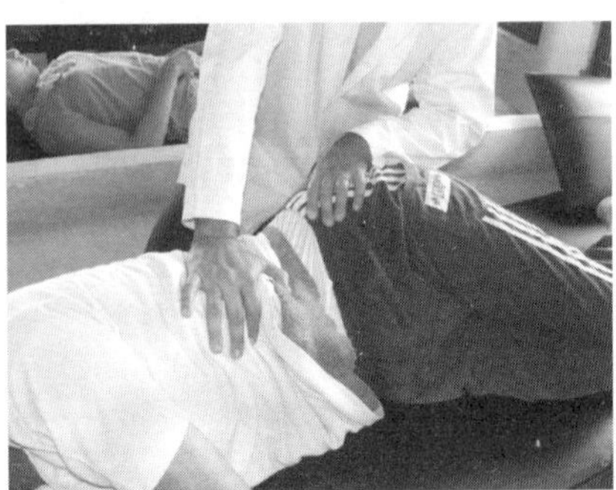

FIGURE 10.60: Posterior depression of pelvis, left hemiplegia

All the above mentioned activities are of utmost importance during entire gait cycle. All the motions occur as a single series and hence, description of individual motion during gait is a futile activity, as the gait is a constant phenomenon and we have divided it into phases for our convenience in explanation.

USE OF THE BALL IN TRAINING LOWER LIMB AND TRUNK IN LYING

The vestibular ball is very useful in training as it provides a dynamic surface to move as well as dynamic support at the same time. Eccentric training and, training for timing of contraction is best done with the vestibular ball. Activities described in this section can be done either on the couch or on the mat. While in the initial stages, it would be difficult for the patient to assume lying position on the mat, the exercises with the ball on the couch can be started right from the beginning. The patient lies comfortably in supine position. A vestibular ball of optimum size is kept below the lower limbs as shown in the Figures 10.61A and B. Care must be taken so that the knee joints of the patient do not fall into hyperextension, for this, knees may be kept in few degrees of flexion. After this the patient is instructed to carry out

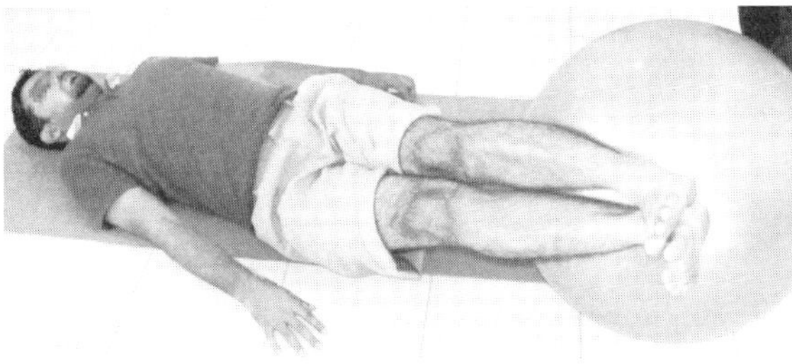

FIGURE 10.61A: Controlled trunk rotation to right using vestibular ball, left hemiplegia

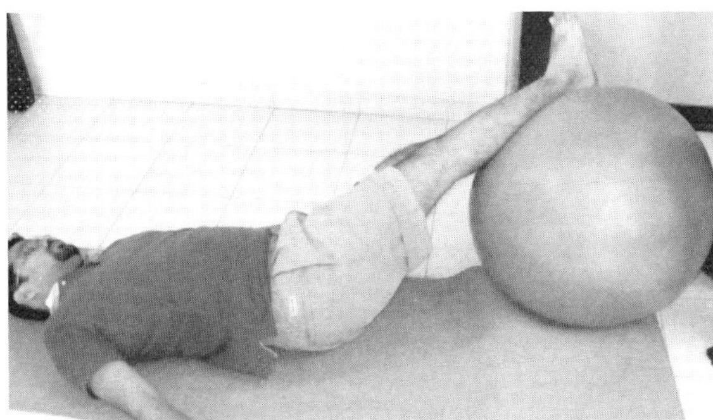

FIGURE 10.61B: Controlled trunk rotation to left using vestibular ball, left hemiplegia

rotation of the trunk by moving the ball to both sides. This activity is helpful in training abdominals and lower limb control. Assistance may be required in the initial stages. Later on, resistance to motion on both the sides can be given manually (Figures 10.62A and B).

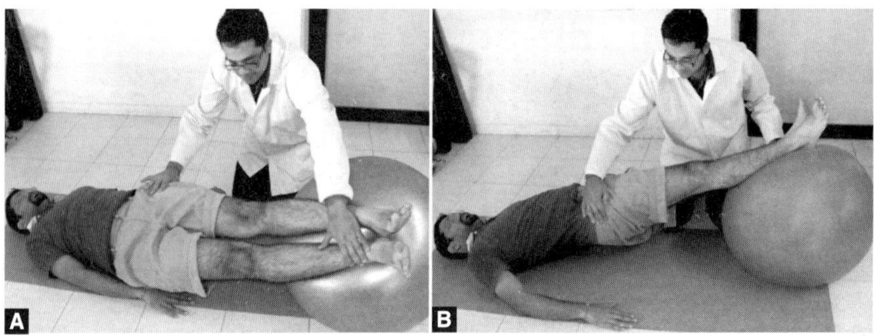

FIGURES 10.62A and B: Controlled trunk rotation with pelvic lifts, left hemiplegia

In the same position of the lower limbs, with the extreme rotation, the patient is asked to raise the pelvis and rotate to same side to aid rotation at higher level.

To gain control of lower limbs, the affected lower limb, left in this case is kept actively stabilized on the ball while the sound limb performs abduction and adduction of hip with knee kept in slight flexion (Figures 10.63 and 10.64). The same procedure can be carried out by the affected limb too.

For progression, a ball is held between both the hands and is held above in elevation as shown in the Figures 10.65A and B. This procedure actively involves the stability of shoulder and thoracic region. The lower limbs are moved alternatively as in previously described activity. Assistance is provided to the affected limb whenever required and limbs are not allowed to fall prey to exaggerated and synergistic patterns of activity. Speed of the movements

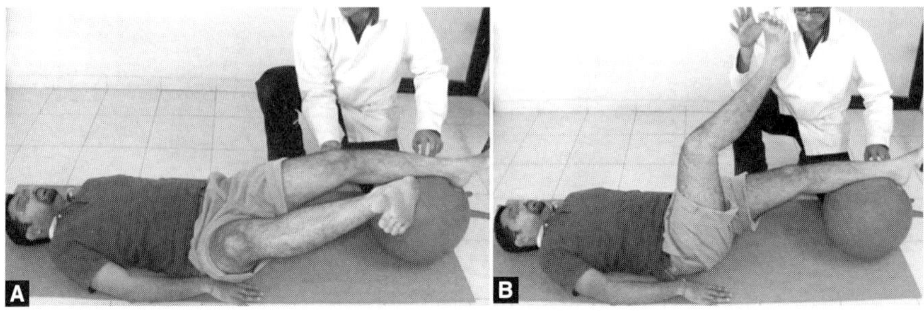

FIGURES 10.63A and B: Movement of sound limb while the ball is controlled by affected limb, left hemiplegia

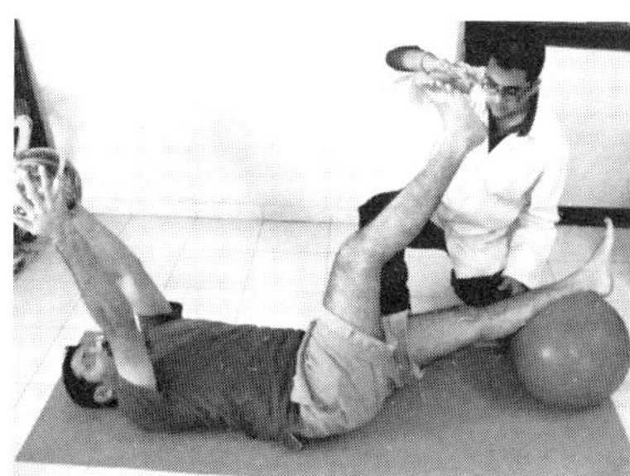

FIGURE 10.64: Movement of sound limb while the ball is controlled by affected lower limb, with a ball held by hands for thoracic and scapular stability, left hemiplegia

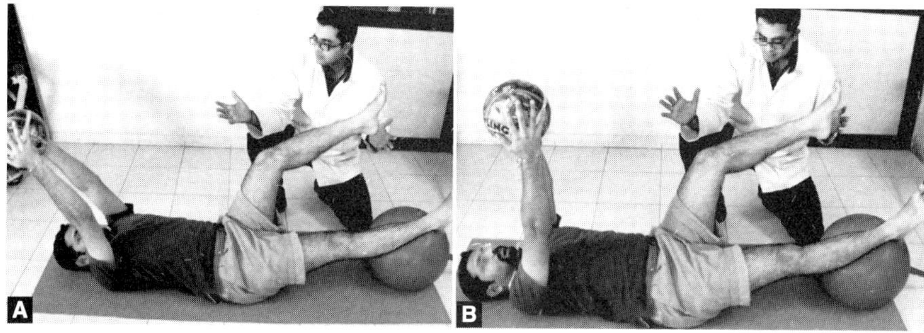

FIGURES 10.65A and B: Movement of affected lower limb while the ball is controlled by sound lower limb, with a ball held by hands for thoracic and scapular stability, left hemiplegia

is kept optimum to avoid hypertonicity. If the patient is unable to move the limb actively throughout the range of motion, 'placing' is done by the therapist and patient is asked to hold the limb in that position as far as possible. Note the size of the ball in above activities. Moving the upper limbs in various directions will aid in training multiple tasks where all four limbs and trunk participate either as movers or stabilizers.

Activities in Sitting

INTRODUCTION

As soon as the general condition of the patient allows, progression from position of lying to sitting is begun. From supine-lying, patient is taken to side-lying on either side. With the support of upper limbs, and taking both lower limbs near the edge of the couch with hip and knee flexed, simultaneous effort is made to raise the body up as well as taking the lower limbs down. Activation of synergistic patterns is prevented by assisting the patient wherever needed and reflex inhibiting patterns like clasping the hands are used along with the flexion of head and neck, trunk, hips and knees to counteract extensor thrust activity.

The usual progression of activities would be:

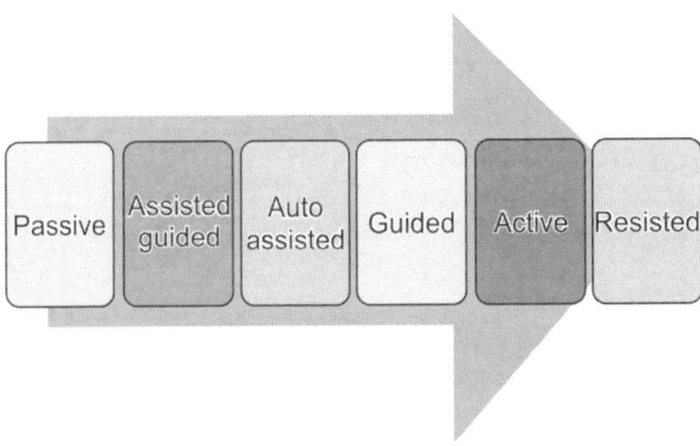

TRAINING OF LYING TO SITTING USING TRUNK

The Figure 11.1 shows the method which is prerequisite to sitting. The patient assumes the crook lying position. By flexing hip and knee further and by flexing the trunk, both the knees are brought near abdomen by contraction

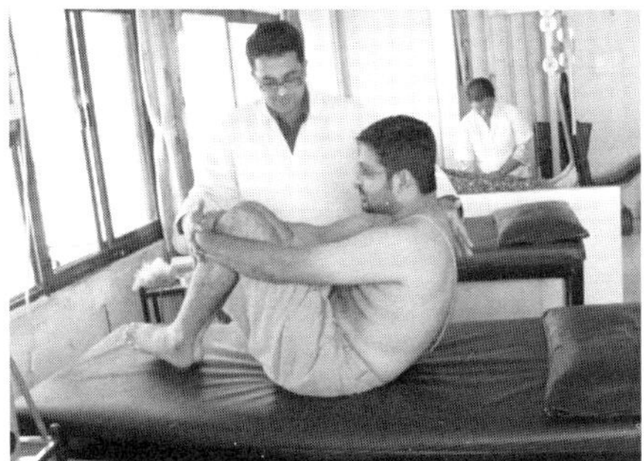
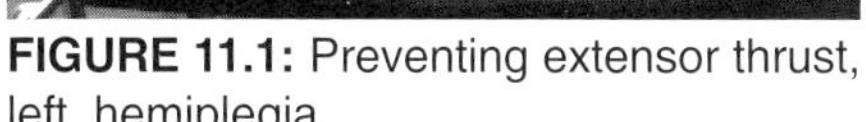

FIGURE 11.1: Preventing extensor thrust, left hemiplegia

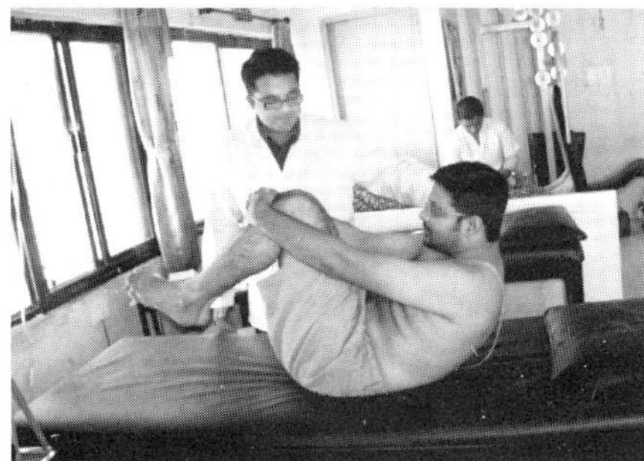

FIGURE 11.2: Rocking back and forth

of abdominal muscles. The patient is assisted to hold both the lower limbs at the knee by both the upper limbs which are clasped around. A gentle rocking of the trunk in flexion is done so that patient assumes a posture as shown in Figure 11.2. Gentle rocking back and forth can be performed to practice this activity. This is a total flexion pattern activity.

The therapist stabilizes both lower limbs of patient at thigh level. By holding both upper limbs, the patient is instructed to actively flex head and neck and trunk. The direction of the movement is controlled by the therapist, which may be flexion of the trunk or flexion with rotation on the side on which the therapist stands. This activity strengthens trunk flexor and oblique muscles. As the patient progresses, he actively stabilizes lower limbs and,

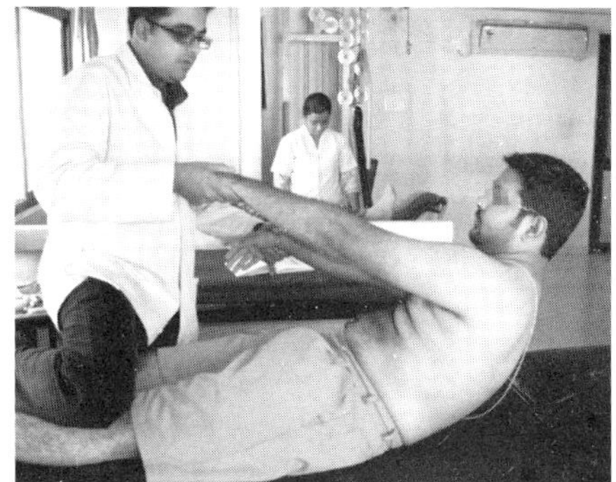

FIGURE 11.3: Abdominal activation, supported, left hemiplegia

assistance from the therapist in flexing the trunk also reduces. The upper limbs are held as shown in the Figure 11.3, for ensuring flexion of thoracic spine also. Care must be taken not to pull hemiplegic shoulder. Eccentric contractions can be trained by controlling the movement by the patient while returning to supine position.

SITTING FROM SIDE-LYING

In addition to promotion of early weight-bearing on the hemiplegic shoulder and hip, this posture also elongates the lateral trunk flexors, which may be spastic. Consider Figure 11.4. The patient can then be assisted in moving the legs over the edge of the bed and pushing up to full sitting position using both arms.

The lower extremity can assist in rolling by pushing off from flexed and adducted, hook-lying position. This encourages an important advanced limb pattern needed for gait- hip extension with knee flexion and also facilitates early weight-bearing in the supine position. An alternate method involves using a proprioceptive neuromuscular facilitation (PNF) chop pattern, which also encourages upper trunk rotation and flexion with upper extremity diagonal movement. The patient can be taught to use the leg to assist in rolling by pulling the hip and knee up and across the body in a flexion pattern (flexion, adduction, external rotation).

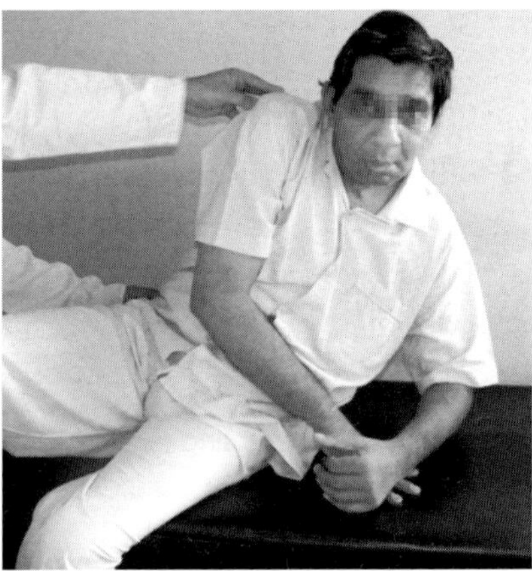

FIGURE 11.4: Lying to sitting with forearm support, left hemiplegia

SITTING IN THE BED

Sitting in the bed for meals is not desirable, but may be necessary to fit in with staffing and ward routine. The half-lying position should never be used, as there is increased flexion of the trunk with extension in the legs and greater risk of pressure sores. The patient should be as upright as possible with the head and trunk in line and his weight evenly distributed on both buttocks. The affected arm is protracted at the shoulder; both hands are clasped together and placed forward on a bed-table. The legs are straight, not laterally rotated.

MOVING SIDEWAYS IN SITTING

In sitting, the therapist can aid the patient in initially maintaining the posture by ensuring proper pelvic alignment (particularly pelvic anteroposterior alignment, so that the patient's foot is flat on the support surface) and by having the patient use extended arms for support. It is important to use the affected arm for support rather than leave it hanging. Gentle resistance can be applied to assist in holding, using techniques of alternating isometrics rhythmic stabilization (Figure 11.5). Gentle

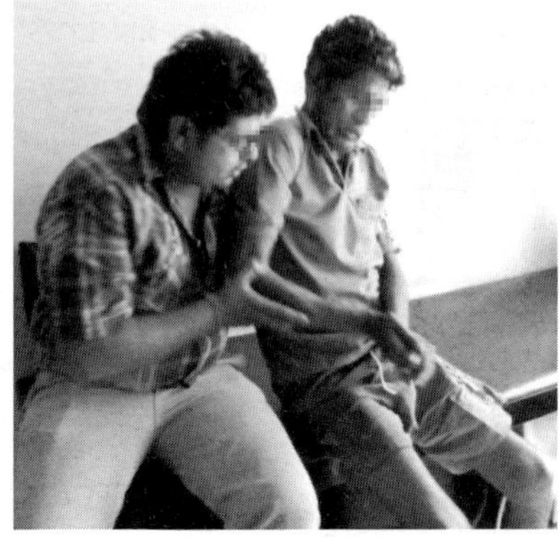

FIGURE 11.5: Shifting sideways in sitting, assisted, left hemiplegia

rocking movements should incorporate moving forward, backward, side-to-side, and in rotatory directions. Transferring sideways on both the sides initially with assistance helps the patient to become mobile early in the process of rehabilitation. Shifting sideways can be done in two ways, i.e. with lower limbs grounded on the floor or without the assistance of the lower limb using lots of trunk activities and lifting both the buttocks up alternatively with the help of upper limbs. "Gluteal walking" sideways without the use of the upper limbs can be used as a progression to this activity.

TRANSFER ACTIVITIES

Lying on the bed is restricted to few hours in a day even when the patient is in the hospital. As soon as the general condition of the patient allows, the patient is shifted to a chair. Sitting in a chair is a functional position and apart from training variety of muscles and patterns of activities, it is moral boosting for the patient. Visual scanning of the environment becomes easy as the head is held upright. Overall perception of the patient also improves.

Much damage can be done to the patient's shoulder as well as to the nurse's or therapist's back during transferring the patient from bed to a chair, if this maneuver is performed incorrectly. It can also be a very frightening time for the patient, if he is suddenly transferred without any explanation or chance to move himself. The following is an easy, safe, therapeutic way of transferring a patient from bed to chair. The chair is placed in position on the affected side and the patient is rolled or assisted on to his affected side. The helper places one hand under the patient's affected shoulder, swings his legs over the edge of bed with her other hand, and brings the patient to the sitting position (Figure 11.6). During this phase, elongation of the trunk occurs, and if a pause is needed to rearrange clothes, etc., the patient can be propped on the affected elbow and take weight throughout it. The patient, with his

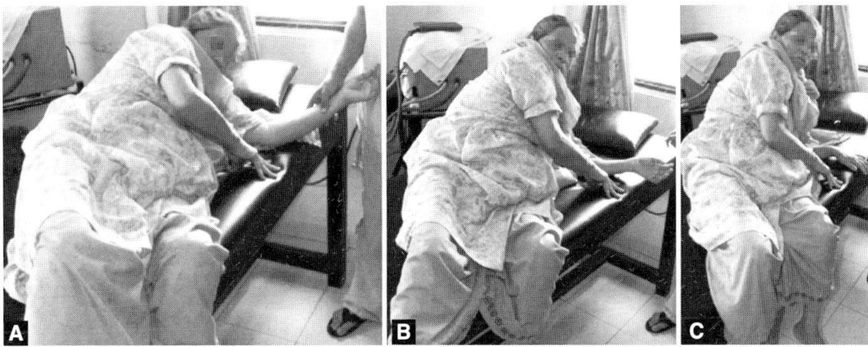

FIGURES 11.6A to C: Sequential lying to sitting, left hemiplegia

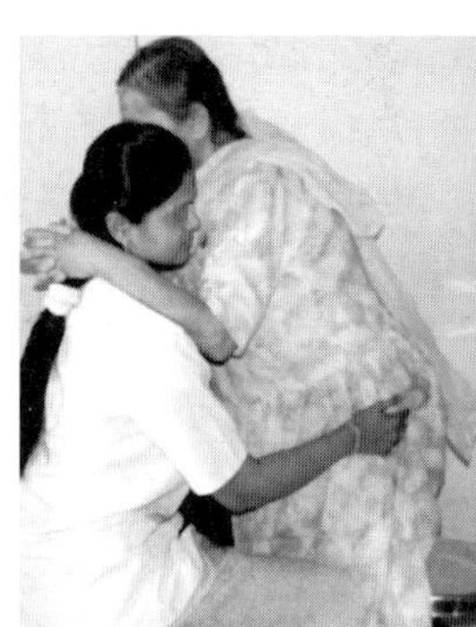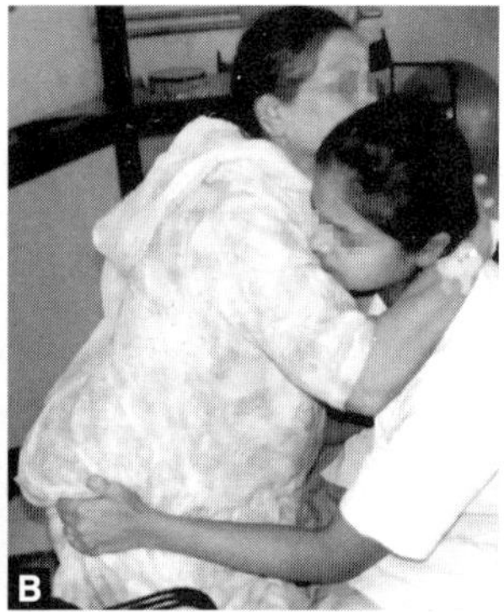

FIGURES 11.7A and B: Transferring from one sitting place to another, assisted, left hemiplegia

hands clasped together in front of him, is helped to move to the edge of the bed. He transfers his weight over to one side and then to the other and moves the opposite hip forward each time as if he was walking on his buttocks. The assistant's arms are placed under the patient's shoulders with her hands over the scapulae while her leg wedges the patient's feet and knees. The patient's arms are placed round the helper's waists or on her shoulders, but he must not grip his hands together. The patient is forward and he is brought to standing by pressure forward and down on the shoulders, so that his weight goes equally through both legs. No attempt is made to lift him up at all. The assistant's weight counterbalance the patient's, and with shoulder and knees fixed, he is pivoted round to sit on the chair (Figures 11.7A and B). Transferring in such a way emphasizes the hemiplegics side and encourages weight-bearing and weight transference to that side.

UPPER EXTREMITY CONTROL

Initial mobility of upper extremity can be achieved by focusing first on scapular motions. Since the typical spastic pattern is one of retraction and fixation, protraction with external rotation should be emphasized. This is typically performed in sitting position as shown in Figures 11.8A and B.

The arm is mobilized forward and the patient is asked to hold this position. If holding is successful, then eccentric and reciprocal movements are attempted. Once initial control is achieved, the posture can be altered to a more challenging one (e.g. active against gravity) and more active control of shoulder and elbow components can be added through an increasing range. The patient should be taught to mobilize the affected arm using hands clasped together (prayer position). The therapist mobilizes the scapula in sitting position as shown in Figures 11.8A and B, by keeping the upper limb cardled and fully supported.

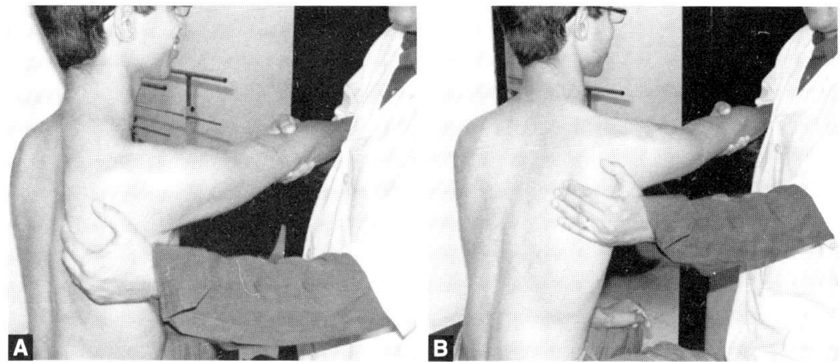

FIGURES 11.8A and B: Scapular retraction and protraction in sitting. Mobilization and resisted workout in same grip, right hemiplegia

After this guided mobility, the patient is asked to carry out this activity actively along with reaching out.

Movements that should be stressed include hand to mouth and hand to opposite shoulder, since these have important functional implications in feeding and dressing. Elbow extension movements combined with shoulder abduction or flexion should also be stressed to counteract the effects of the dominant flexion synergy. The quadruped posture provides the greatest challenge for upper extremity weight-bearing but may be too difficult for some hemiplegia patients. An alternate posture would be sitting, weight-bearing on an extended arm on a stool in front, as shown in Figure 11.9 or modified plantigrade. Control should progress form initial holding in the posture to controlled mobility using rocking movements.

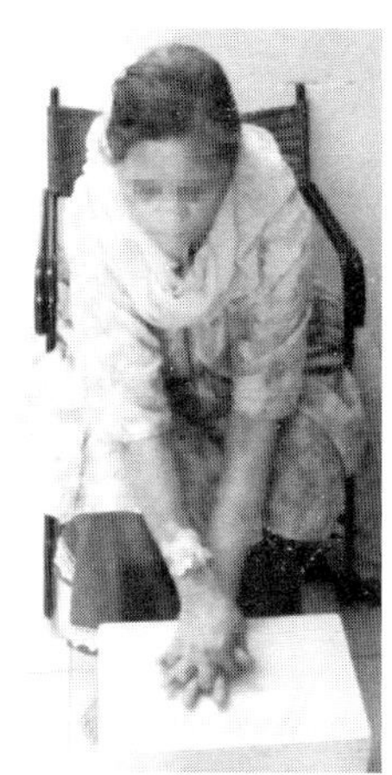

FIGURE 11.9: Bilateral upper limbs held in clasped position and affected side is kept supinated in rip, left hemiplegia

CONTROL OF QUADRICEPS IN LONG SITTING

This activity is used to gain control of extensors of knee i.e., quadriceps in sitting position. The patient assumes long sitting position as shown in Figures 11.10A and B. The affected lower limb is flexed at the knee about 15 to 20 degrees. The therapist stabilizes patient's foot in dorsiflexion by his thigh as shown. The patient is instructed to carry out knee extension gradually and with control. The patient continuously watches the moving patella. The patient

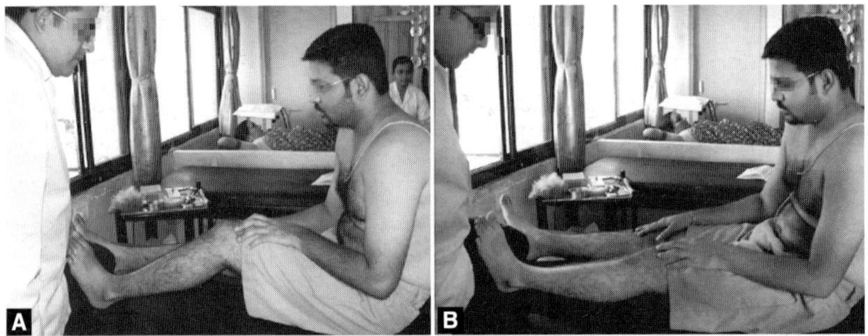

FIGURES 11.10A and B: Controlled knee extension in long sitting with foot stabilized, left hemiplegia

may put his hand on quadriceps muscle for added proprioception. This activity also trains gastrocnemius as well as soleus to some extent. As per the synergistic pattern, it may be thought that planter flexors of ankle may not need attention as they are already spastic. But in the contrary, the spastic plantar flexors have no or little active control in sitting and standing, which is required for getting up and walking.

The patient is assisted to come into long sitting position with affected knee kept extended or slightly flexed. The patient keeps both upper limbs on legs, respectively and while flexing the back, they are slided onto the legs. Note the contraction of back flexor muscles as the extensor muscles of back gradually relax in Figure 11.11. Lateral movement of the trunk on either side by keeping both upper limbs together on the couch can also be practiced.

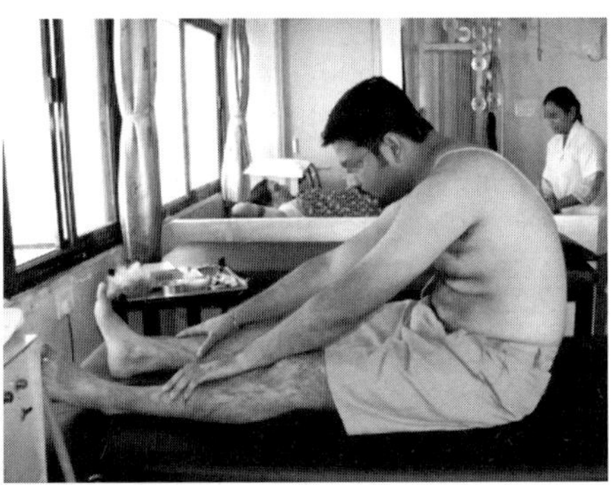

FIGURE 11.11: Counteracting extensor thrust of back in long sitting, left hemiplegia

INHIBITION OF EXTENSOR THRUST

The patient's affected leg is crossed over the sound one and is held in full flexion and lateral rotation with the foot and toes in full dorsiflexion, until it will stay in position on its own (Figure 11.2). Maintain inhibition at the foot

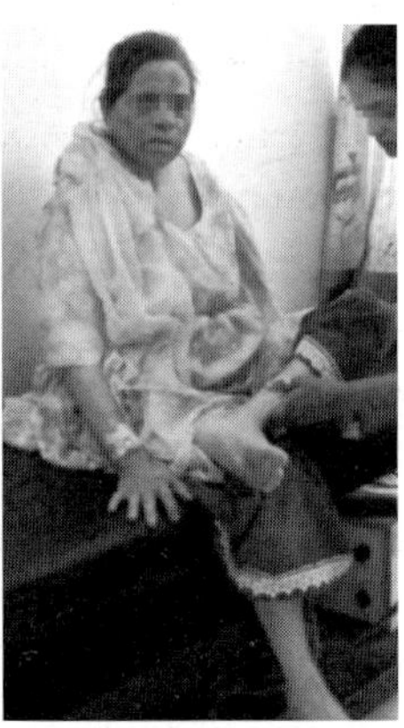

FIGURE 11.12: Crossover of affected leg to counteract extensor thrust of lower limb, left hemiplegia

and ask the patient to uncross his leg and lower it, making it feel light and to raise it once more across the other leg.

To prepare for walking, teach the patient to move the legs without moving the trunk, one leg at a time, asking to make it feel light by taking the weight himself. They must maintain control while the leg is lowered onto the bed. The patient is asked to keep his trunk still and not to lean back throughout the activity.

WEIGHT SHIFTS IN HIGH SITTING

As the patient is propped up in high sitting position, assessment of weight-bearing on both the ischial spine is checked for. For the ease of viewing lateral folds of trunk, slight amount of neck flexion may be done. Figure 11.13 shows increased lateral folds on left side which is affected. The same position can be used for correction in the posture and for training forward flexion of the trunk.

Note the transition from back flexion in Figure 11.13 to back extension in Figure 11.14. Slump and straightening of back is a good postural exercise in making the patient understand pelvic tilts. Figures 11.15 and 11.16 show the training of anterior and posterior pelvic tilt in sitting position.

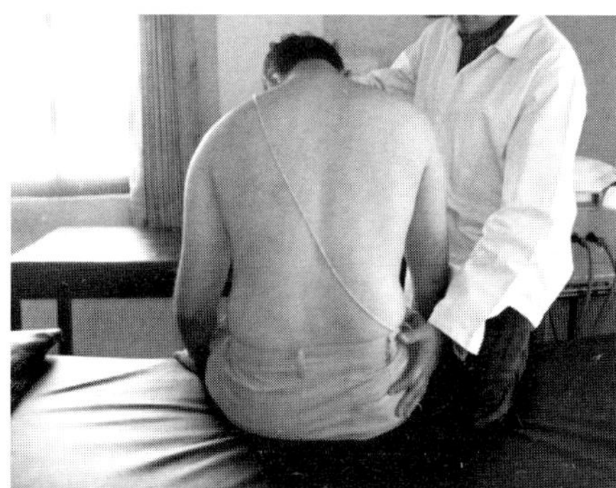

FIGURE 11.13: Assessment of posture in sitting for equal weight-bearing, left hemiplegia

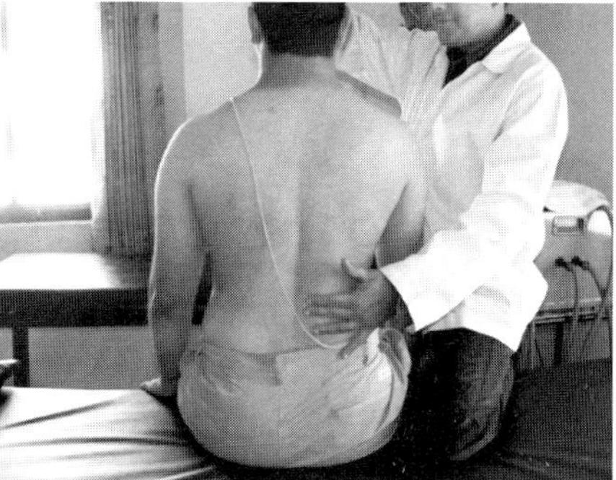

FIGURE 11.14: Back extension in sitting from flexion

Anterior pelvic tilt associated with increase in lumbar lordosis as pointed out in the Figure 11.15.

Posterior pelvic tilt is associated with obliteration of lumbar lordosis and contraction of abdominal muscles (Figure 11.6). These exercises are taught to the patient to carry out several times in a day.

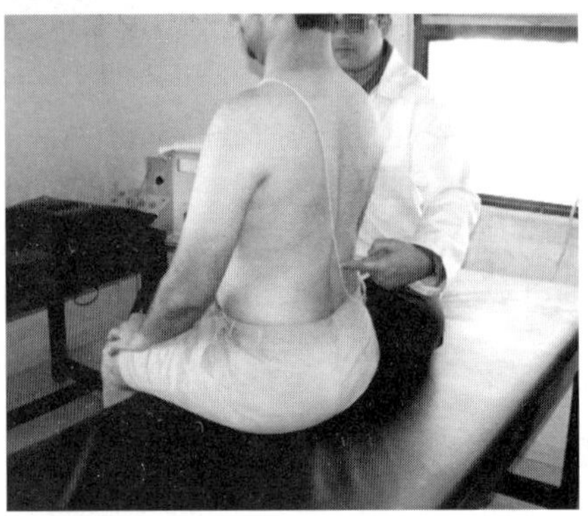

FIGURE 11.15: Anterior pelvic tilt in sitting

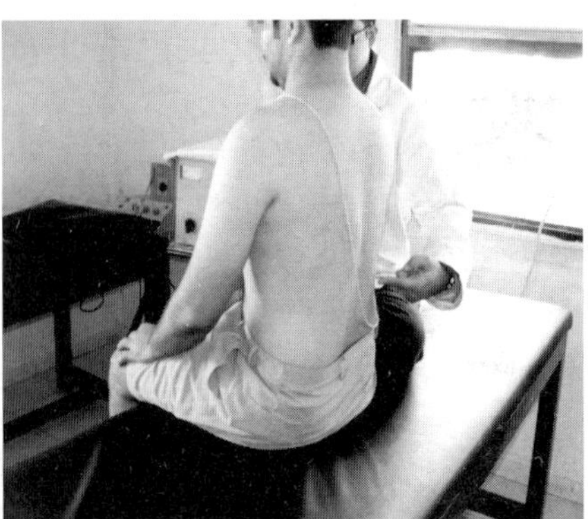

FIGURE 11.16: Posterior pelvic tilt in sitting

SIMULTANEOUS ACTIVATION OF UPPER LIMB AND TRUNK

After the practice of tilts, rotation of the trunk is started. As shown in Figure 11.17, the affected upper limb is held in adduction, flexion and few degrees of internal rotation at shoulder with flexion of elbow, so that the hand rests on opposite clavicular region. The sound arm cradles the affected arm so that it does not drop off. Rotation of trunk in few degrees of flexion is gained by instructing the patient to take the tip of elbow (olecranon) towards downwards and to the left or right. Note the shifting of the weight on the affected side ischial tuberosity.

Gradually, the cradling from the sound arm is reduced and it is kept free to move actively in the direction of the rotation of the trunk.

Practice of abdominal activity along with stabilization of thorax in sitting position is carried out by moving the sound upper limb while the affected upper limb is kept on the right clavicular region as shown in Figure 11.18. Note the flexion of the trunk which is gained by posterior pelvic tilt. In the initial stages, this activity is of particular importance in gaining dynamic posture control on sitting position. The sound upper limb position aids in increasing the leverage.

Patient is instructed to move the affected (left in this case) elbow towards opposite knee while the sound upper limb is maintained as shown in Figure 11.19. Note the movement of trunk in flexion and rotation. Also note that the patient is constantly aware about the direction of the motion.

The sequence of the movement shown in Figures 11.20A and B is used in gaining primary motor control of upper limb in sitting position. As seen in the previous activities where the affected upper limb was either cradled

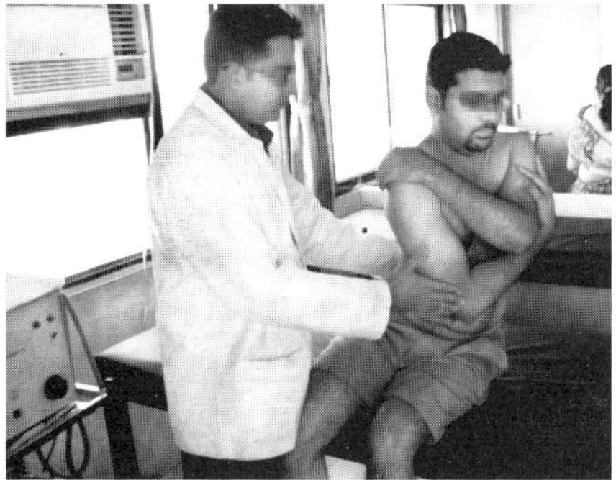

FIGURE 11.17: Rotation of trunk with the upper limb in RIP, left hemiplegia

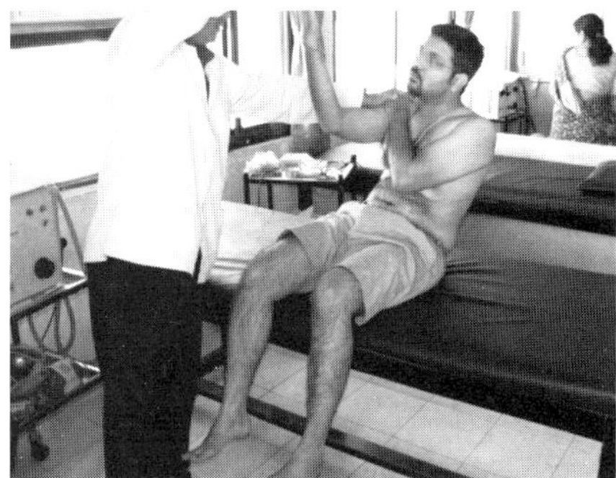

FIGURE 11.18: Active placing of sound upper limb, while affected limb is stabilized, left hemiplegia

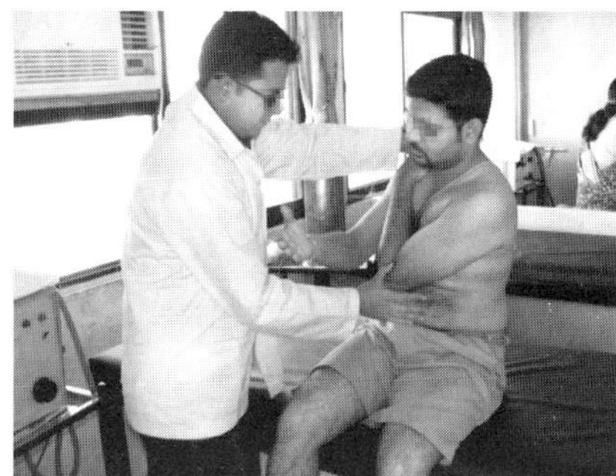

FIGURE 11.19: Placing with added flexion-rotation of the trunk to the right, left hemiplegia

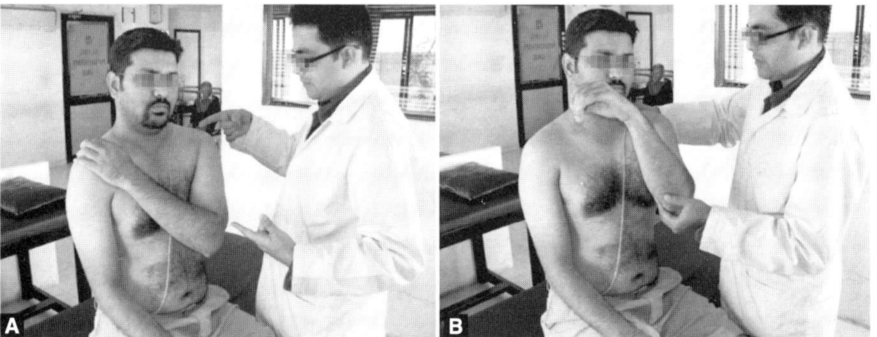

FIGURES 11.20A and B: Active movements of left upper limb and placing it back, left hemiplegia

by the sound limb or was supported by therapist, is now gradually left on its own. Patient uses active effort in keeping the upper limb in the position. The hand is lifted up from resting position by contraction of external rotation of shoulder and is kept back slowly. The therapist may have to assist at the elbow to prevent exaggerated abduction of the shoulder. Note the position of the right hand of the therapist which is stabilizing the scapula as shown in Figure 11.20B. This activity trains the movement of scapula protraction, shoulder adduction with external rotation and this position is also a precursor to controlled elbow flexion with supination of forearm.

WEIGHT-BEARING THROUGH UPPER EXTREMITIES

The patient is instructed to keep both upper limbs at one side with weight-bearing on both palms as shown in Figure 11.21. The therapist assists in keeping affected palm on the couch by extension and abduction of fingers and thumb and extension of wrists. Affected elbow is not allowed to drop in hyperextension i.e., in a locked position. Controlled flexion of elbow in the weight-bearing position is done and patient comes back to the starting position once again. This close chain activity is carried out mainly by the contraction of triceps and is useful in counteracting the flexor synergy. Rotational component of the trunk will physiologically reduce the flexor tone.

Figures 11.22A and B show dynamic activity on both the sides as explained above.

Figure 11.23 shows weight-bearing on affected limb sideways. Here, note the weight shifted on affected ischial tuberosity. As the patient shifts the weight towards affected side, the trunk on that side elongates. This is a true method of weight-bearing; if done

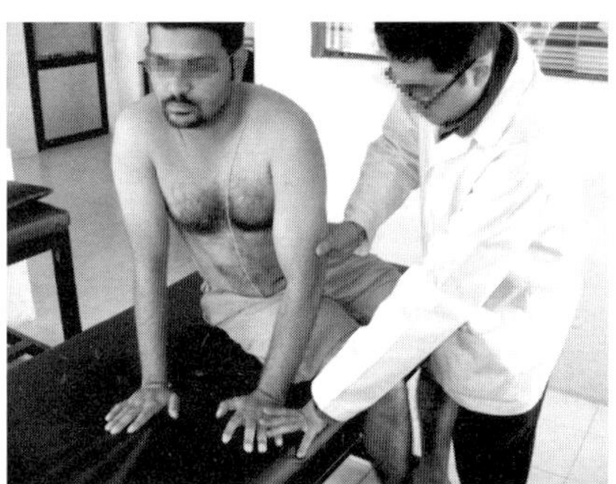

FIGURE 11.21: Weight-bearing through upper limbs sideways, left hemiplegia

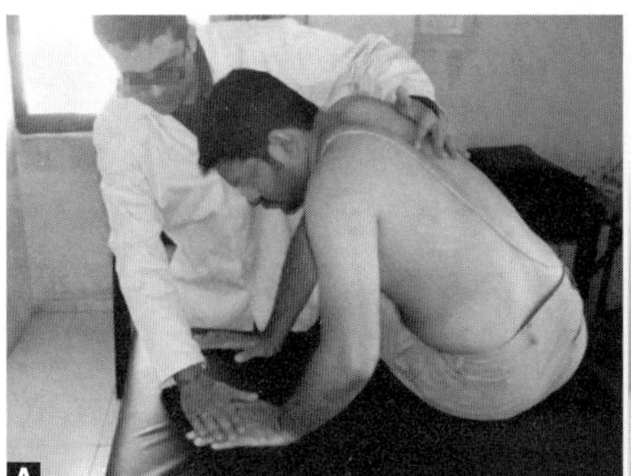

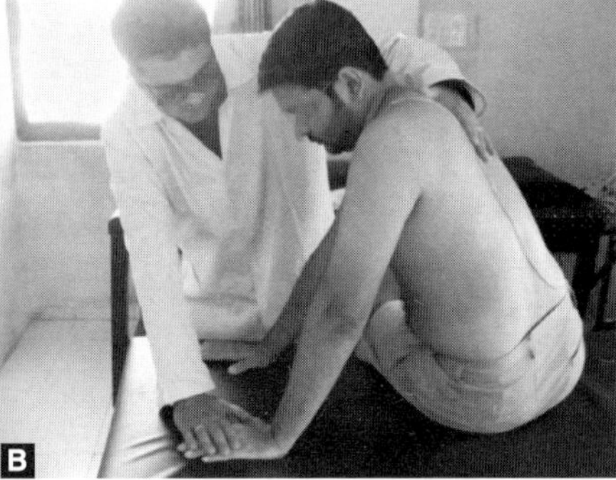

FIGURES 11.22A and B: While weight-bearing sideways, gradually flexing and extending elbows

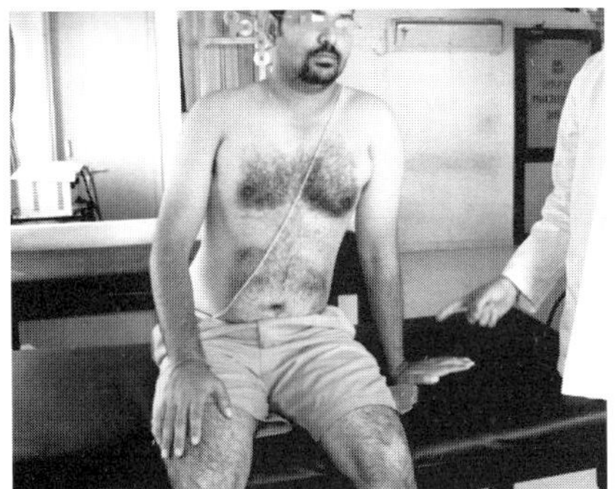

FIGURE 11.23: Conventional weight-bearing through affected upper limb, left hemiplegia

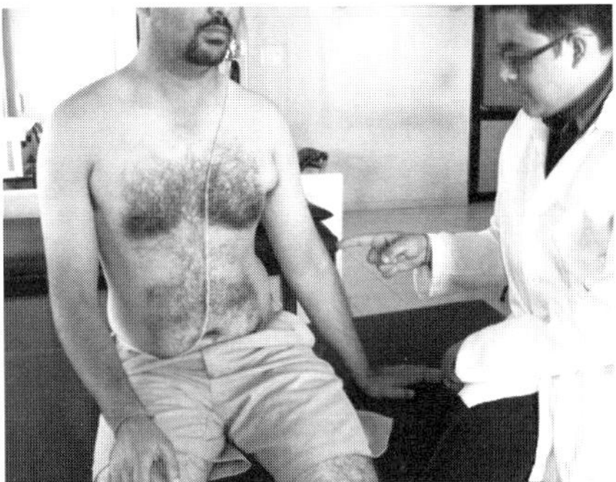

FIGURE 11.24: Incorrect method of weight-bearing

incorrectly, the trunk on affected side will flex which will result into increased stiffness of trunk and decreased weight-bearing on upper limb. Figure 11.24 shows the incorrect method of weight-bearing.

UPPER EXTREMITY PLACING

Active motor control activities of the upper limb can be started once dynamic balance reactions and weight-bearing improves. There are many methods by which this goal can be achieved. Activities which promote active control of the muscles that are antagonists to the synergistic patterns, are used either individually in initial stages or as combined movements as the patient progresses. The method of 'placing' is used in which the therapist places the upper limb of the patient in a desired pattern of activity and the patient is instructed to hold that position. Figure 11.25 shows placing in following pattern: shoulder flexion, abduction, external rotation, elbow partial flexion, forearm supination, wrist in neutral extension, fingers extended and thumb extended and abducted. Assistance may be given at few levels, as shown in Figure 11.25, assistance is given to keep the arm externally rotated and forearm supinated (by holding the thumb).

Training of shoulder adduction with external rotation along with the upper limb in reflex inhibiting posture can be achieved by pressing a moderately thick pillow under the axilla on both the sides. The therapist holds the affected upper limb in the following position: shoulder externally rotated, elbow extended, forearm supinated,

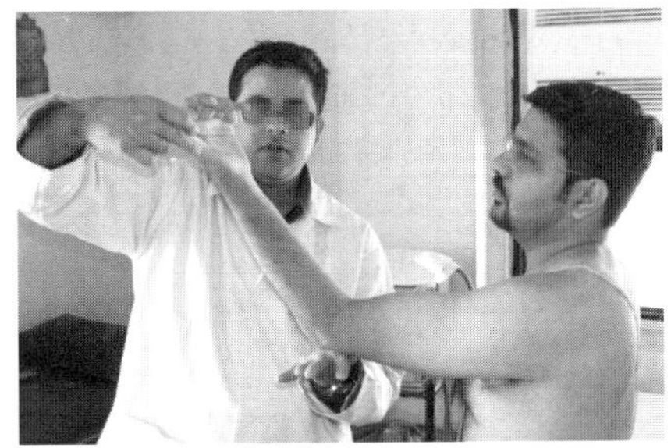

FIGURE 11.25: Active-assisted placing of affected upper extremity, left hemiplegia

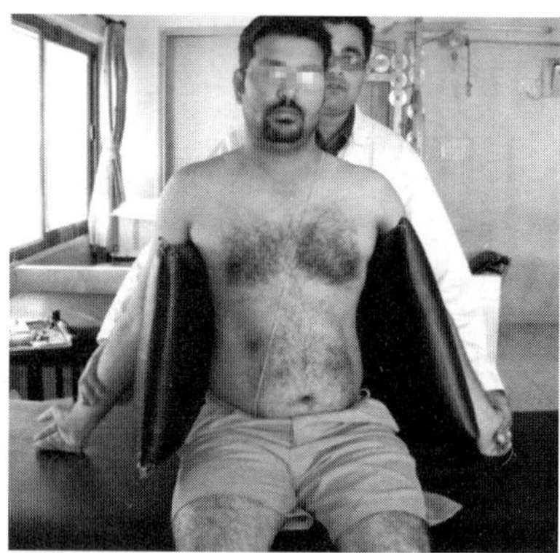

FIGURE 11.26: Pillow compressions to train shoulder adduction with external rotation, bilateral pattern, left hemiplegia

wrist extended, fingers extended and thumb extended and abducted, as shown in Figure 11.26. Sound upper limb may be held actively in this position or the therapist may guide the movement. The patient is then asked to compress the pillows with their arms. This activity is useful for training shoulder adduction with external rotation while forearm is supinated. This activity has functional implication on the movements of upper limb in front of the body, e.g. eating, wiping the face, etc.

DYNAMIC BALANCE REACTIONS

Moving more dynamically on the couch readies the patient to face challenges in the environment at functional level. Transferring the weight completely to the affected ischial tuberosity can be achieved by assisting the patient's affected upper limb in abduction of 90 degrees at shoulder and shifting towards affected side. Note the compensatory hip internal rotation on the sound side where the affected side hip externally rotates in Figure 11.27. Also note the dorsiflexion and eversion of the foot on normal side. The same activity can be performed by taking weight on sound side for gaining benefit of compensatory activity on the affected side throughout the kinematic chain.

The above mentioned exercise can be progressed by decreasing the assistance and allowing the patient to move the affected limb more actively. When the patient is moving actively, the sound upper limb counteracts the force of movements towards gravity by taking a center of gravity within the base of support. Please note the movement of trunk side flexion towards sound side (right side in this case) in Figure 11.28.

In the patient where weight shift towards affected side is difficult due to any reason, the technique shown above is implemented. The therapist sits on the affected side of the patient and holds the rim of the pelvis as shown in Figure 11.29A with both hands, one at back, another in front. The therapist

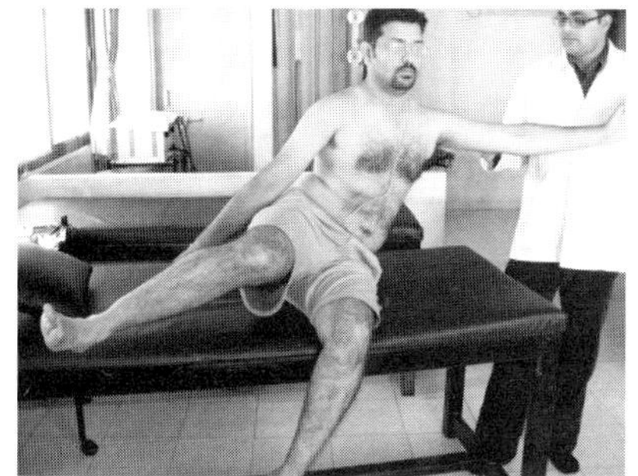

FIGURE 11.27: Dynamic balance reactions sideways in sitting, left hemiplegia

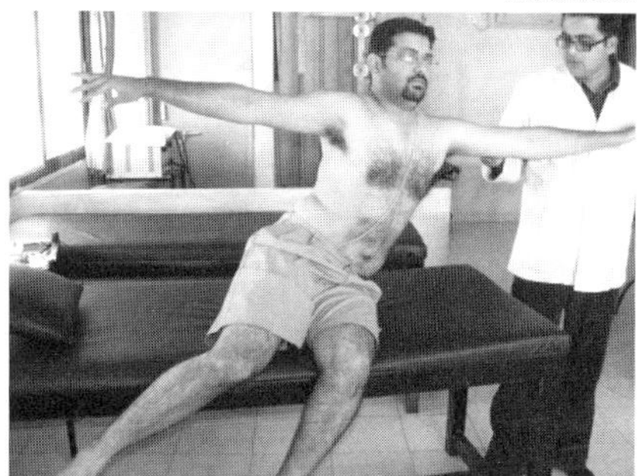

FIGURE 11.28: Moving more actively and dynamically

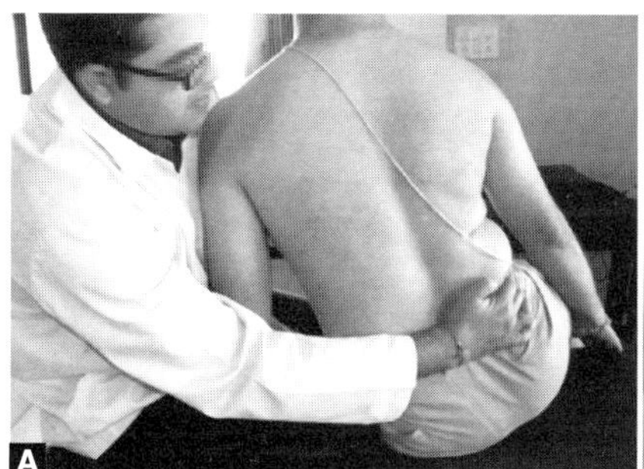

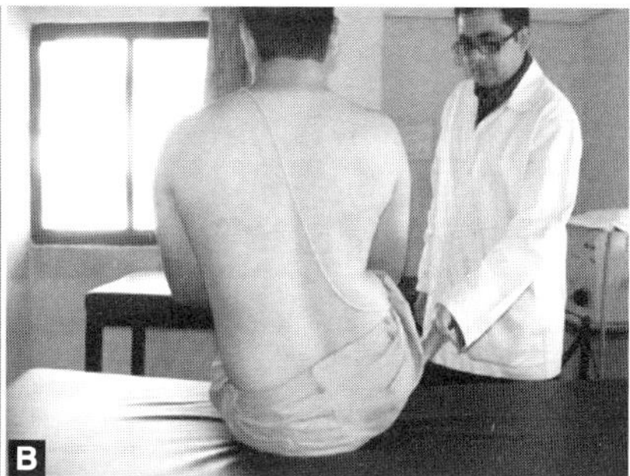

FIGURES 11.29A and B: Assisted and active lateral pelvic tilts, left hemiplegia

elongates the trunk on that side and inhibits any flexion in the arm. The patient's good leg is then free to be raised in the air. The body-weight is shifted over the sound side, and the head is placed in position if it is not right automatically. Side flexion of his trunk on the affected side is facilitated by giving pressure at the waist with one hand and encouraging lifting the buttock clear of the bed. The movement is repeated in a rhythmic manner until automatic head and trunk righting occurs to both sides.

The therapist then instructs the patient to lift the sound ischial tuberosity off the couch while he pulls the pelvis up and towards himself. Note the elongation of the trunk on the affected side while the trunk side flexes on the sound side in Figure 11.29B.

The therapist then decreases the assistance and can just guide by holding the affected upper limb in scaption as shown in Figure 11.30A.

Facilitate increased balance reactions of the head, trunk and upper limbs by lifting both legs together and rotating them to either side. Alter speed and position to obtain the required reactions in the rest of the body. The affected arm should assist balance in a similar way to the sound arm and not pull into flexion (Figure 11.30B). The patient is instructed to hold this shifted position for longer duration for progression. If the effort on the part of the patient increases, hypertonia may result on the affected side. To counteract

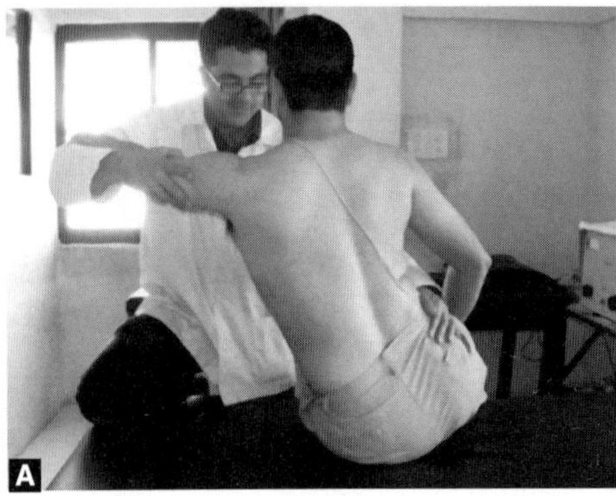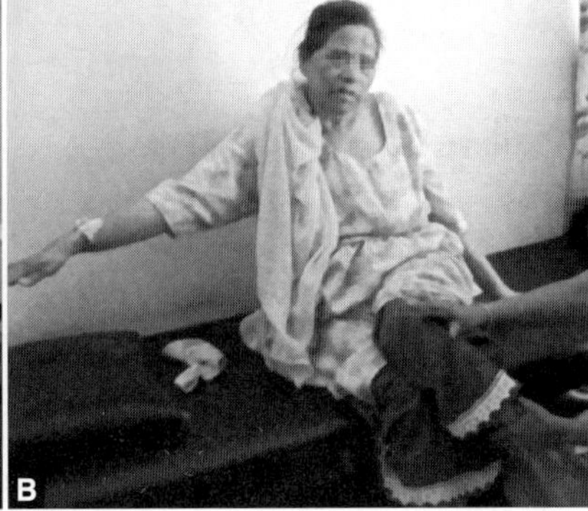

FIGURES 11.30A and B: (A) Affected side weight-bearing on ischial spine, left hemiplegia, and (B) Dynamic balance reaction with guiding lower limbs, left hemiplegia

this, either the effort on the part of the patient is reduced or assistance by the therapist is increased.

MOVING LOWER LIMB

Active movements of lower limb associated with the activation of abdominal muscles has an added advantage of counteracting synergistic patterns throughout the lower half of the body whereas upper body adapts automatically. A unilateral flexion of affected hip can be practiced while the pelvis is posteriorly tilted. This movement elicits activity of tibialis anterior and toe flexors which can be prevented by keeping the hip adducted and internally rotated.

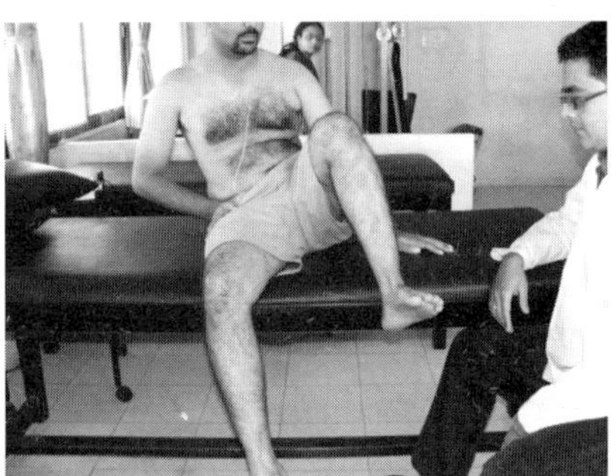

FIGURE 11.31: Moving lower extremity in flexion along with trunk flexion activation, left hemiplegia

Patient is instructed to take the affected knee towards opposite side chest. Active relaxation of tibialis anterior and other foot muscles is practiced by the patient along with the hip movements. Progression can be made by moving both the upper limbs and holding this position as shown in Figure 11.32. Note the contraction of lower abdominals in Figure 11.31 and also note the contraction of upper and lower abdominals both in Figure 11.32. Patient's attention is always focused on the quality of the moving lower limb.

Similar activity can be performed by the sound limb also. This gives an added advantage of weight shift towards affected side. Thus, active lower limb movements on both the sides encourage obliques and transversus abdominis (Figure 11.33).

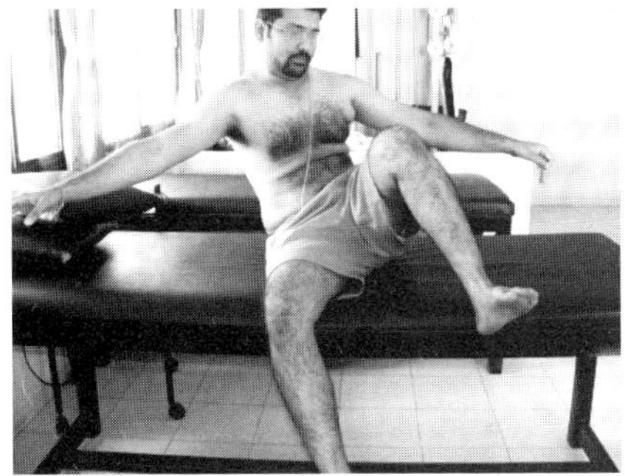

FIGURE 11.32: Lower limb flexion along with movements of upper extremities, left hemiplegia

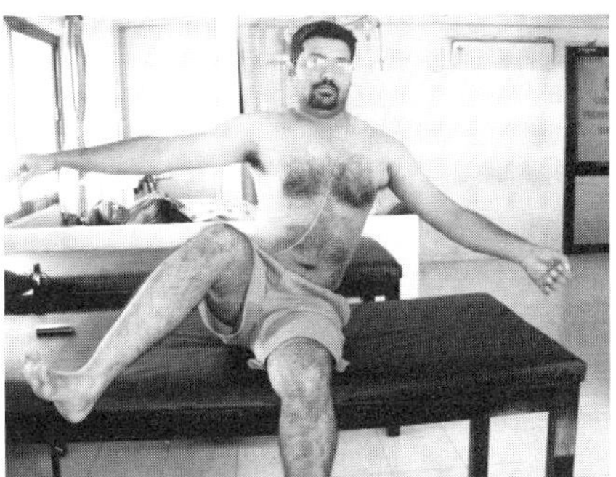

FIGURE 11.33: Flexion of sound side lower extremity, left hemiplegia

WEIGHT SHIFT ON ELBOWS, SIDEWAYS

The patient takes weight on elbow on affected side with trunk on that side elongated. Figure 11.34A shows incorrect method of weight-bearing in which the trunk side flexes on the affected side. This can be prevented by giving the assistance to the lateral pelvic tilt and side flexing the trunk towards sound side (Figure 11.34B). The progression of the activity can be done by asking the patient to rock forwards and backwards, axis being at elbow.

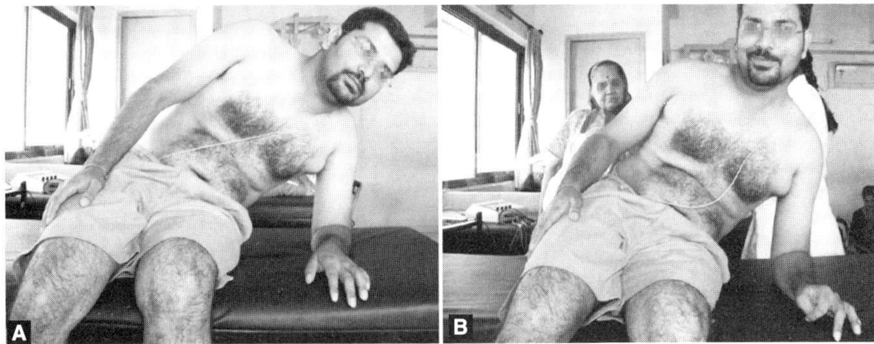

FIGURES 11.34A and B: Weight-bearing on affected elbow: (A) incorrect method and (B) correct method

SITTING IN THE CHAIR

A better sitting posture can be obtained in an upright chair. The chair should be of sufficient height to allow the patient's hips, knees and ankles to be approximately at right angles when he sits well back in the chair. His head and trunk are in line with the body-weight evenly distributed over both buttocks. His hands are clasped and placed well forward on a table in front of him (Figure 11.35).

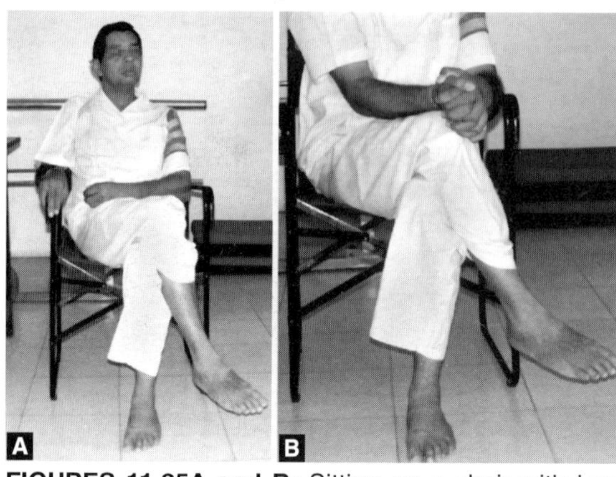

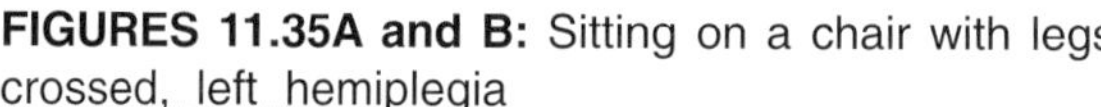

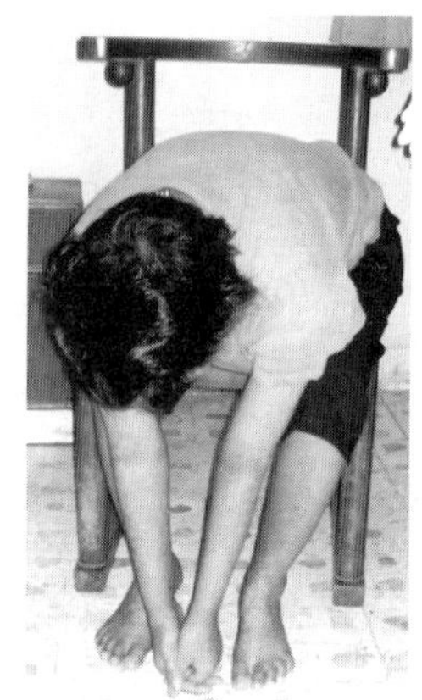

FIGURES 11.35A and B: Sitting on a chair with legs crossed, left hemiplegia

FIGURE 11.36: Flexion of trunk while sitting on chair with clasped hands

With the hands clasped in front, and elbows extended, the patient can practice reaching out to either side, forward and down to the feet (Figure 11.36).

WEIGHT TRANSFERENCE ON AFFECTED UPPER LIMB WITH REACHOUTS

The hand is placed flat on the bed or plinth and with one hand under the axilla and the other supporting the elbow (Figure 11.37A). The therapist draws the patient toward the elongating trunk at the same time. Weight transferring on the affected upper limb can be enhanced by reaching out by the unaffected upper limb towards the affected side as shown in Figure 11.37B. The therapist may support the elbow of the patient to prevent exaggerated flexion or extension.

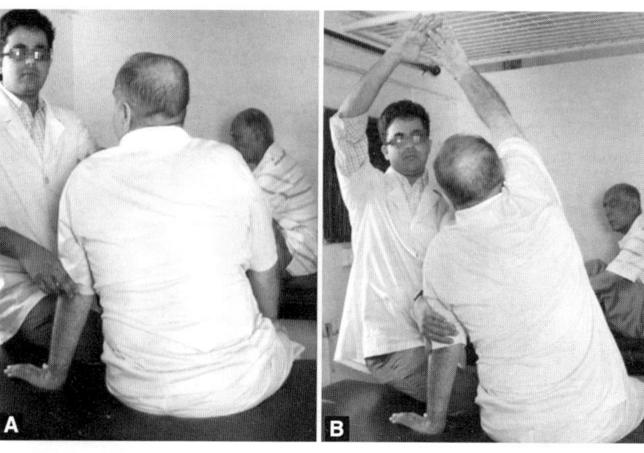

FIGURES 11.37A and B: Weight-bearing on affected side while reaching out with sound side, left hemiplegia

The patient may cross over the other to completely transfer the weight on the affected side ischial tuberosity. Reaching out can also be carried out with affected upper limb in various directions that train optimum weight shifts. Note Figures 11.38A and B, where during reachouts, the affected side trunk elongates along with complete weight-bearing on affected side ischial tuberosity.

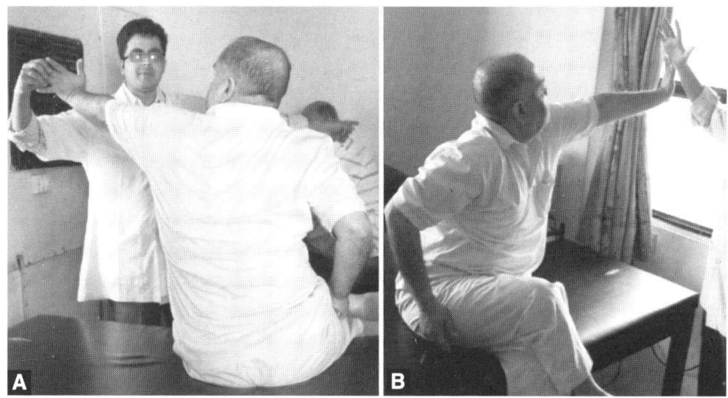

FIGURES 11.38A and B: Reachouts with affected upper extremity with legs crossed, left hemiplegia

MOVING IN SITTING POSITION

While one leg remaining flexed, make the patient transfer the weight on to the hip of the underneath leg and lift the other buttock off the bed. Facilitate flexion of the trunk with pressure at the waist (Figure 11.39). Repeat the same activity to both sides. The patient must be moved in sitting without

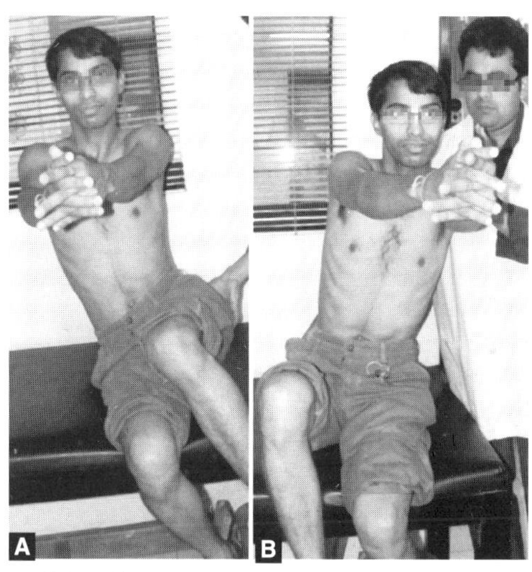

FIGURES 11.39A and B: Gluteal walking, right hemiplegia

using the hand. The patient is taught to shuffle or walk on the buttocks forwards and backwards and later sideways. Help is given by placing one hand under each hip or thigh and then rock and move from side to side.

WEIGHT TRANSFERENCE THROUGH THE ARMS BEHIND

Both arms are taken carefully behind the patient with the hands being supported on the therapist's hands. Extension is facilitated by using a sharp push-pull action up through the arms until they support his weight (Figure 11.40). Progress is made by shifting the weight from one side to the other without bending the elbows.

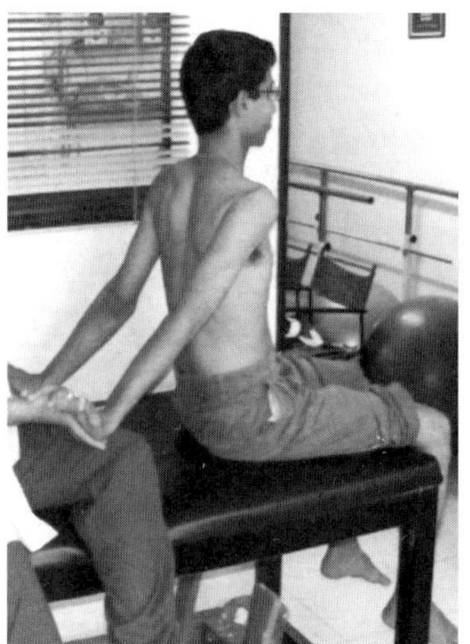

FIGURE 11.40: Weight-bearing behind, right hemiplegia

NECK STRETCHING

All the movements of neck need to be stretched and strengthened in sitting position as it is a functional position. Stretching of sternocleidomastoid on both the sides is best done in sitting position with the patient on the chair or a stool and therapist standing behind (Figure 11.41). Stretching of upper trapezius is also vital. Neck posture due to insufficient sternomastoid is often distorted. There may be a difference in strength of clavicular and sternal fibers. Note Figure 11.42.

In Figure 11.42 of patient with right side hemiparesis, note the difference in contraction in clavicular and sternal fibers of sternocleidomastoid. Right side sternal fibers are not activated at rest but they participate, though weakly,

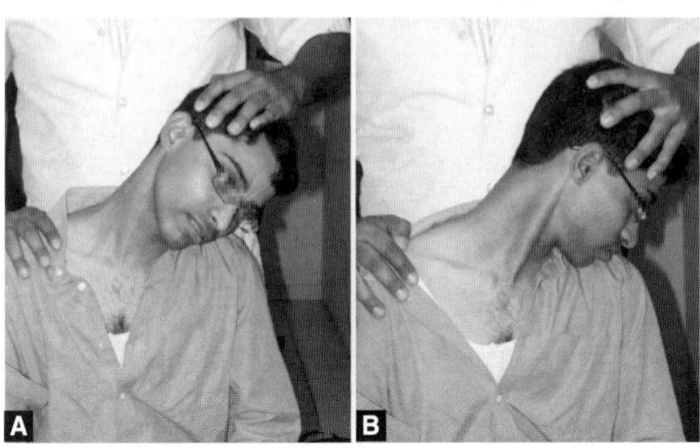

FIGURES 11.41A and B: Neck stretching, right hemiplegia

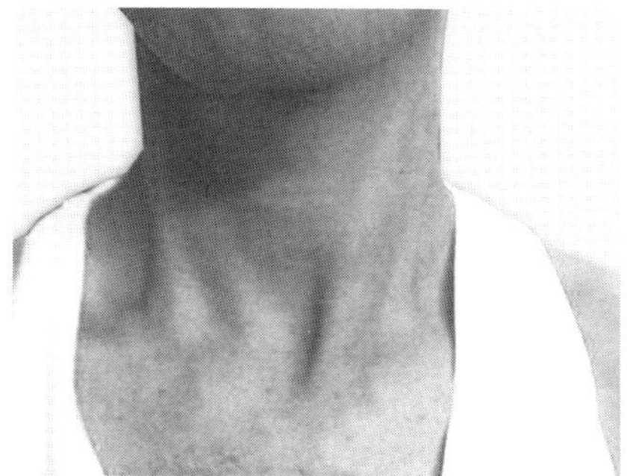

FIGURE 11.42: Asymmetrical activation of sternal and clavicular fibers of sterno-cleidomastoid muscle, right hemiplegia, at rest

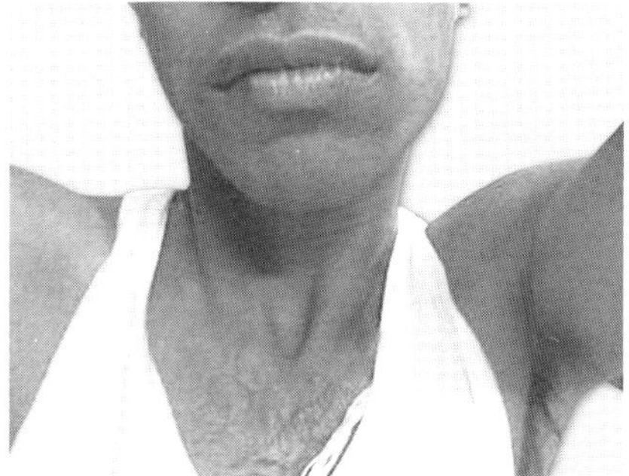

FIGURE 11.43: Asymmetrical activation of sternal and clavicular fibers of sternocleidomastoid muscle, right hemiplegia, during activity of upper extremities

when attempting shoulder elevation as seen in Figure 11.43. Note the deviation of the chin towards sound side, i.e. rotation of neck towards sound side and side flexion towards affected side. Also note the exaggerated contraction of upper trapezius on affected side.

Training of hand function should emphasize forearm, wrist, and finger movements independent of shoulder and elbow motions. Excessive shoulder adduction, elbow flexion, pronation, and finger flexion are the typical spastic patterns that must be counteracted. Voluntary release is generally much more difficult to achieve than voluntary grasp, and inhibitory techniques may be necessary before extension movements are successful. Prehension patterns should be practiced and manipulation of common objects attempted. The therapist needs to observe these movements carefully and to assist the patient in eliminating those aspects of performance that interfere with effective control.

ACTIVATION OF WRIST EXTENSORS

Activation of wrist extension is best done in sitting position where the patient is watching the movement throughout. Brushing is done at the start of the treatment as it has a latency period for its effect on contraction of the muscles. Optimum speed for brushing is selected and is carried out at the extensor surface of the forearm upto the dorsal aspect of distal end of the fingers, as shown in Figure 11.44. Other activities then follow.

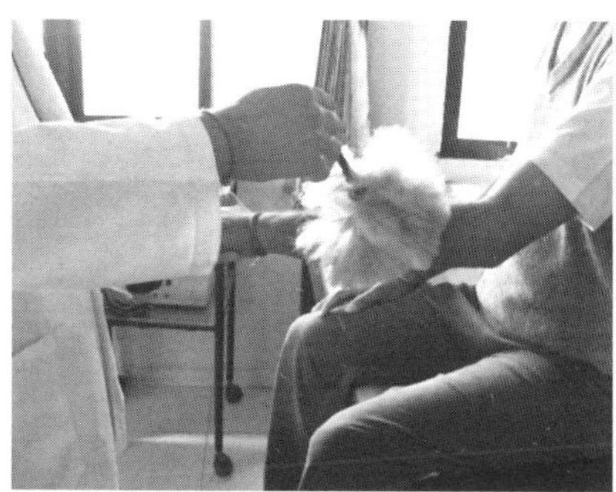

FIGURE 11.44: Brushing for long extensors of wrist and fingers, left hemiplegia

A scrubber can be used which provides a different texture for elicitation of the extensor muscles. Immediately after a quick stroke, patient is asked for active wrist extension. This technique has proved to be highly effective and hence, can be used frequently. As with any sensory activation, number of repetitions is kept to 4–5 strokes to avoid sensory adaptation.

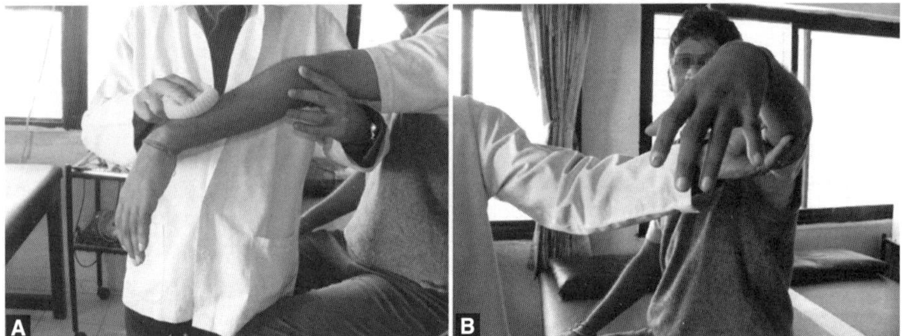

FIGURES 11.45A and B: Scrubber for facilitation of wrist and fingers extension, left hemiplegia

Figures 11.45A and B show the activation of long extensors of forearm and reciprocal relaxation of the flexor muscles of wrist and fingers immediately after using a brush and a scrubber. This reciprocal relaxation can be used in favor of wrist and fingers extension. Patient is asked to keep attention on raising tips of fingers rather than wrist extension as it can be done by flexion of fingers as in tenodesis; which is an unwanted action as it increases tone of flexor digitorum superficialis and profundus muscles.

SHOULDER ACTIVITIES

Activities of shoulder in sitting position require the shoulder to move in flexion without an exaggerated response from abductor muscles. Figure 11.46A shows an active attempt to lift left hemiplegic upper limb. Due to synergistic activities

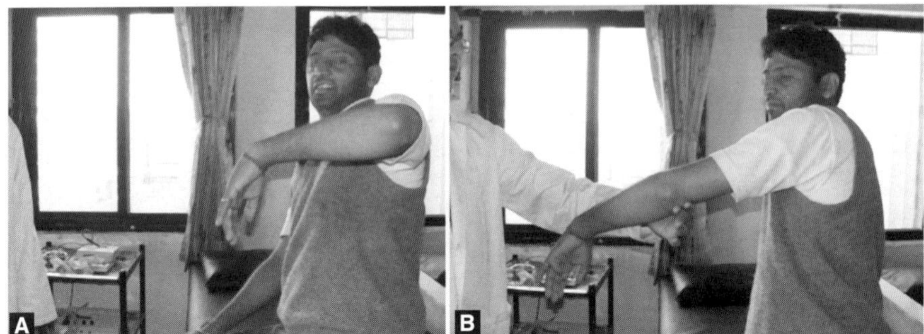

FIGURES 11.46A and B: Synergistic patterns of left upper extremity on active effort, left hemiplegia

the upper limb goes in the following pattern: shoulder abduction, internal rotation with elbow flexion. The more the patient puts his efforts in raising the upper limb, the more synergistic it gets. To prevent this, assistance from the therapist in guiding the movement in desired direction is mandatory.

Many a times for patient with hemiplegia, even the slightest amount of movement is encouraging, even if it may be in synergistic pattern. Thus, the therapist may not always discourage the patient from carrying out that activity but teaches him a proper method, e.g. activities with clasped hands or using minimal assistance as in guiding the motion.

PREPARATION FOR HAND ACTIVITY

Rehabilitation of upper limb functions post hemiplegia is one of the most challenging aspects for the treating therapist. Adequate head and neck control, scapular stability and mobility, thoracic and lumbar stability, shoulder external rotation and forearm supination are vital in gaining control over wrist and fingers. Nevertheless, activation of all the aforesaid parts is done in unison. Many activities overlap each other for one final aim of gaining motor control in upper limb. These activities help in making the patient independent.

With the patient sitting in chair, the therapist stands on the affected side with one hand controlling the scapula and the other hand resisting abduction of affected shoulder in scaption position. Isometric contraction in this angle is helpful in eliciting long extensors of forearm. Patient is asked to extend wrist and fingers as best as they can, while the therapist maintains the resistance. Overhead shoulder flexion with elbow extension also elicits contraction of wrist and fingers extension. As patient tries to extend the wrist and fingers, a brisk stroke by the therapist is given for facilitation. After releasing the resistance, the patient is asked to extend wrist and fingers while the therapist holds the affected upper limb in front of the patient's body as shown in Figure 11.47.

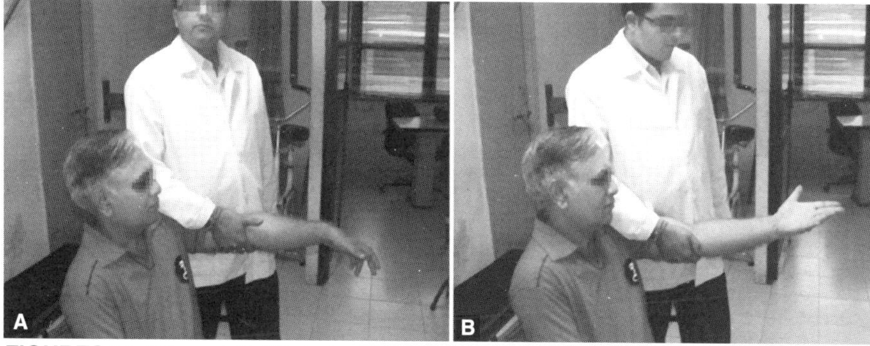

FIGURES 11.47A and B: (A) Active wrist and fingers extension in sitting, left hemiplegia and (B) active supination of forearm with upper extremity in front, left hemiplegia

Patient is then asked to supinate the forearm while the therapist holds the upper limb in external rotation from the shoulder. Patient also concentrates on keeping the palm open.

If the patient is unable to extend the fingers, the grip which is shown in Figure 11.48A is used. Here, the therapist is holding the patient's wrist so that the force of muscular contraction is concentrated on extending the fingers. Therapist may have to flex the wrist initially to use the length tension relationship of long extensors. Similar grip is used for supination of forearm. This movement can be resisted to gain abduction and extension of thumb.

Figure 11.48B shows good extension of fingers actively with the therapist holding patient's forearm in supination. Note the uncontrolled fanning of all the fingers. Patient is instructed to keep fingers in adduction. Note Figure 11.49A given below in which the patient attempts although incompletely to adduct the fingers.

Figure 11.49B shows the use of a rubber band to control fanning of fingers. The band can also be used in extending the fingers as the band would help

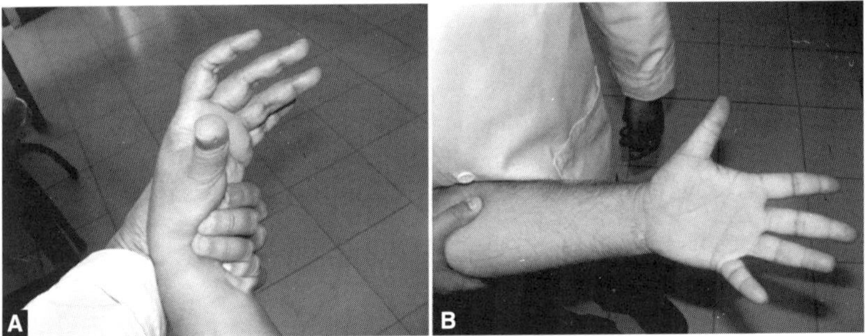

FIGURES 11.48A and B: (A) Grip for opening of fingers and extension abduction of thumb, left hemiplegia and (B) grip for assisted supination for fingers extension, left hemiplegia

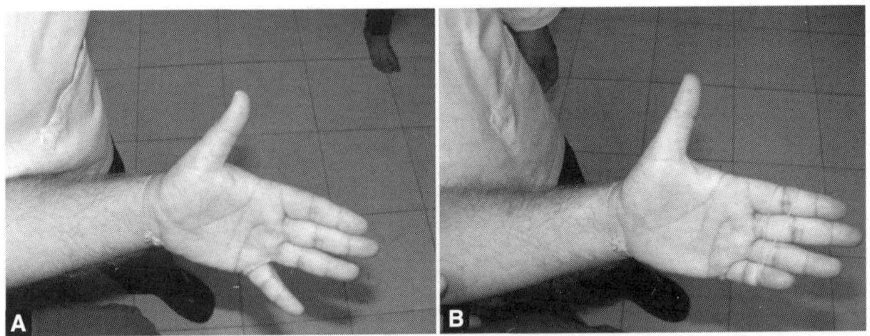

FIGURES 11.49A and B: (A) Active adduction-extension of fingers, left hemiplegia and (B) use of a rubber band in assisting fingers adduction

in uniform movements of all fingers. The band can also be used for giving resistance as and when required.

FOREARM SUPINATION AND ELBOW FLEXION

Patient performs activities of elbow, wrist and fingers with the upper limb in front supported adequately by a firm pillow. Figure 11.50 shows active supination of forearm. For the patient who is unable to carry out the movements themselves, assistance (self or by therapist) can be given in the same position. Resistance to supination movement at later stages can be carried out using the same position.

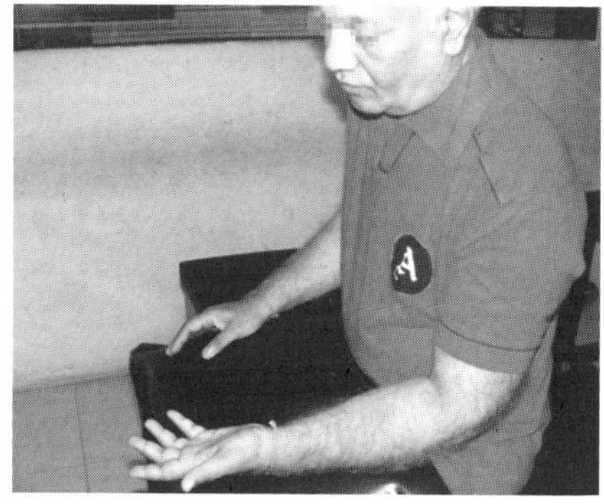

FIGURE 11.50: Active supination supported by a pillow, left hemiplegia

Once the supination of forearm is achieved, the elbow can be selectively flexed keeping the forearm supinated. This movement is useful in functional activities like wiping the face, eating etc. shoulder should be kept in adduction and external rotation to avoid unnecessary and exaggerated movement of the arm. If this position is not achieved and maintained actively, the therapist may assist to keep the arm stabilized by holding lower end of humerus against the chest wall.

Figures 11.51A and B show the abduction and external rotation of shoulder while the patient is attempting hand to mouth activity. The patient may be asked to stabilize the affected arm with sound arm at elbow as shown in Figure 11.52.

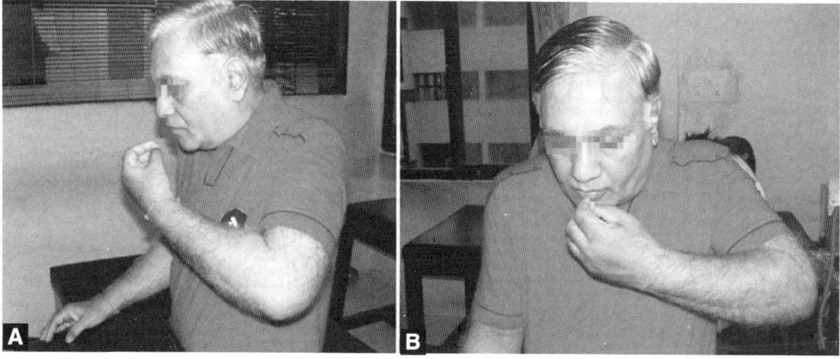

FIGURES 11.51A and B: (A) Hand-to-mouth side view and (B) hand-to-mouth front view, note the position of arm, left hemiplegia

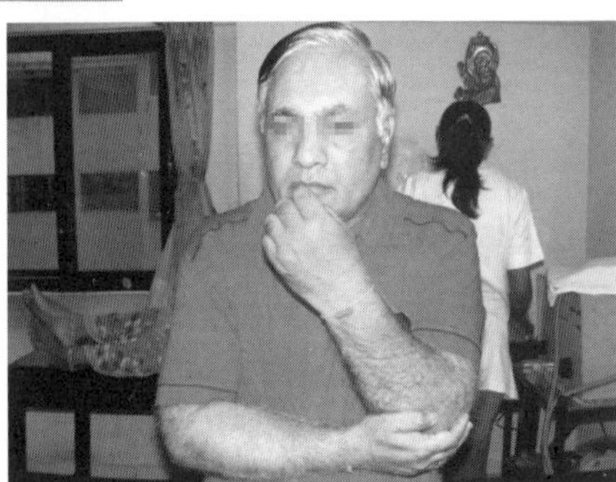

FIGURE 11.52: Self stabilization of arm while performing hand to mouth, left hemiplegia

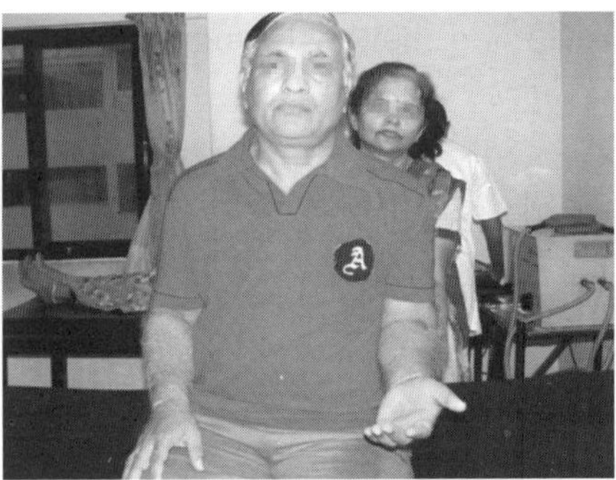

FIGURE 11.53: Active-assisted shoulder external rotation with elbow flexion, left hemiplegia

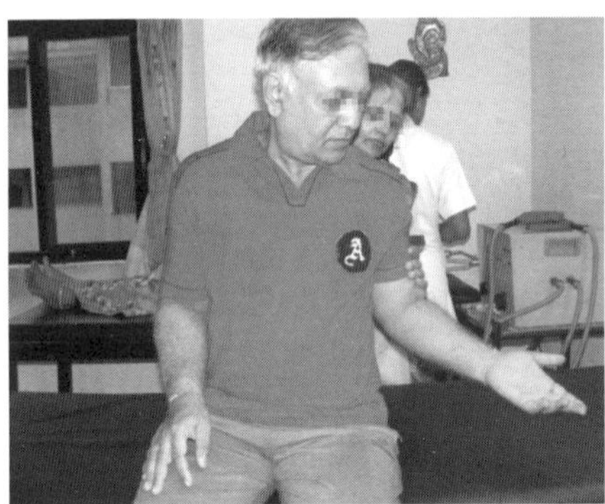

FIGURE 11.54: Active external rotation with minimal assistance

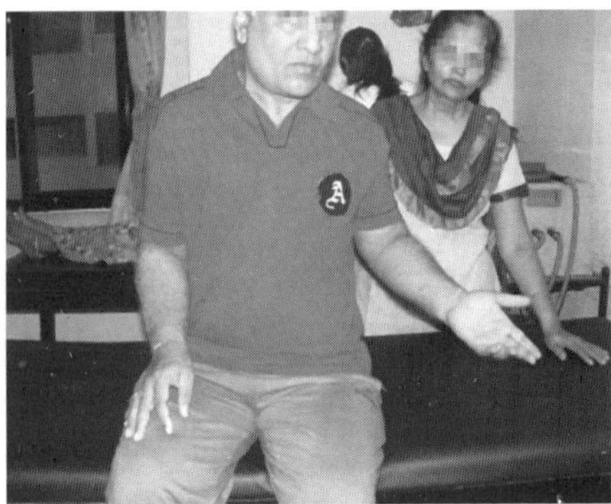

FIGURE 11.55: Active shoulder external rotation

SHOULDER EXTERNAL ROTATION ACTIVITIES

Active external rotation of affected shoulder with adduction along with elbow in flexion in sitting position is practiced as shown in Figure 11.53. The therapist may assist the patient in keeping the arm close to chest wall so that the effort of the patient is concentrated on external rotation of the shoulder only. Later on, this assistance can be taken off and patient can selectively perform the activity of shoulder external rotation with adduction.

Figure 11.54 shows active external rotation movement of shoulder while elbow is flexed and forearm supinated. Note the assistance given from behind the patient. Gradually, assistance is reduced and patient is asked to maintain the position. Note the Figure 11.55.

USE OF ELASTIC BAND IN APPLYING RESISTANCE

As soon as possible, resistance to all possible movements can be given by a use of elastic band. Initially, very light resistance can be given. Though

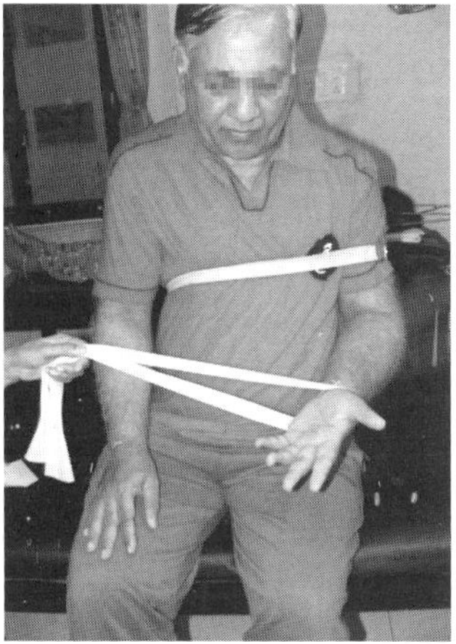

FIGURE 11.56: Resisted external rotation using elastic band

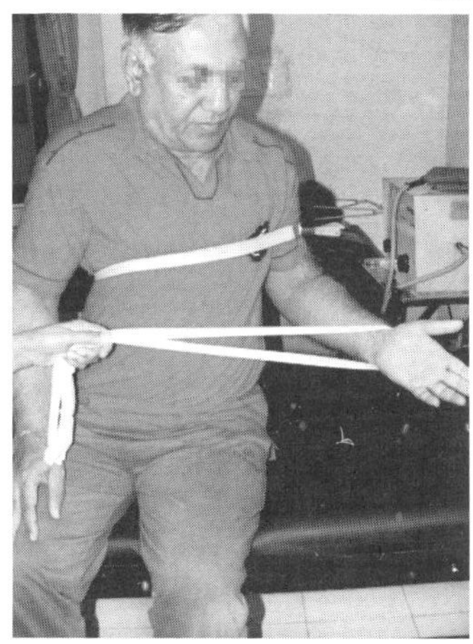

FIGURE 11.57: End position of external rotation of shoulder

manual resistance given by the therapist is the best form of resistance, the use of elastic band gives the liberty of using resistance by patient at home too. Note the stabilizer band attached to patient's affected arm in Figure 11.56. Patient attempts pulling the elastic band in direction of external rotation of shoulder, while the assistant holds the elastic band firmly in opposite direction to the direction of motion at 90 degrees. Figure 11.57 shows the end position of the activity.

Similarly, movements of elbow flexion and extension can also be resisted using the elastic band. If hypertonia results post activity, caution is advised. *See* Figure 11.58.

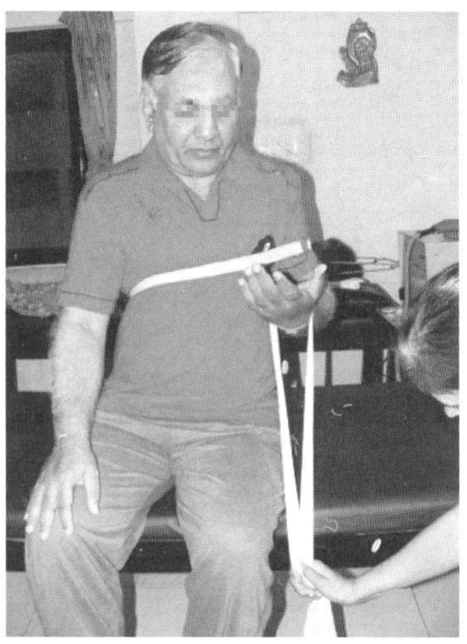

FIGURE 11.58: Resisted elbow flexion using elastic band, left hemiplegia

USE OF A BALL IN APPLYING RESISTANCE

A slightly deflated ball can be very useful in applying resistance to desired movements. Many purposeful movement combinations and activities and can be designed for individual use. Some of the activities are described here.

Figure 11.59 shows the use of ball in resisted activity of shoulder adduction while the therapist maintains the arm in external rotation and forearm supinated. The patient is asked to press the ball against the lateral chest wall and hold that position for as long as he can.

Ball can be pressed between both hands which will also improve proprioception along with strength of muscles. Care must be taken not to allow synergistic activity to take over. Adequate guiding may be required at some instance for maintaining the quality of movement.

By pressing the ball between the hands and with pressure over the root of the affected palm (Figure 11.60), there is an elicitation of wrist and fingers extension. Figure 11.61 shows the extension of the fingers with pressing the ball. Note the assistance given by the therapist at the level of the wrist to guide the movement in a right direction. Patient's affected side is left.

Ball can be pressed in different directions for gaining various results. The hands may completely mold the ball for hand functions to improve. Assistance from the therapist in moulding can be given initially till the patient achieves it himself (Figure 11.62).

Figures 11.63A and B show a different position in bearing the weight on root of the palm with use of a ball. Here, the patient uses serratus anterior with elbow in few degrees of flexion in applying the pressure while the therapist directs the force in a proper way.

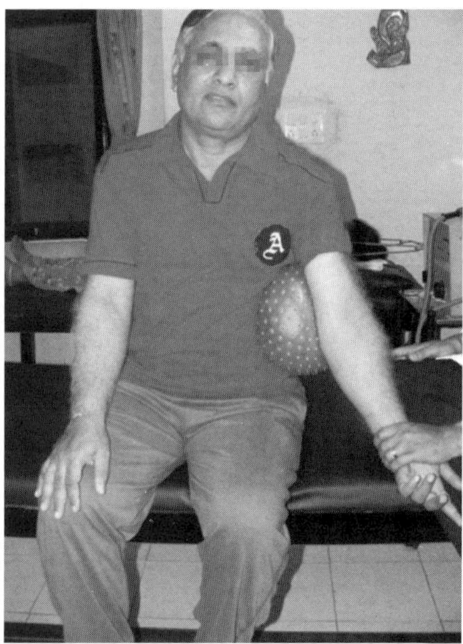

FIGURE 11.59: Resisted shoulder adduction using a ball, left hemiplegia

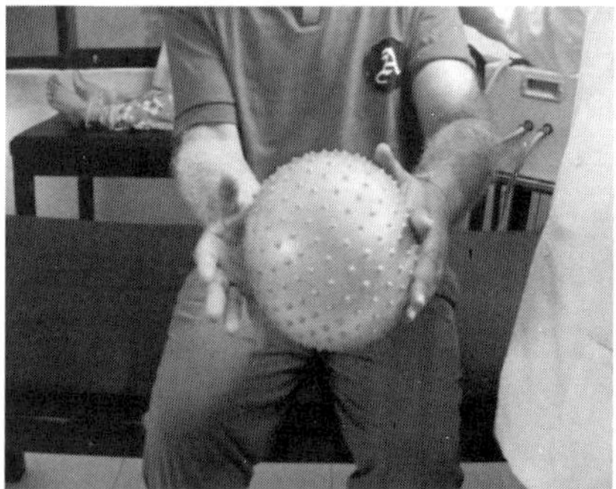

FIGURE 11.60: Ball pressing with both hands, left hemiplegia

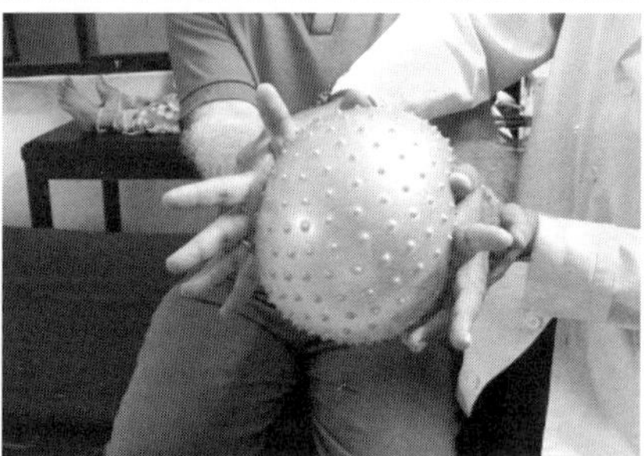

FIGURE 11.61: Assisted ball pressing with the root of palm for facilitation of wrist extension, left hemiplegia

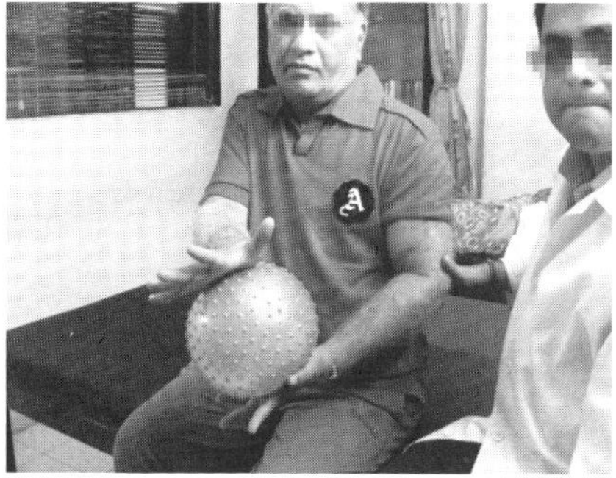

FIGURE 11.62: Ball pressing with affected forearm in supination, left hemiplegia

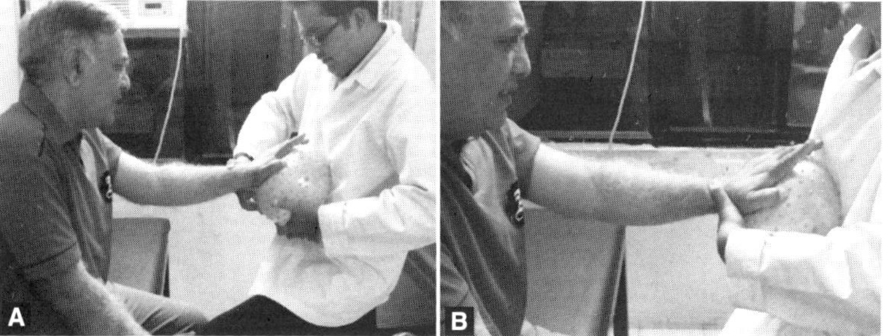

FIGURES 11.63A and B: Ball pressing in front, left hemiplegia

USE OF STRETCH REFLEX

Use of stretch reflex in finger and wrist extension can be used as shown in Figures 11.64A and B. A quick movement of flexion of wrist and fingers is done and the patient is asked to extend them immediately. The same grip, as shown in Figures 11.64A and B, is used to resist the movement of wrist and fingers extension.

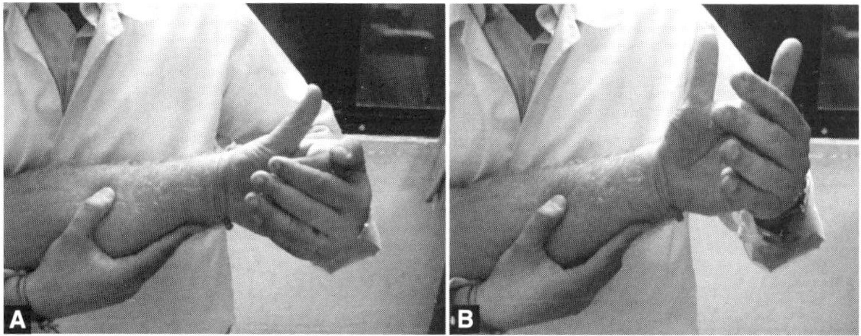

FIGURES 11.64A and B: Stretch reflex for fingers extension, left hemiplegia

USE OF BILATERAL UPPER LIMB ACTIVITIES

To train the affected upper limb, the use of sound limb is very useful because all the movements of sound side can influence the affected side. Hence, the training for the affected side is started by moving the sound limb first. The patient registers this movement in the brain and then mirrors it to the affected side. In this method, lot of visual and auditory cueing is used by the patient as well as by the therapist. Patient is taken in sitting position with both the upper limbs in front of the body and in line of the vision. Activities of forearm, elbow, wrist and fingers can be readily done in this position. Figures 11.65A and B show the sequence of forearm supination and pronation training. Guidance by the therapist can be given, as and when required.

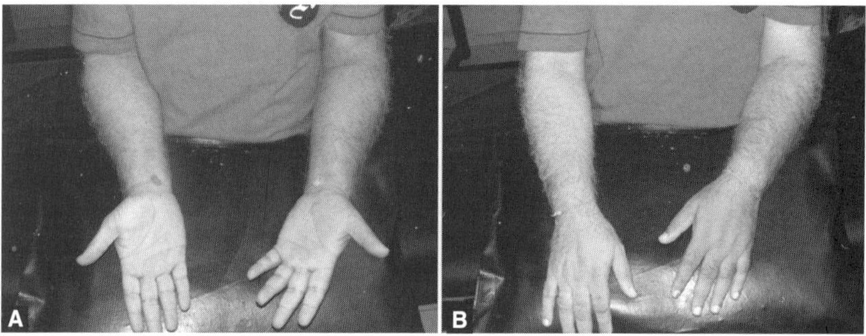

FIGURES 11.65A and B: Bilateral symmetrical pattern of pronation and supination, left hemiplegia

Bilaterally asymmetrical pattern of activities can be started when the patient has mastered the symmetrical patterns. Figures 11.66A and B show the pattern of pronation and supination, asymmetrical in both the forearms.

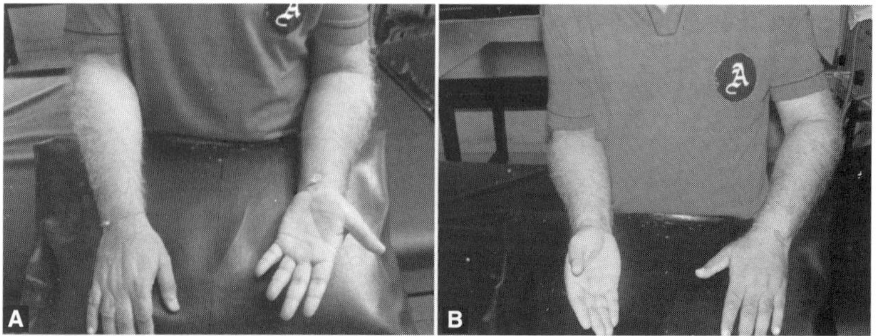

FIGURES 11.66A and B: Bilateral asymmetrical pattern of pronation and supination

Note the sight abduction and internal rotation of affected left shoulder while attempting pronation of forearm.

MOVING THE HAND

Modification and progression of the very famous 'clasp hand' activity is shown in Figures 11.67A and B. Both the hands are kept in a 'namaskar' position as shown in Figure 11.67A. This position reduces the flexor tone of the long flexor muscles. After optimum reduction of the tone is achieved, wrist extension with the fingers kept in extension, is practiced. A rubber band can be attached to all the fingers to keep them together and aid in finger motion. *See* Figure 11.68.

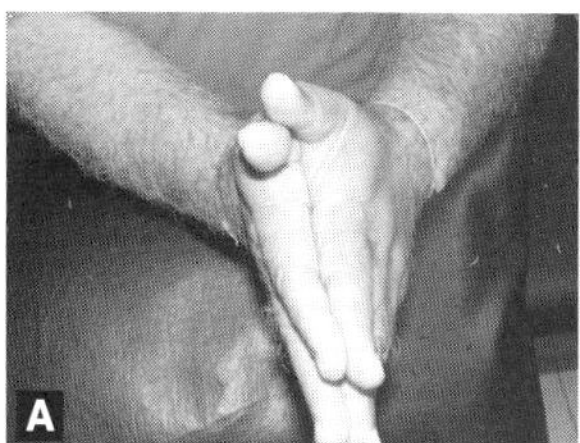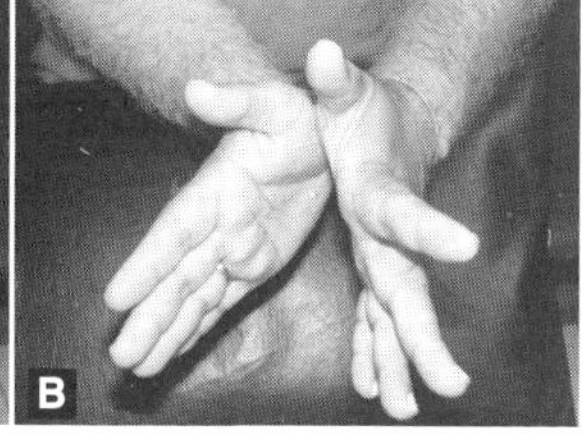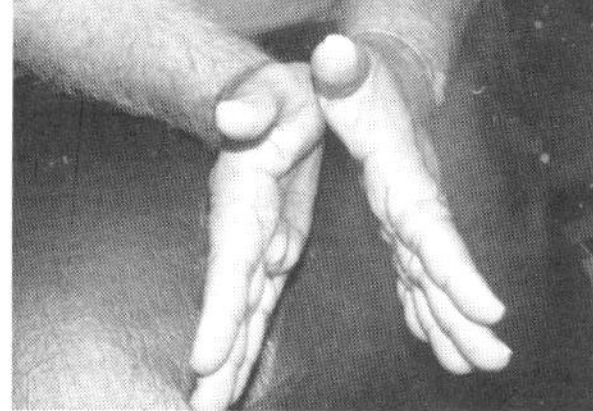

FIGURES 11.67A and B: Bilateral wrist and fingers extension, left hemiplegia

FIGURE 11.68: Use of a rubber band to prevent abduction of fingers, left hemiplegia

Extension and abduction of thumb is practiced in the position explained above.

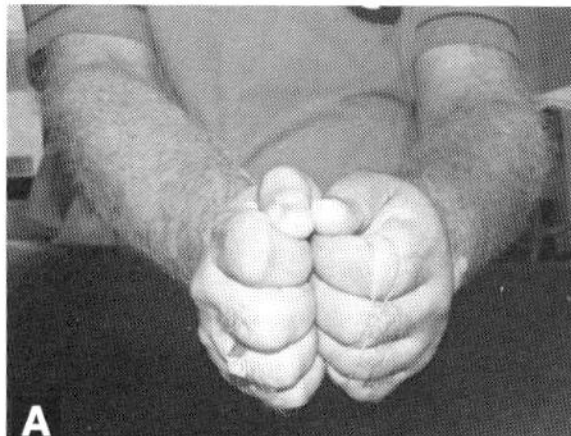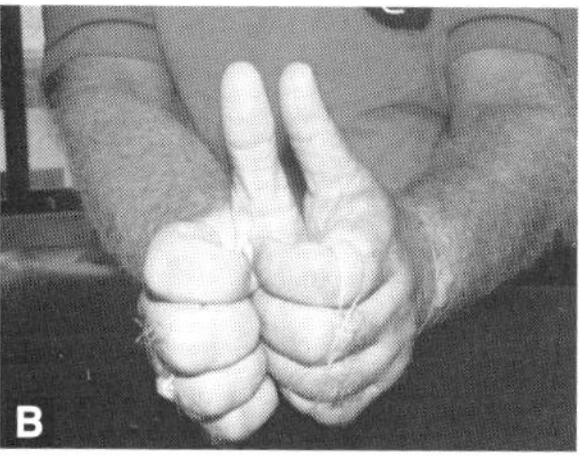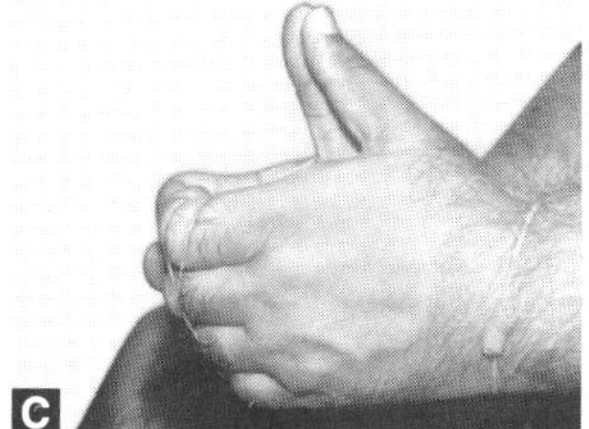

FIGURES 11.69A to C: Bilateral abduction and extension of thumb with fingers flexed; note the use of rubber band for fingers, left hemiplegia

Note Figures 11.69A to C, in which the patient attempts bilateral extension and abduction of thumb with the fingers held in flexion. The use of a rubber band can be useful as explained before. Assistance from the sound thumb can be done by the patient if active movements are inadequate in same position. Use of brushing, icing, myofacial release and other techniques can be used for activation of abductor pollicis longus and extensor pollicis longus and brevis.

Practice of fingers extension and flexion can be performed after stabilizing the wrist and forearm with sound hand as shown in Figures 11.70A and B.

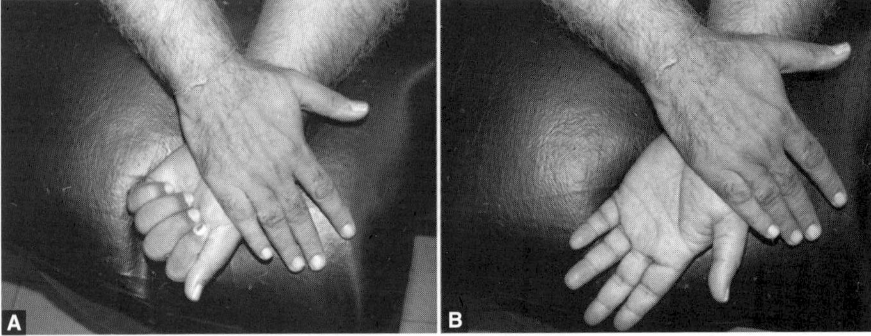

FIGURES 11.70A and B: Active extension of fingers with forearm supinated by sound limb, left hemiplegia

By fixing lower end of radioulnar joint in supination, the patient attempts flexion of fingers very gradually and gently. The patient opens up fingers as far as possible, and the position is held as long as possible. Initially, assistance from the therapist may be required in opening up the fingers. A conical-shaped object can be placed in patient's palm with the narrow portion held towards the ulnar side and the broad portion towards the radial side. Use of the cone is helpful in eliciting finger extension.

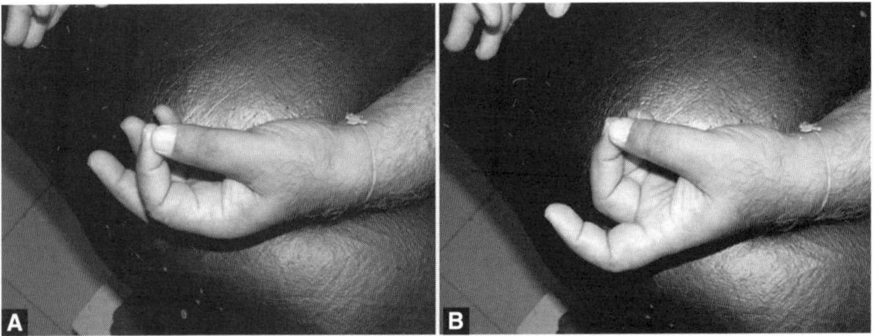

FIGURES 11.71A and B: (A) Thumb to index finger; (B) thumb to middle finger

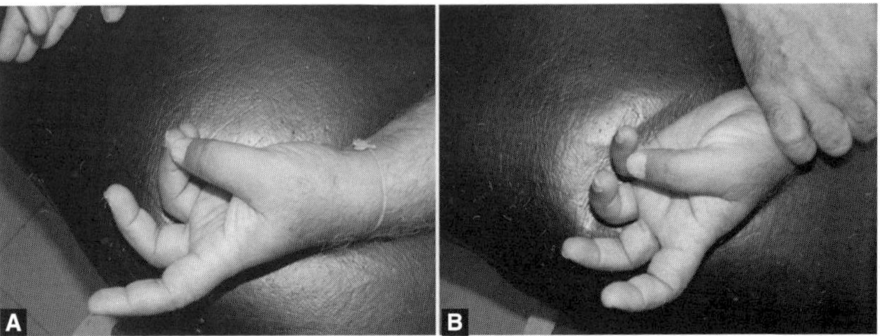

FIGURES 11.72A and B: (A) Thumb to ring finger and (B) thumb to little finger

As shown in Figures 11.71 and 11.72, approximation of tip of the thumb to tip of all the fingers is first practiced with assistance. As the dexterity of the movement improves, assistance can be gradually decreased and active movements are encouraged.

ACTIVITIES ON VESTIBULAR BALL

Anticipatory postural adjustments can be challenged by having the patient perform voluntary movement that have a destabilizing effect. For example, the therapist can utilize static-dynamic activities of PNF chopping or lifting patterns or cone stacking activities. Dynamic surfaces like the wobble board, foam wedge and vestibular ball can be used for the dynamic surface balance training. Once initial control is achieved, the patient is ready to practice more dynamic balance activities. The therapist should have the patient explore his or her limits of stability (LOS) through low-frequency sway. Thus, the patient learns how far in any one direction he or she can move, while typically maintaining upright stability. Patients with hemiplegia typically demonstrate reduced voluntary sway with more weight being directed on the sound side than on the affected side. The therapist will, therefore, need to stress symmetrical postures, as well as, activities that overcompensate, shifting the weight more on to the affected extremities. Gentle perturbations can be used to displace the patient's center of mass (COM) and stimulate postural adjustments. The therapists can also have the patient sit or stand on a movable support surface, thereby stimulating adjustments through displacement of the base of support (BOS). For example, a gymnastic ball or equilibrium board can be used. The patient learns to actively control posture while the device is moved, or while the patient actively moves the device.

A vestibular ball of optimum size is selected so that the patient's hip and knee flexed at around 90 degree and both the soles of feet touch the ground comfortably. Ball is slightly deflated to increase the friction of the ball to the surface and thus, ensuring a slightly larger base of support. A suitable floor mat is used to prevent skidding. Preferably the patient should sit on the ball facing a mirror for visual bio feedback. At first, the patient is made to sit on the ball as a part of orientation program. Adequate support may be required initially to decrease the fear of falling off the ball. Once the fear is reduced, assessment of the balance can be done in a correct manner. Usually, sitting steadily on the ball with equal weight-bearing on both the sides requires assistance from the therapist. The therapist may kneel on either side or behind the patient. Assisted weight shift in different directions can be started once the patient stabilizes on the ball.

Figure 11.73 shows correct position of sitting on the ball.

Figures 11.74A and B shows posterior shifting of weight assisted by the therapist. Figure 11.74A shows the therapist assisting from behind. This position is easier for the patient as he feels more secure. Figure 11.74B shows the therapist holding the patient from distal end of femur which can be used as a progression of the activity stated before. In either of the case, strong contraction of abdominal is required to maintain the balance. To workout obliques of abdominals, diagonal patterns of activity are used i.e, shifting of the weight posteriorly and to the right or left and anteriorly in either directions. Note Figures 11.75A and B.

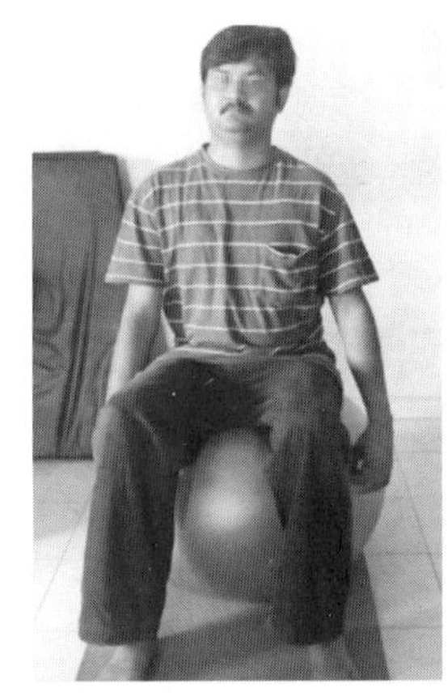

FIGURE 11.73: Orientation in sitting on a ball, left hemiplegia

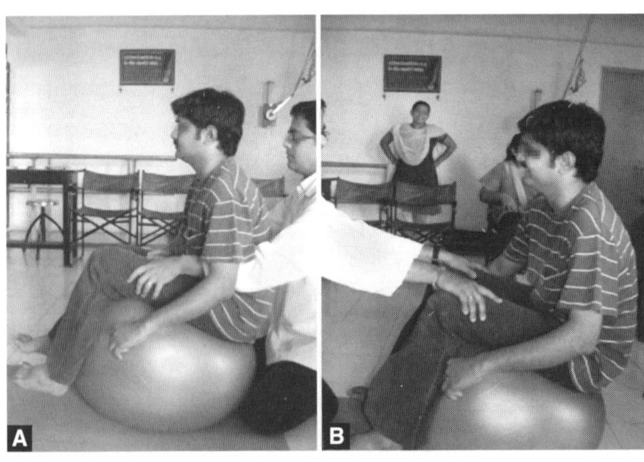

FIGURES 11.74A and B: (A) Posterior weight shifts on ball, assistance from behind left hemiplegia, (B) posterior weight shifts on ball, assistance from front, left hemiplegia

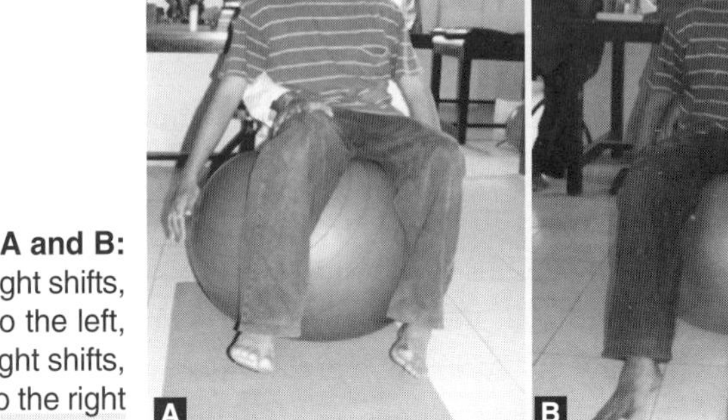

FIGURES 11.75A and B: (A) Diagonal weight shifts, posteriorly and to the left, (B) diagonal weight shifts, posteriorly and to the right

As the patient gets used to these positions, active movements in either directions with the feet on the mat can be started.

Figure 11.76 shows active shifting on sound side. Patient's affected side is left.

All these activities can also be resisted from pelvis by the therapist. Initially, unidirectional movement can be resisted, i.e., forward and backward shifting and lateral shifting to the right and to the left. Resistance to the diagonal movements can be used as a progression.

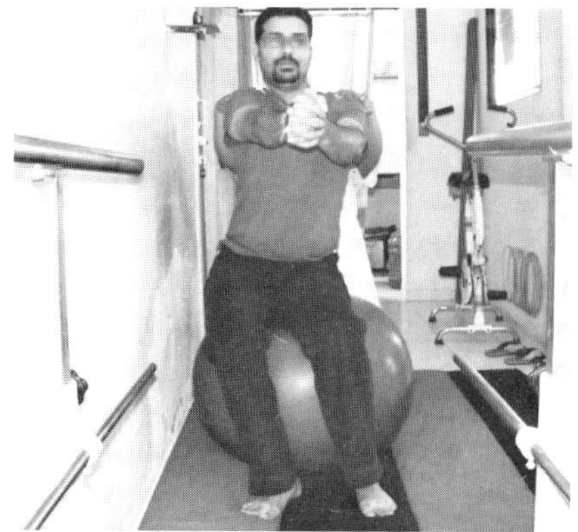

FIGURE 11.76: Lateral pelvic shifts on ball, left hemiplegia

Figures 11.77A and B show the resisted workouts for forward and backward shifting.

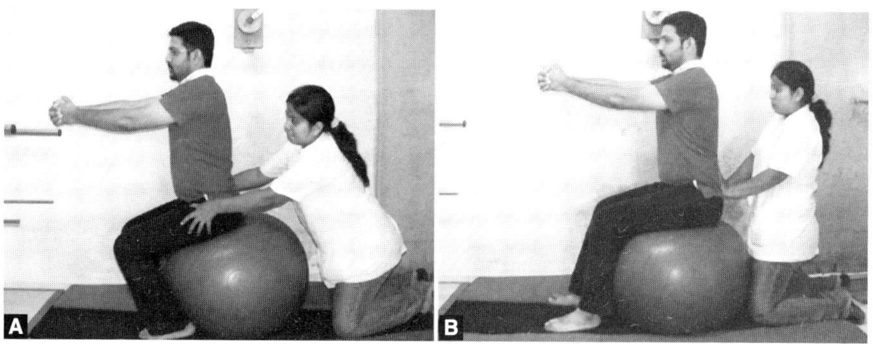

FIGURES 11.77A and B: (A) Resisted forward shift, and (B) resisted backward shift

The patient is asked to clasp both the hands and bring them in front of the body to stabilize the thorax (Figure 11.78A). Gradually, the patient is asked to lift the sound leg up in the air as shown in Figure 11.78B and maintain the balance. Then, affected leg is lifted up actively in a similar fashion and balance is maintained as shown in Figure 11.78C.

As the patient achieves the maintenance of posture with single leg on the ground, the leg can be crossed over on the other leg and reaching out can be practiced in various directions to improve dynamic postural control and overall proprioception (Figure 11.79).

Figures 11.80A and B show the affected lower limb (left) crossed over on the sound lower limb. Once the posture is maintained, reaching out with affected upper limb can be started in anti-synergistic postures.

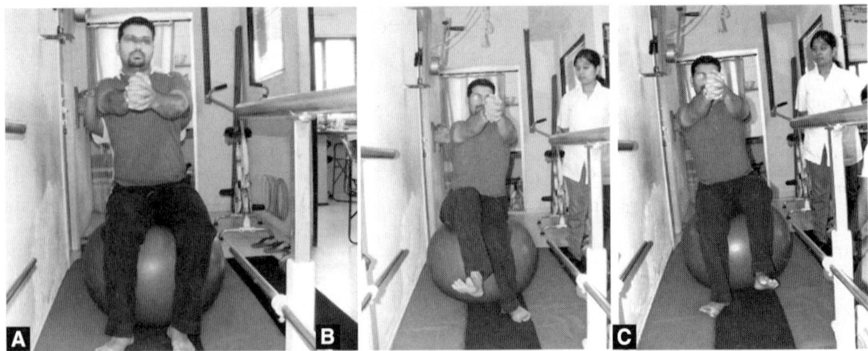

FIGURES 11.78A to C: (A) Maintaining balance with clasp hands, (B) raising sound limb up, left hemiplegia, and (C) raising affected limb up, left hemiplegia

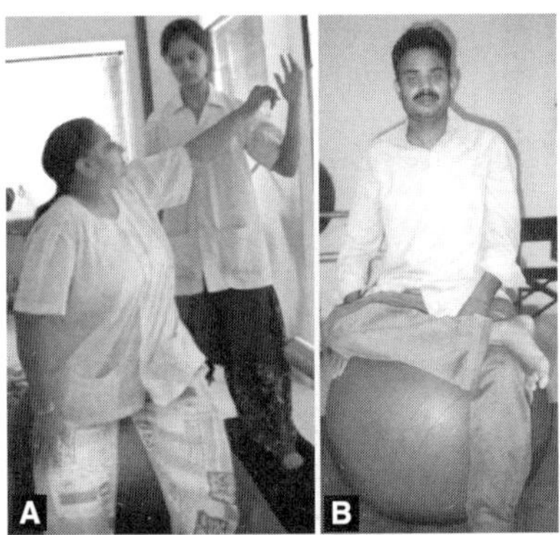

FIGURES 11.79A and B: (A) Reachouts with affected upper extremity, left hemiplegia, and (B) balancing with legs crossed

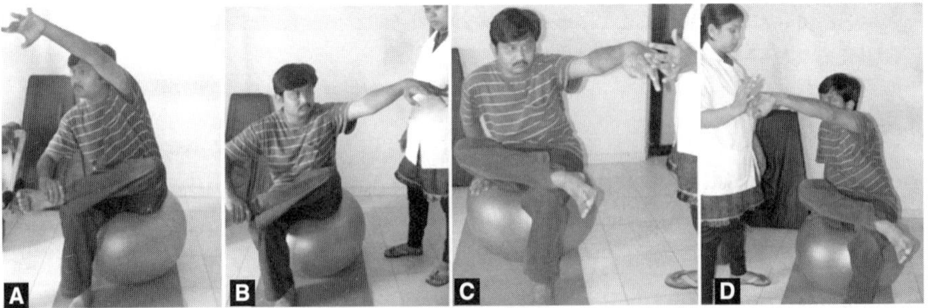

FIGURES 11.80A to D: (A and B) Affected leg crossed over sound leg, reach outs with affected upper extremity, left hemiplegia and (C and D) sound leg crossed over affected leg, reach outs with affected upper extremity, left hemiplegia

Figures 11.80C and D show crossing over of sound lower limb (right) on the affected side. In either case, the reaching out can be done by both the hands clasped together, if active control of the affected upper limb is insufficient to complete the movement.

Sit-to-stand transitions should be practiced, with an emphasis on symmetrical weight-bearing on both the lower limbs and controlled responses of the hemiplegic side as shown in Figure 11.81. Trunk rotation can be increased by having the patient stand up and shift the pelvis to one side or the other before sitting down. Arms should be clasped and held straight ahead during this activity. A vestibular ball can be used in variety of ways; the patient can sit on the ball and carry out hand functions as shown in the Figure below. Dynamic postural control can be maintained effectively, while the patient can perform other functional tasks.

See Figure 11.82; here, the patient has put the affected right upper extremity in reflex inhibiting posture supported by a table in front while sitting on a ball. As a part of progression in balance training, the patient is taken in a crossed leg position on a vestibular ball as shown in Figure 11.83.

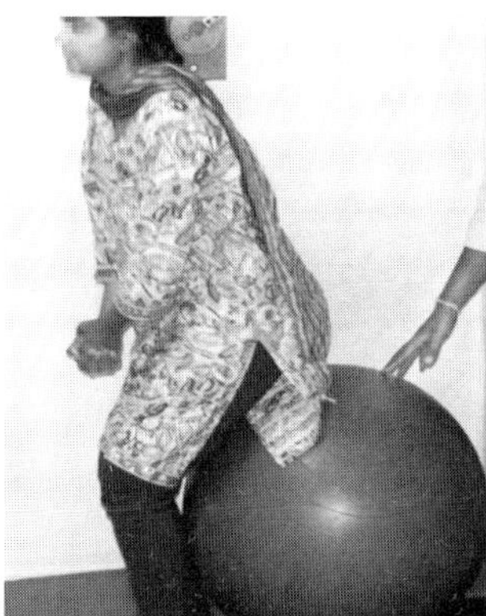

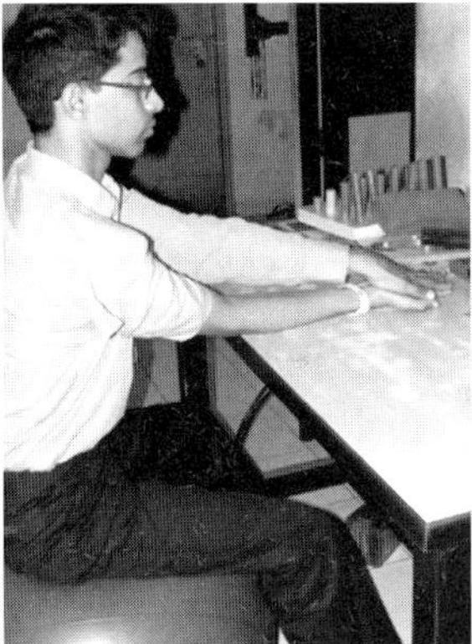

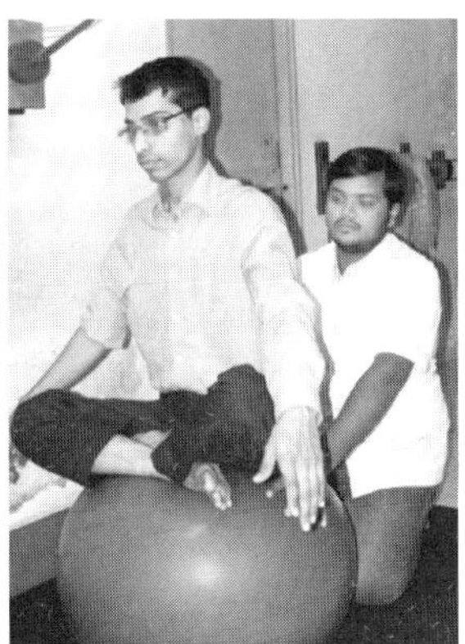

FIGURE 11.81: Sitting to standing

FIGURE 11.82: Affected upper extremity held in reflex inhibiting posture while sitting on a vestibular ball, right hemiplegia

FIGURE 11.83: Crossed leg sitting on a ball, supported, right hemiplegia

For sitting crossed leg on the ball, the patient is given adequate support from behind and asked to relax upper limbs as much as possible. After this position is maintained for sometime, gentle movements in forward and backward directions are started. The therapist holds the patient's pelvis and assists in the movement while the patient maintains the upright position. Strong contraction of trunk muscles is required to maintain the posture on the ball. Diagonal patterns can later be added as shown in Figures 11.84A and B. Backward and to the right, backwards and to the left, forwards and to the right and forwards and to the left are the diagonal patterns which can be incorporated in the list of activities. Note the reactions of both upper limbs in these Figures.

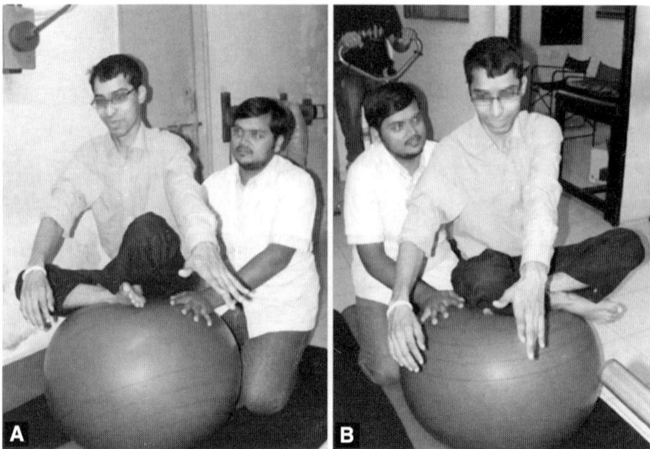

FIGURES 11.84A and B: Diagonal patterns while sitting cross-legged on the ball, right hemiplegia

Patient's affected side is right and movements of both the upper limbs counteract the movement of the trunk to maintain the center of gravity.

While sitting on the ball, affected side upper limb activities in PNF patterns can be started as shown in the Figure given below. The pattern of flexion, abduction and external rotation can be trained and later on can be resisted as shown in Figures 11.85A to C and Figures 11.86A and B. Adequate guiding from the therapist may be required at distal or proximal level to ensure quality of the movements.

The pattern of extension, abduction and external rotation is shown in Figures 11.86A and B.

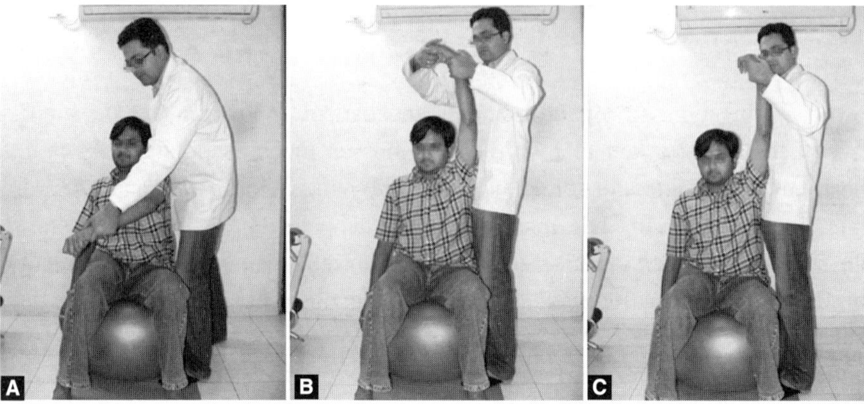

FIGURES 11.85A to C: PNF patterns on vestibular ball, flexion-abduction-ER, left hemiplegia

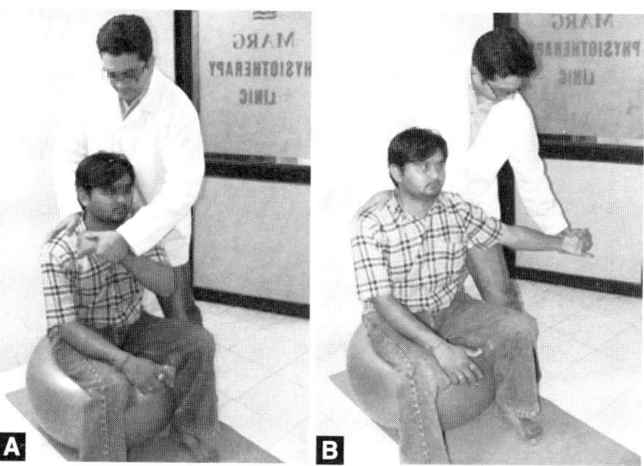

FIGURES 11.86A and B: Extension-abduction ER pattern, left hemiplegia

The patient can carry out ball catching and throwing activities while seated on the ball which trains dynamic postural control and aids in dynamic postural stabilization. Please note Figures 11.87A and B.

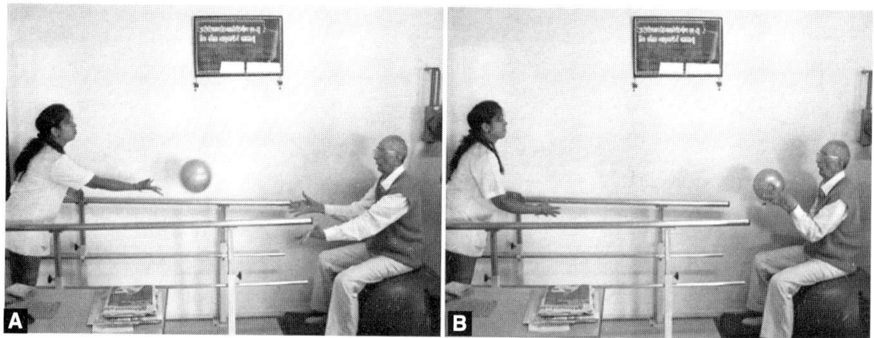

FIGURES 11.87A and B: Ball catching while on vestibular ball, left sensory stroke

■ Supine on ball

The patient can be taken supine on the ball with adequate support. The patient is first made to sit on the ball and is asked to take steps forward one by one gradually, while still maintaining contact with the ball till the patient's upper back rests on the ball as shown in Figure 11.88A. Adequate support is required so as to prevent the patient sliding off the ball. The patient is then asked to maintain the pelvic position in upward direction and assistance may be given by the therapist if the patient is unable to hold this position. For further workout of stabilizer of the thorax, both the upper limbs of the patient are flexed up to 90 degrees from shoulder. Side to side movements of the upper trunk can be carried out, while keeping the feet firmly on the ground to strengthen the rotator of the trunk and training the advanced balance reactions (Figure 11.88B). As a progression to this activity, one by one, lower

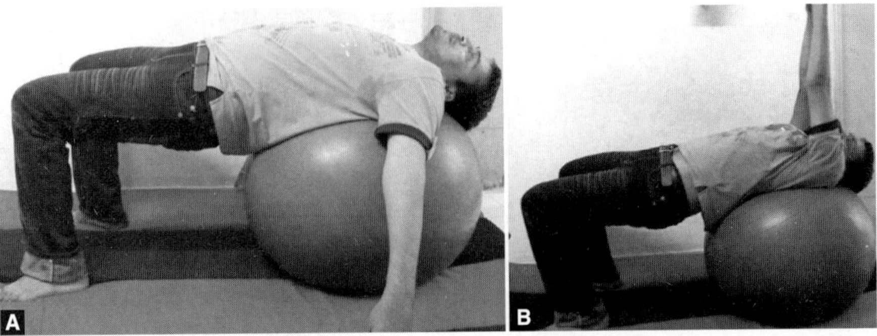

FIGURES 11.88A and B: (A) Supine on a ball, raising the trunk, left hemiplegia and (B) supine on a ball, raising the trunk, raising the upper limbs, left hemiplegia

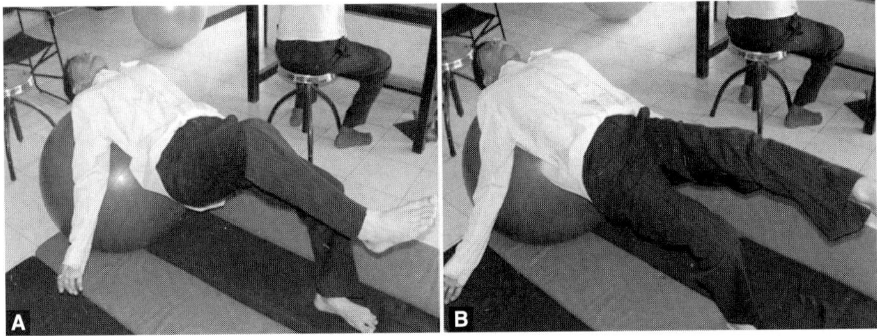

FIGURES 11.89A and B: (A) Unilateral bridging on sound limb while supine on ball, right hemiplegia and (B) unilateral bridging on affected side while supine on ball

limbs can be raised up in the air thus maintaining the entire weight only on a single lower limb (Figure 11.89).

■ Turning on Ball

Practicing quarter and full turns can be taught to a well-recovering patient as shown in Figures 11.90A to D. The patient is helped to turn to either side by using both the upper limbs as lever. While half turning, both the feet are kept firmly on the ground. Weight is taken on the lateral aspect of the trunk and the patient is asked to breathe in and out normally but slowly.

During the practice of three-fourth turns on right side, the patient flexes his right lower limb as shown in the Figure 11.90D. The left lower limb crosses over to the right side. Both the upper limbs can be clasped together or can also be kept separate but in line as shown. Gradually, the patient pivots the weight on the lateral aspect and then to the anterolateral aspect of the right trunk. The patient can also be taken prone on the ball by extending the above mentioned procedure till both the hands of the patient rest on the mat. All these activities require enormous amount of skill and control for

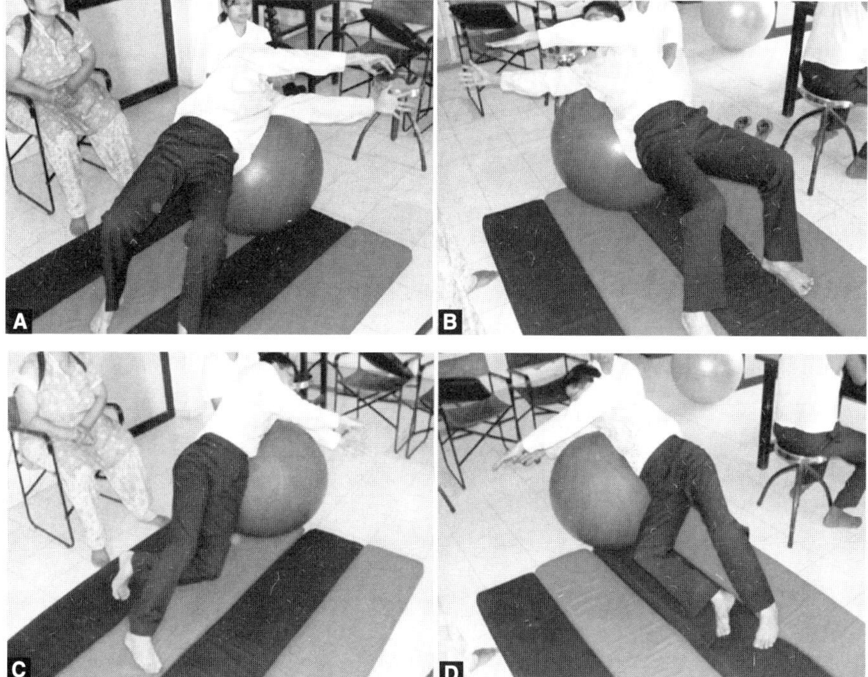

FIGURES 11.90A to D: (A) Half turn to the sound side, left hemiplegia, (B) half turn to the affected side, (C) three fourth turn to the sound side, (D) three fourth turn to the affected side

the patient. Till then, the therapist supports the patient full and gradually decreases the support as and when required. Increased effort and lack of dynamic balance reactions increase muscle tone of the patient and hence, if any increase in tone is noticed after completion of the exercises, these may be discontinued or effort on the part of the patient is reduced by proper assistance by the therapist.

■ Prone on Ball

In the kneeling position with the ball in front, the patient places both the upper limbs on the ball with elbow kept in extension (Figures 11.91A and B). If due to spasticity, this position cannot be maintained individually, than the patient can clasp hands and can keep them on the ball. While keeping the trunk in side flexion, the patient is asked to move the ball forwards as much as possible. The ball can be moved sideways to the left and right, also maintaining the forward position by contraction of abdominal muscles. The patient then can be taken prone on the ball with weight on extended upper limbs. Weight shift to one side and onto the single upper limb and wheel barrow are the activities which can be performed while prone on ball.

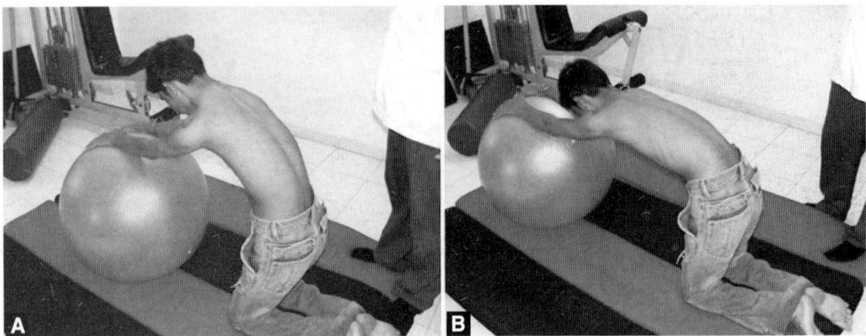

FIGURES 11.91A and B: Training flexion of trunk in kneeling position with the use of a ball

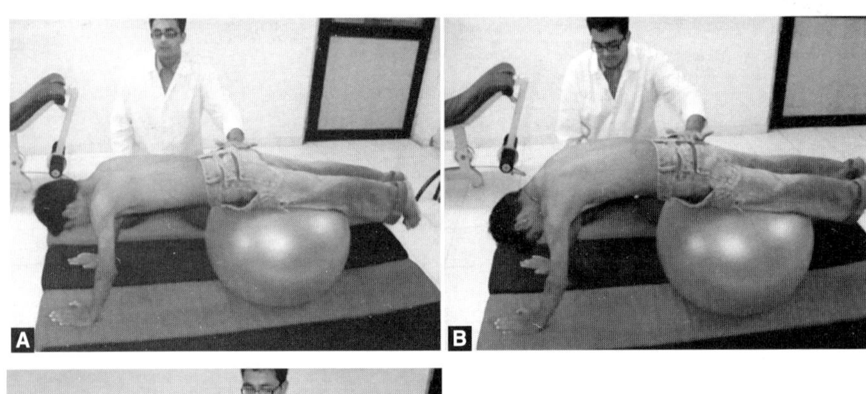

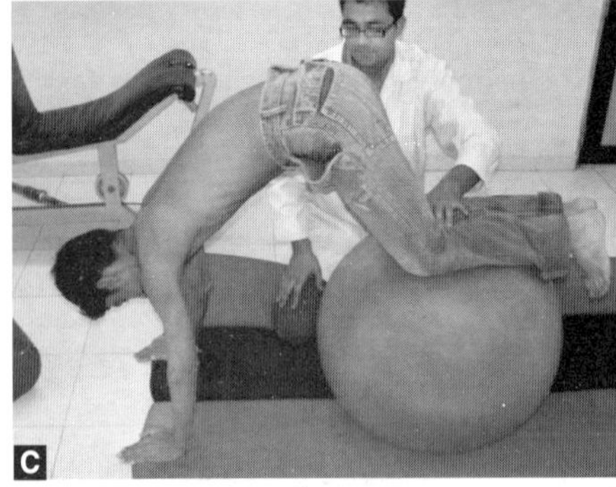

FIGURES 11.92A to C: (A) Prone on ball with weight-bearing on hands, (B) raising the trunk, abdominal muscle activation, (C) flexing the trunk fully, weight on knees and hands

From prone position on the ball, patient can slide forward on the ball till the thighs rests on the ball (Figures 11.92A and B). By flexing the trunk, weight can be shifted to the knees which are also flexed and now are resting on the ball (Figure 11.92C). This activity is a total flexion pattern activity on the trunk with complete weight-bearing on the upper limbs while shoulders are flexed.

Bilateral hip and knee flexion can be attempted with the ball placed under both knees. This activity trains lower abdominal muscles, hip flexors and knee flexors and counteracts the extensor thrust response. After flexing both the

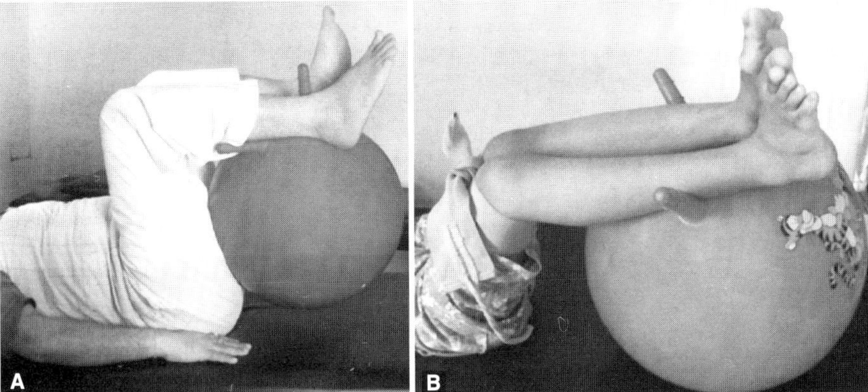

FIGURES 11.93A and B: (A) Bilateral hip knee flexion in lying position using a ball, (B) trunk rotation using a ball, note a band tied at thighs to prevent uncontrolled abduction of hips

lower limbs and taking the ball off the couch, rotation to the left and to the right can also be practiced (Figure 11.93A). If during initial stage, the patient is unable to keep the knees together, a strap tied to both the thighs will prevent falling off the limbs apart in abduction (Figure 11.93B).

FOOT MOVEMENTS

Sitting position can also be used in training movements of foot, toes and as a prerequisite of weight-bearing on affected lower limb in standing. Figure 11.94 shows activation of peronei muscles using quick ice. Application of the ice to the lateral aspect of the leg elicits the contractions of peronei muscles.

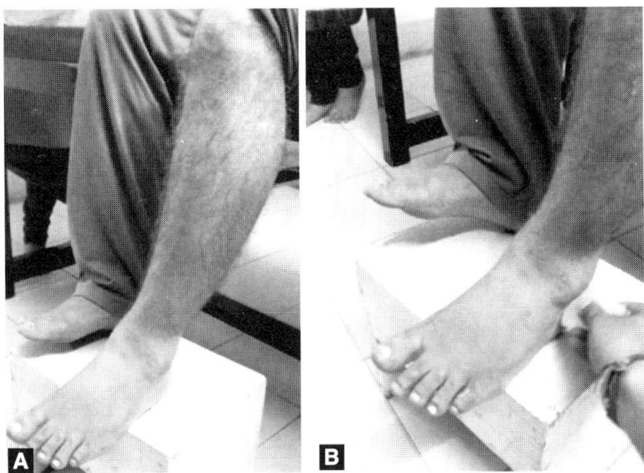

FIGURES 11.94 A and B: (A) Attempting active dorsiflexion with eversion, left hemiplegia, (B) attempting the movement after application of ice

Usually, the therapist holds one ice cube and briskly strokes the lateral side of the leg from fibula head to little toe, two to three times. During stroking, the patient is asked to dorsiflex and evert the affected ankle. Movement can be performed on unaffected side also to facilitate the movement on the affected side further.

ACTIVITIES ON MAT

Mat is the best suitable for variety of activities as it is safer for the patient. Activities like rolling, going to prone position and kneeling are best done on the mat. Patient is taken on the mat and rolling is practiced on both the sides. The patient is then taken to sitting position.

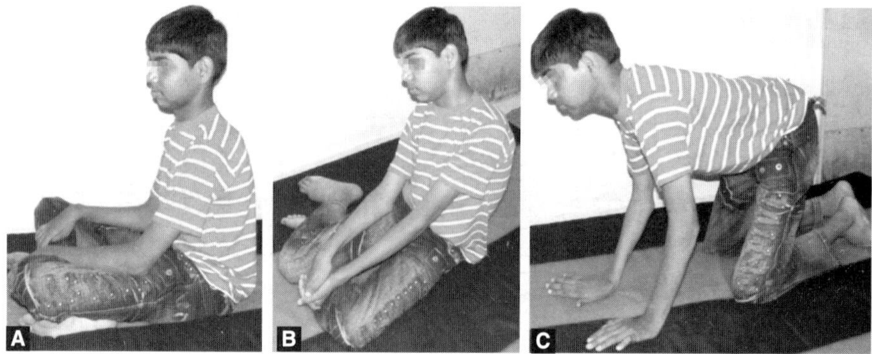

FIGURES 11.95A to C: Sequence of sitting-side sitting-prone kneeling, right hemiplegia

Side sitting with the support of the upper limbs is practiced. Side sitting is the starting position for prone kneeling (Figure 11.95). The therapist first holds the patient from the pelvis with both hands and the hands of the patient may hold the therapist for support. The therapist then pivots the pelvis so that the patient takes the weight on the knees. The hands are then are extended and put on the mat where the weight is taken on palm of hands while the elbows are extended. This is prone kneeling (Figure 11.95C). Variety of activities of reach outs and weight shifts can be performed in this position. Arms and legs can be raised alternatively and weight shifts are practiced.

From the prone kneeling position, one leg is taken in front for the half kneeling. The half kneeling can be practiced with taking both the legs in front one-by-one. Reach outs can be practiced as a progression. Half kneeling is a prerequisite for standing and if the patient has to go down to the floor or has to get up from the floor, the sequence would be: sitting—side sitting—prone kneeling—kneeling—half-kneeling—standing, and reverse (Figures 11.96A to E).

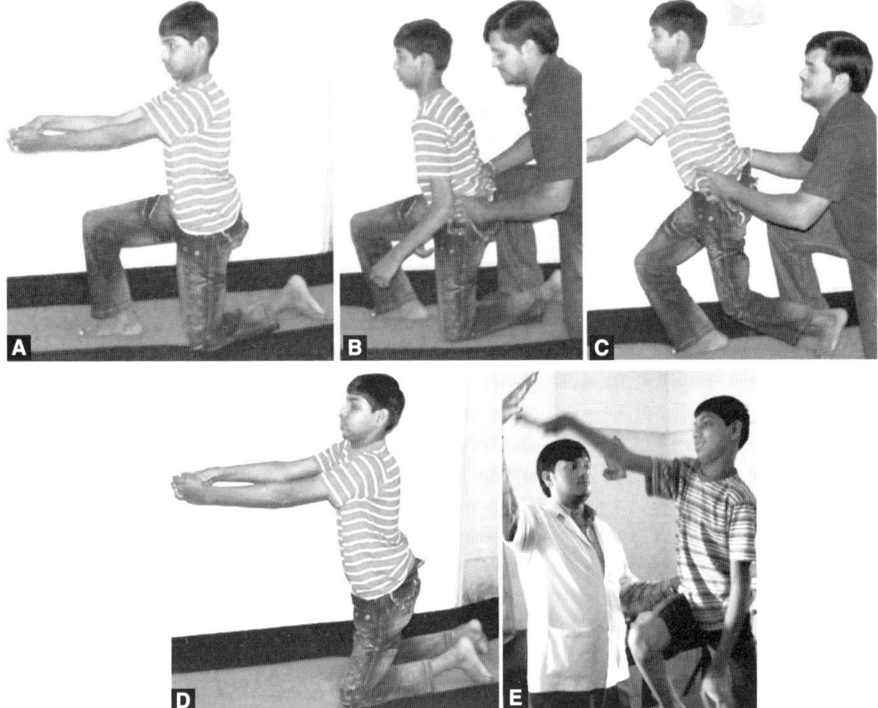

FIGURES 11.96A to E: (A to C) Sequence of half kneeling, half standing—standing, (D) kneel walking, and (E) reachout in kneeling, right hemiplegia

Activities in Prone Kneeling

Various activities which can be carried out in prone kneeling are shown in Figures 11.97 to 11.99.

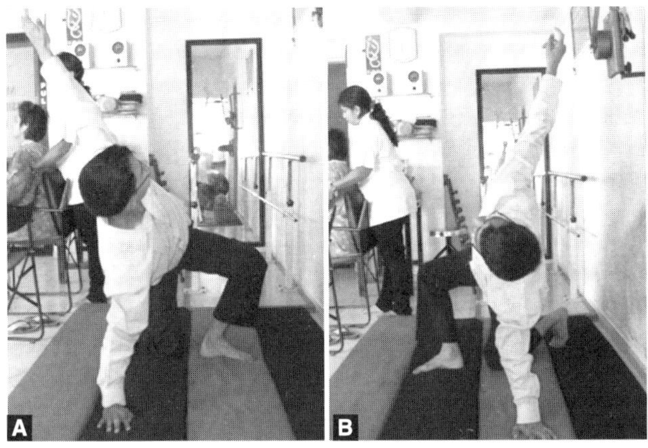

FIGURES 11.97A and B: (A) Unilateral prone kneeling with weight on affected upper extremity, right hemiplegia, and (B) unilateral prone kneeling with weight on unaffected upper extremity, right hemiplegia

From prone kneeling position, the patient can take the weight on the affected side (right in this case) while the sound upper limb is taken up by carrying out horizontal abduction at shoulder and trunk rotation to the left side. The sound lower limb is kept in external rotation at hip and flexion at knee while putting the foot on the ground as shown in Figure 11.97A. Similar position can be attempted on the other side also.

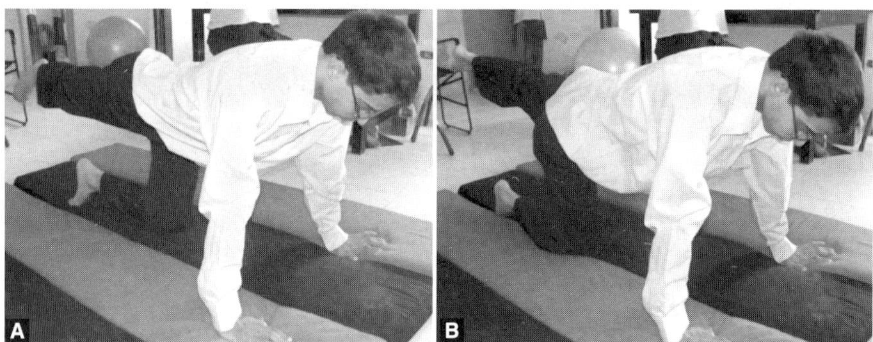

FIGURES 11.98A and B: (A) Prone kneeling with right lower extremity extension, right hemiplegia, (B) prone kneeling with left lower extremity extension, right hemiplegia

In prone kneeling position, the patient can attempt unilateral backward extension of the lower limb one by one while maintaining posterior pelvic tilt. Care is taken not to force the leg abruptly into extension. While one leg is in extension, the opposite side upper limb can also be lifted up one by one on each side as shown in Figures 11.99A and B.

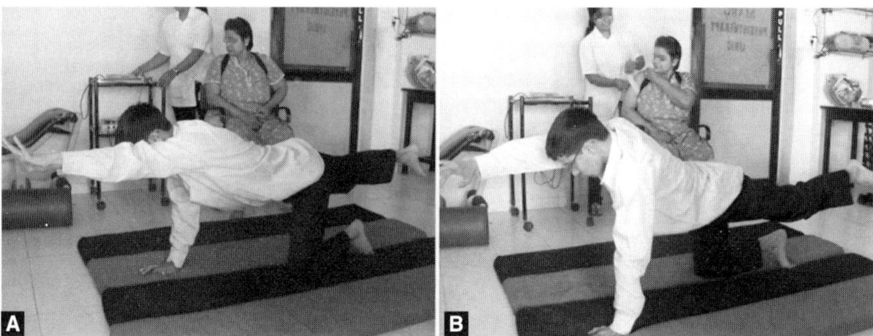

FIGURES 11.99A and B: Contralateral upper and lower extremity movements in prone kneeling

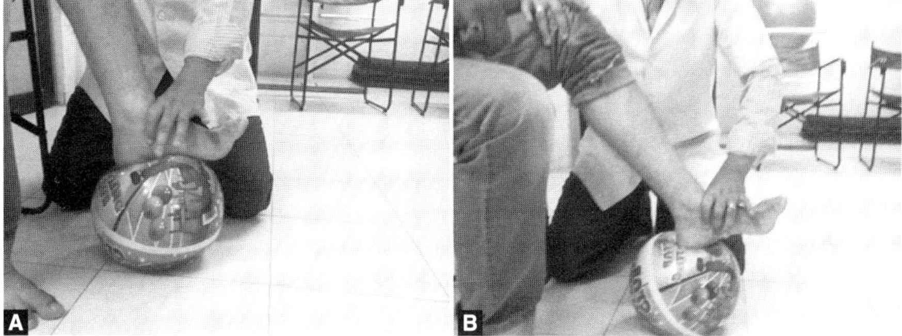

FIGURES 11.100A and B: Facilitation of ankle dorsiflexion with the use of a ball

TRAINING FOR DORSIFLEXION OF FOOT

Training for dorsiflexion in initial stages is easier with the knee in flexion. A pattern of hip flexion with knee flexion in sitting elicits reflex activity of ankle dorsiflexors. However, this activity is a mass pattern and may not be useful functionally. For the functional use as in walking, dorsiflexion of ankle is necessary with knee extension for heel strike. Thus, gradually a combination of activity which uses controlled extension of knee and dorsiflexion of ankle is used. Affected foot of the patient is placed on 4 inches high ball while the patient is seated on the chair. The patient is asked to extend the knee while the ball is slided forward by the foot, taking the weight on the heel. As the patient takes the weight on the heel, dorsiflexion of ankle is elicited. The therapist may resist this forward movement by placing the hand near distal end of tibia. *Note* Figures 11.100A and B.

SPECIFIC ACTIVITIES FOR PATIENTS WITH SENSORY INVOLVEMENT

Patients of stroke with sensory involvement pose a challenge to the treating therapist as all the motor responses are dependent upon the sensory stimulation. Nevertheless, in many patients, the motor movement recovery may be good enough but there may be residual sensory perception involvement. Lack of kinesthetic and proprioception sense require the therapist to stimulate other intact sensory systems of the body like vision and hearing. The following patient has a stroke on the right side of the brain resulting into left sided kinesthetic sense and superficial and deep sensory loss with near normal

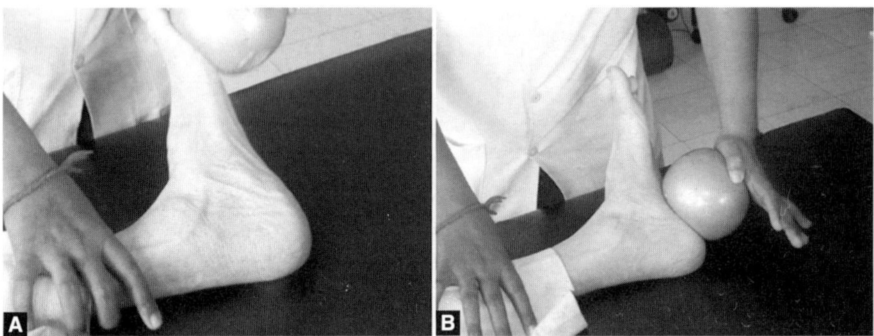

FIGURES 11.101A and B: Deep pressure being applied to the sole of foot using a medicine ball

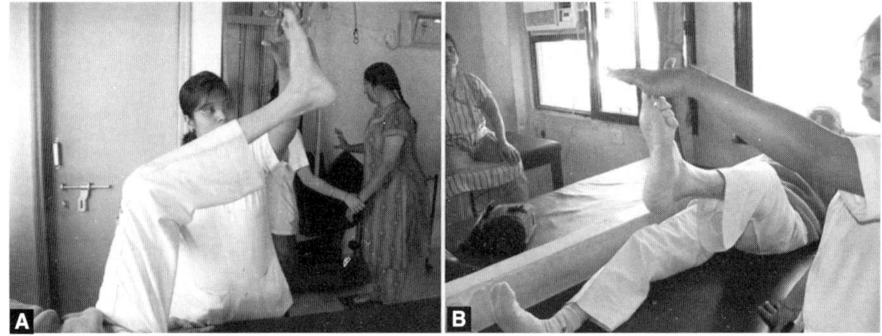

FIGURES 11.102A and B: Multiple angles isometric holds with objective activity, left hemiplegia

motor strength. Deep pressure applied all over the body on the affected side and also to the sound side with a medicine ball and application of vibrations with the hand held vibrator is used, prior to the treatment to improve the awareness (Figure 11.101). All the activities are carried out with the patient looking at the part being treated.

Various angle isometric holds of the limbs will improve the stability of the limbs and will also impart increased postural awareness in space. The therapist can ask the patient to touch a specific mark with the limbs to improve coordination (Figure 11.102).

The therapist asks the patient to touch the tip of finger of the affected side to the tip of therapist's finger to improve coordination and awareness in space. The therapist can then ask the patient to give a clap at various angles to train controlled rapid movements of upper limb. These activities are playful and hence, patients can get training without any stress of performing.

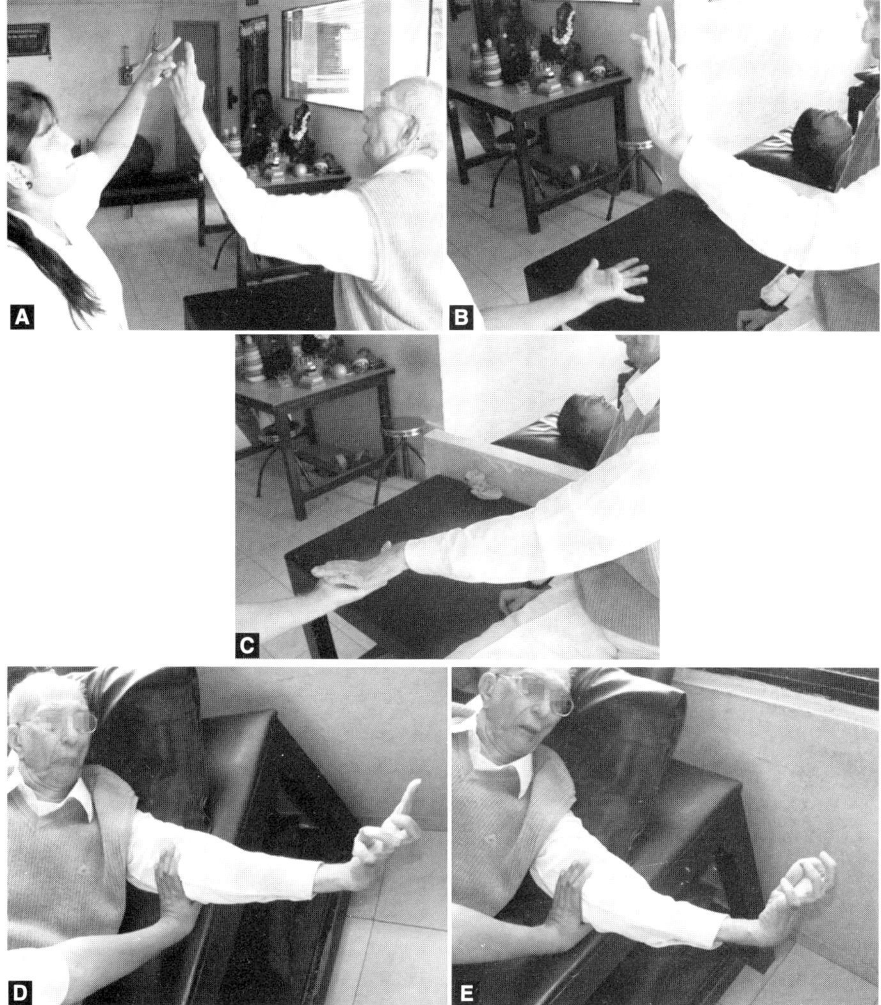

FIGURES 11.103A to E: (A) Finger-to-finger touching for coordination, left hemiplegia, (B and C) palm-to-palm (giving a clap), left hemiplegia, (D and E) self thumb to finger in side-lying, left hemiplegia

Activity of the hands like touching the finger tips to the tip of the thumb can be done with the patient looking at the hand and fingers which are moving. Note Figures 11.103D and E in which, while the patient is attempting the finger activities, the wrist remains in flexion due to dystonic posture of the affected upper extremity. A verbal cue to keep the wrist extended usually counteracts this problem.

Use of both the upper limbs is advocated in training of simple tasks as the movement of the sound side facilitates the contraction of the involved

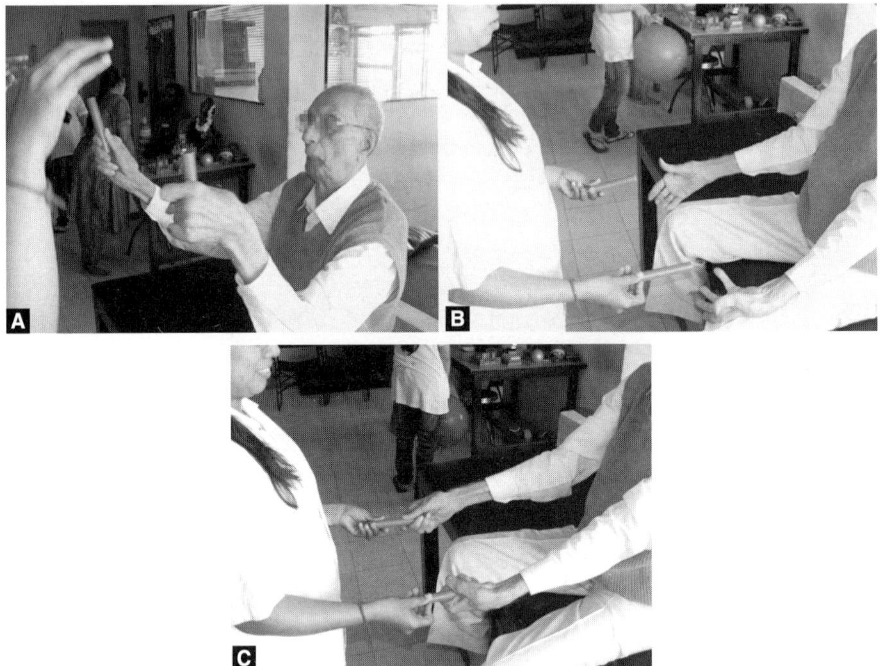

FIGURES 11.104A to C: Holding objects bilaterally at various angles, left hemiplegia

side. Figures 11.104A to C show the holding of simple objects with both the hands at various angles of upper extremity. Note that the left side is the affected side in this case. Also note that the patient constantly looks at the task at hand.

■ Coordination Activities of Upper Extremity

Coordination activities of both upper limbs can be carried out best in sitting position. Please note the series of Figures (Figures 11.105 and 11.106), in which the patient is having left-sided hemiplegia with incoordination and gross sensory involvement. For the same reason, visual feedback becomes highly important. Patient assumes a sitting position and bilateral symmetrical and asymmetrical patterns are used. Also note that postural instability may occur if the lower limbs of the patient are not touching the ground. In such cases, sitting on a chair with back support and with the patient's feet touching the ground becomes a better position. The patient is asked to carry out alternate activity of pronation and supination of forearm and can gently tap the pillow kept in the lap while performing this task. Patient can also perform

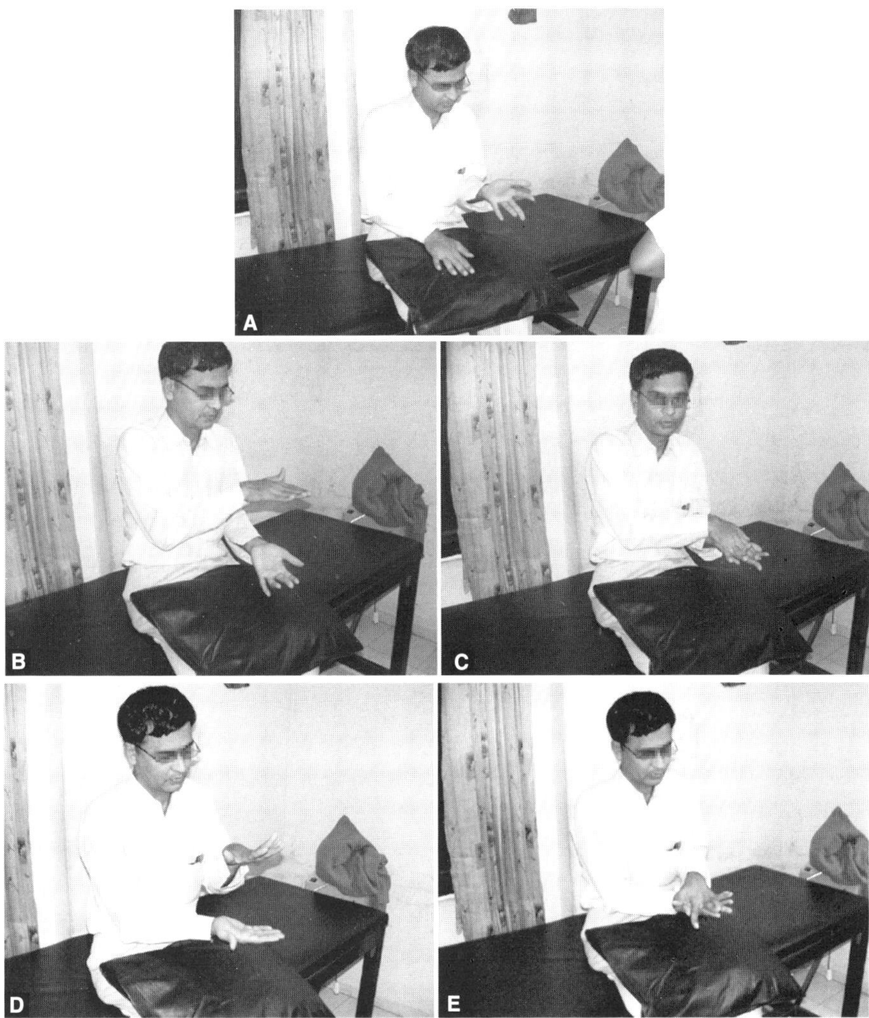

FIGURES 11.105A to E: (A) Alternate pronation and supination, left hemiplegia and (B to E) clapping with alternate hand on top, left hemiplegia

bilaterally symmetrical and asymmetrical activity of pronation and supination of forearms, flexion and extension of elbows, tapping of palmar and dorsal surface of hands, shoulder flexion and extension, etc., in a rhythmic pattern. Use of beats of music can be effectively used in gaining a desired rhythm of activity.

Figures 11.105A to E show controlled clapping in various ways.

Figures 11.106A to D show classic finger to finger and finger to nose activities which can be carried out with eyes opened, progressed to eyes shut.

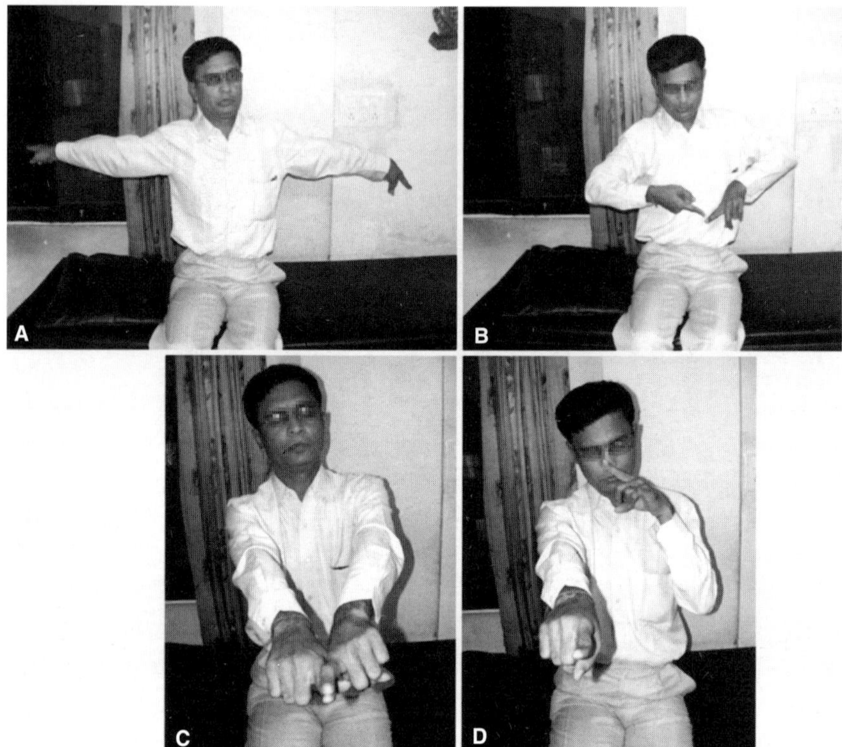

FIGURES 11.106A to D: (A and B) Finger to finger, left hemiplegia, (C and D) finger to nose, with eyes closed, left hemiplegia

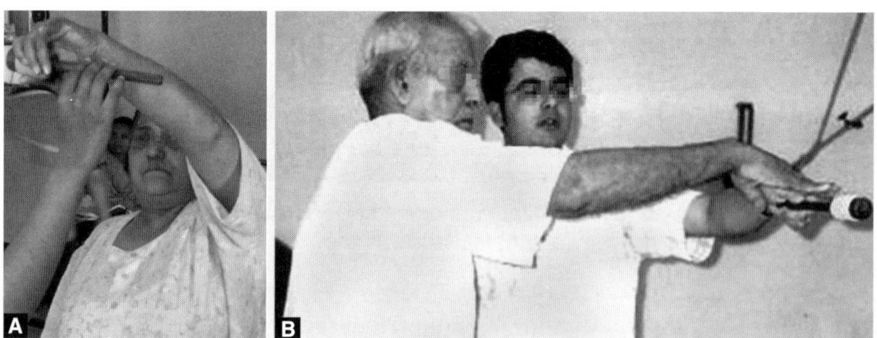

FIGURES 1.107A and B: Object holding at various levels, functional task, left hemiplegia

ACTIVITIES FOR RECOVERING ARM

Progression of activities for upper extremity is carried out as and when indicated. Gradually, goal-oriented activities like reaching out and functional tasks are carried out (Figures 11.107A and B).

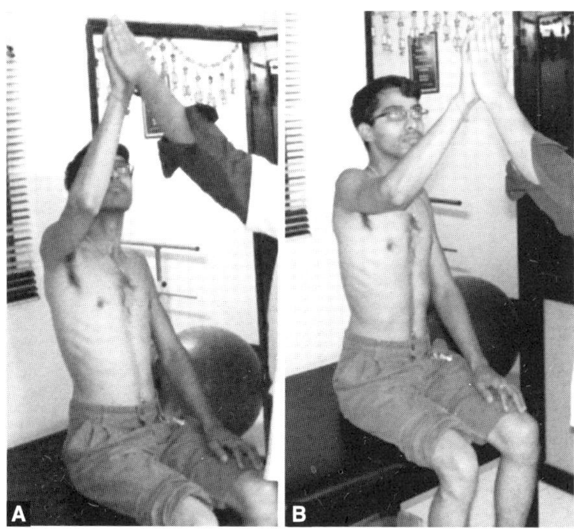

FIGURES 11.108A and B: Mirroring movements of right upper extremity, right hemiplegia

Mirroring of Movements

Figures 11.108A and B show the guiding of the upper limb movements where the patient follows the the palm of the therapist. Initially, the patient may keep the contact of his palm with the palm of the therapist and follow it wherever it is taken. As active movements start developing, patient may no longer touch the therapist's palm but can follow therapist's palm by keeping a few centimeters distance. Patient is asked to keep the distance between the palms fixed throughout the movement. This activity is also useful in training coordination and proprioception. This activity can be done on both the sides also. The therapist challenges the patient by involving many combination of movements which involves multiple joints at various angles. Quality of the contractions is fantastic in the goal-oriented activities. When patient is unable to finish a movement, guiding can be carried out. The guiding is only done for the brain to learn a pattern of activity. Once it is learned, more active movements are carried out. If prototype exercises are not translated to functions, these activities become useless. It is not so that all the prototype exercises are useless, but they have to be stopped when patient is ready to carry out the functional activities independently. The patient may use the help of the sound side in completing the task initially. The ultimate aim of the therapy is to make the patient functional in all the disciplines of their lives.

Functional Activities

Sitting position becomes an ideal platform in carrying out training of various functional activities like grooming, dressing up, hand activities, arranging jigsaw puzzles, stacking the beads and rings, arranging playing cards, putting on

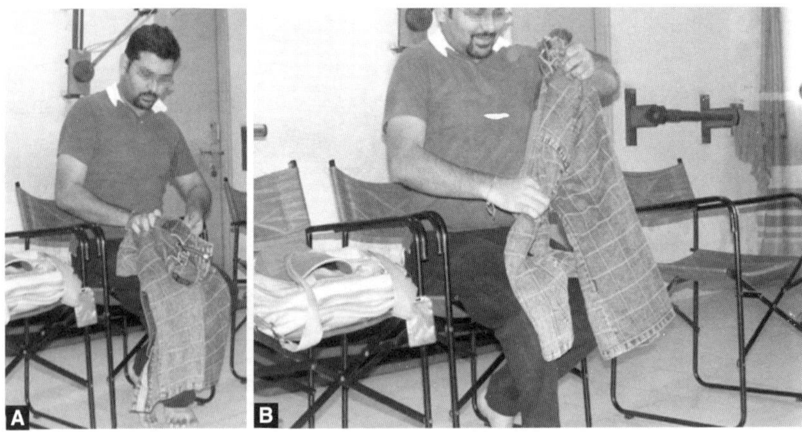

FIGURES 11.109A and B: Arranging clothes, left hemiplegia

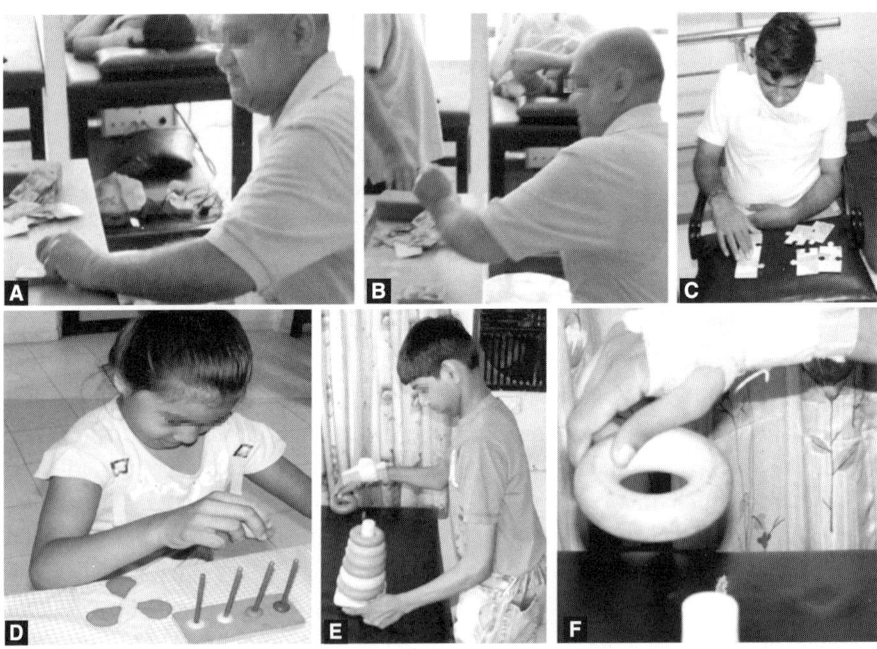

FIGURES 11.110A to F: (A and B) Arranging playing cards, left hemiplegia and (C) arranging jigsaw puzzle with unaffected hand, left hemiplegia, (D) arranging beads in abacus, cerebral diplegia and (E and F) stacking rings, proper grip with the use of splint, left hemiplegia

socks and footwear, reading, watching television and socializing, etc. (Figures 11.109 and 11.110).

Training of hand function should emphasize forearm, wrist, and finger movements which are independent of shoulder and elbow motions. Excessive shoulder adduction and abduction, elbow flexion, pronation of forearm, wrist and finger flexion are typical spastic patterns that must be counteracted. Voluntary release is generally much more difficult to achieve than voluntary grasp, and inhibitory techniques may be necessary before extension movements are successful. Prehension patterns should be practiced and manipulation of common objects attempted. The therapist needs to observe these movements carefully and to assist the patient in eliminating those aspects of performance that interfere with effective control.

Judicious use of a splint may be required in keeping the wrist position in few degrees of extension in carrying out hand functions, till the patient actively maintains the position. Rubber bands may also be useful in maintaining position of fingers, as already described above. It should be noted that active stability achieved by patient's own muscular control is better than passive stabillization achieved by the use of splints.

FUNCTIONAL TRAINING

Functional mobility training, begun during the acute phase, should be continued and extended. Prone walking on upper limbs while patient is on a appropriately sized vestibular ball will elicit strong contractions in stabilizer muscles of each joint of upper extremities on both sides. Consider the Figure 11.111, the patient is encouraged to keep the pelvis posteriorly tilted by strong contractions of abdominal muscles, this position trains proprioception of affected uper extremity using the kinematic chain of the upper and middle section of the body, wonderfully. Care must be observed regarding the position of elbow and the wrist. If this position is used before tone of the muscles is optimum, there is a risk of injury to either of the joint. In initial stages, therapist can support the patient's affected elbow and wrist joint manually. A variety of activities and postures can be utilized. Additional postures such as prone on elbows, side sitting, kneeling, and half kneeling can be utilized, although they may not be appropriate for older patients (Figure 11.112). Patients should also be instructed in strategies for getting down to and up from the floor. Therapists need to provide

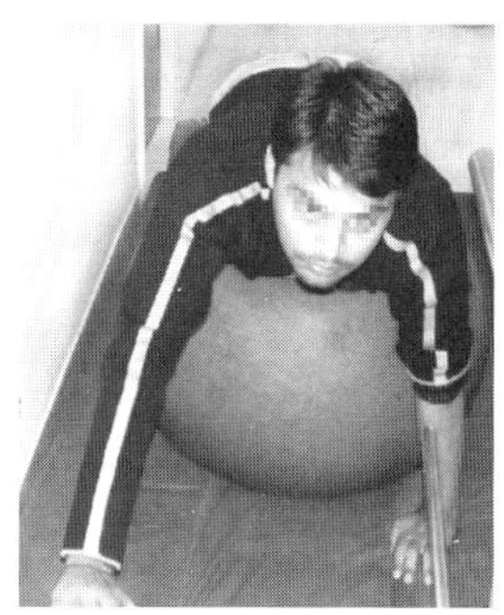

FIGURE 11.111: Prone walking with upper limbs, on a vestibular ball, left hemiplegia

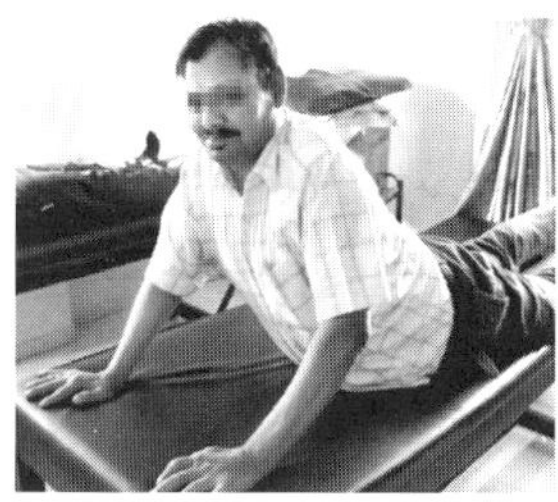

FIGURE 11.112: Prone on extended arms, left hemiplegia

an adequate amount of support, while allowing the patient to relearn, control through active processing of movement. Varying the contexts (changing the environment) is important in ensuring adaptability and generalizability of responses.

Training in activities of daily living is usually directed by the occupational therapist. Continuity between therapies is important to ensure that activities are being done consistently and in the most efficient manner. The reference for all training should be the patient's home environment and normal daily activity. Energy conservation techniques should be incorporated into the patient's daily plan.

Activities in Standing

INTRODUCTION

Correct weight bearing at an early stage provides good afferent stimulation to the brain and is the most effective way of normalizing muscle tone. Preparation for walking can be carried out adequately in an area of one square meter. It is of less benefit to practice walking with a patient who is unable either to take weight on his affected leg or bring it forward in a reasonable normal manner unless these can be facilitated. The same applies to someone who already walks with a poor gait pattern because repetition reinforces the experience of incorrect movement which in time actually contributes to a reduction in ability. It is better to assess the difficulty carefully and practice relevant activities. That is the reason why before walking, activities in standing are aptly practiced and mastered. Till proper weight bearing on the affected lower limb is achieved, patient may not be allowed to walk with an abnormal gait pattern unless absolutely necessary.

TRAINING FROM SITTING TO STANDING

Standing up from High Bed or Plinth

The patient wriggles to the edges of the bed and puts his affected leg to the floor without his foot pushing. If necessary, mobilize his foot by pressing down over the front of his ankle to ensure that his heel is on the ground and that dorsiflexion is possible. The therapist assists the lower limb of the patient from the knee and ensures that the knee joint does not buckle and at the same time, does not snap in hyperextension (Figure 12.1). The therapist can place one hand on

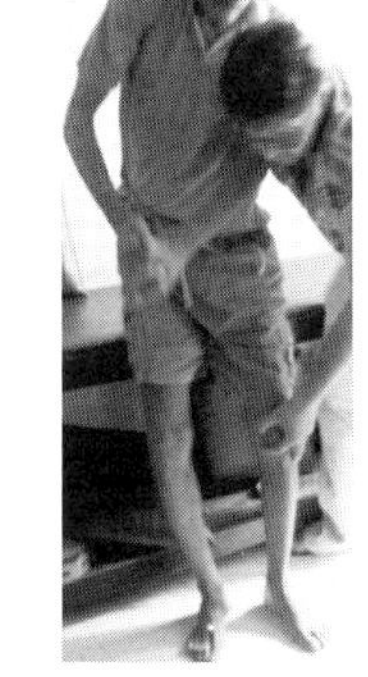

FIGURE 12.1: Sitting to standing from a plinth, with assistance to affected side knee joint, left hemiplegia

the knee as described above and other may encircle the trunk for maintaining trunk alignment as shown in the Figure 12.1. The patient may keep both the hands clasped together to prevent synergistic movements of affected upper extremity. If the patient is unable to fix the affected foot on the ground, it may pose a danger, as it can slide making the patient imbalanced. To prevent this, the therapist can put one of the feet on patient's foot. This activity can be performed many a times so that patient as well as patient's caretakers learn it properly and it can be carried out throughout the day.

Standing from a Chair

Training of standing up in a scientific method from sitting in a chair is taught to the patient, as the correct method reduces the amount of effort by the patient and hence, increases the effectiveness and efficiency. These methods also employ correct muscles in normal patterns of activities and hence, even the functional activity of standing up becomes therapeutic. Under circumstances where a hemiplegic patient is left alone to get up by himself without help or instruction of the therapist, usually, the extensor thrust response of the lower limb as well as the trunk will takeover, making the patient exert the force in the posterior direction. Due to this force production in posterior direction, the patient will move backwards while attempting to get up from sitting. The center of gravity moves posteriorly, out of base of support and hence, there are increased chances for the patient to fall off. Even the chair will move backwards due to force exerted by the knees. To counteract this, first of all, the patient is taught to reduce extensor thrust of trunk. For this while, the patient is seated on a chair, trunk forward bending, with arms hanging down, is taught. Patient's lower limbs are kept firmly on the ground and hip is kept at neutral as far as the rotation is concerned. Figure 12.2A shows the dropping of the affected hip (left) in internal rotation and increased side flexion of the trunk on the hemiplegic side. This is avoided by correct holds by the therapist initially and then by active holds by the patient (Figure 12.2B).

Figure 12.2C shows the correct position of the affected lower limb, left in this case. Trunk of the patient is bent symmetrically and well-forward so that the center of gravity shifts well forwards and in line of the direction of standing. The lower limbs are kept flexed from the knees more than 90 degrees to counteract the quadriceps thrust. The ankles are thus aligned in close chain dorsiflexion as tibia moves forward on the talus in this starting position. Once the patient is bent well forwards, the shift of center of gravity will automatically elicit the movement of standing.

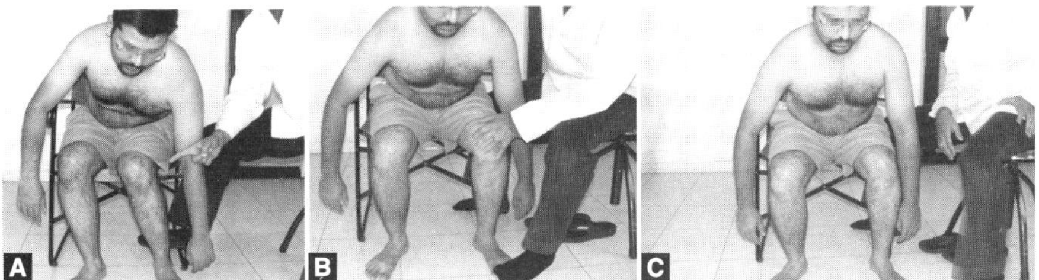

FIGURES 12.2A to C: (A) Forward bending in sitting, hip falling in internal rotation, (B) forward bending in sitting, thigh supported, (C) forward bending in sitting, thigh in neutral, active, left hemiplegia

The patient's feet are placed together with the affected foot slightly behind the sound one to ensure good weight bearing as standing approaches. The patient leans forward until head is vertically in front of the feet and stands without pushing up with the hand (Figure 12.3). If the trunk and arm retract too much at first, the patient can assist standing by pushing the arms out in front with hands clasped together. When returning to sitting, the affected foot remains behind and head is kept well forward while his bottom is placed far back in the chair. The patient should not put a hand down on the chair as this spoils the symmetry and alters the weight-bearing. Instead, the patient should look behind and back, until there is a correct alignment with the chair. Therapist may assist the patient for lifting the pelvis up from the chair in a symmetrical manner. The therapist sits on a level surface on the affected side of the patient and one hand stabilizes the lower end of femur (at the knee) and other hand may be kept on or below the sacrum (Figure 12.4). The patient is then asked to get up gently keeping the weight on both the

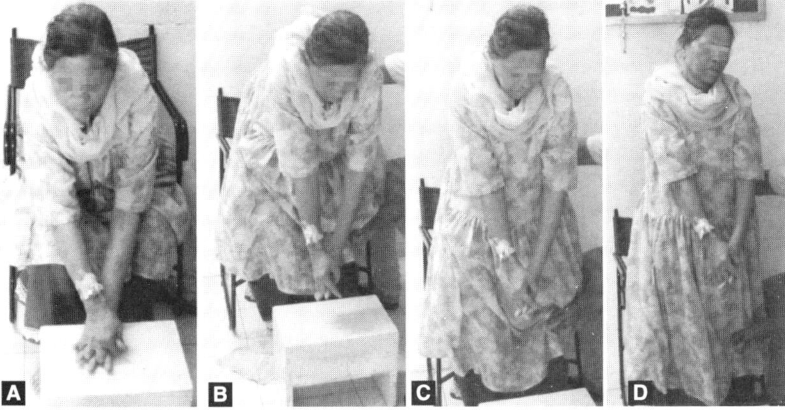

FIGURES 12.3A to D: Active-assisted sit to stand from a chair, right hemiplegia, note the stabilization of trunk and knee by the therapist, front view

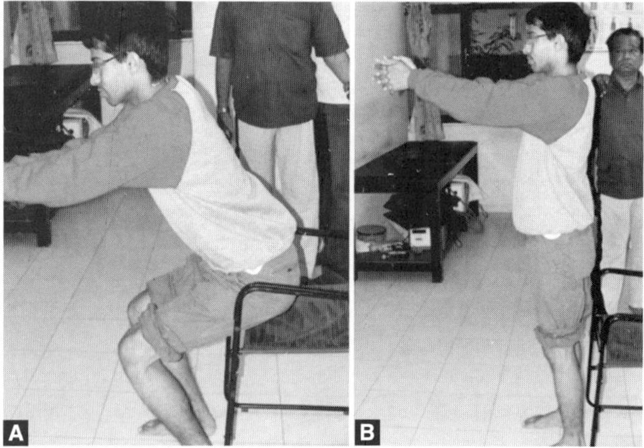

FIGURES 12.4A and B: Sit to stand, active, right hemiplegia, side view

lower limbs equal. At the same time, the therapist asks the patient to contract the gluteal muscles, so that the femur's upper end is engaged so that the hip extends. This movement will assist in knee extension without the extensor thrust. A gentle tap on the affected side gluteal muscles, at the time of getting up, will facilitate the movement of hip extension. Therapist's one hand can control the knee extension and prevent exaggerated knee extension and snapping

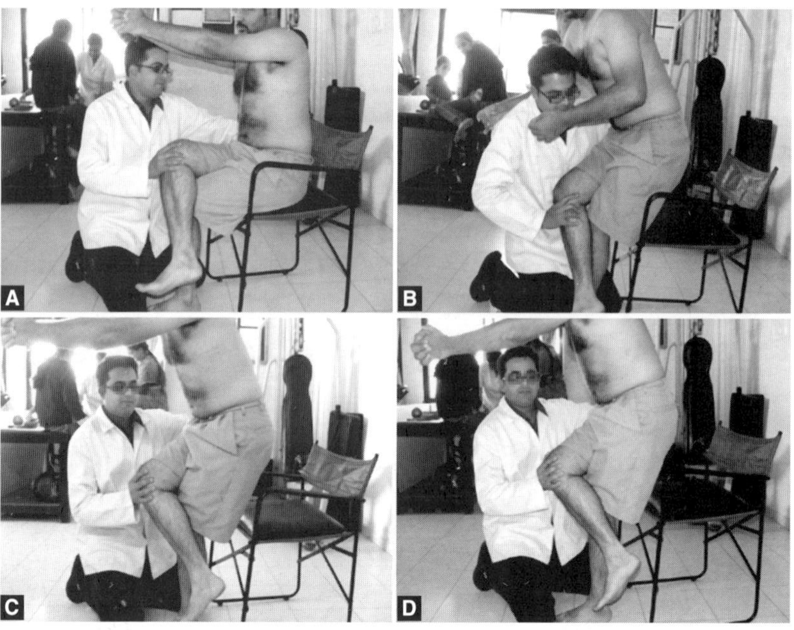

FIGURES 12.5A to D: (A) Crossing sound limb over affected limb, (B) attempt to stand with weight only on affected lower limb, wrong method without upper limb clasping, (C and D) correct method of standing with clasp hands and weight well forwards left hemiplegia

of the knee in hyperextension. All the way through, if the patient is able to brace up the abdominals actively, it will help in keeping the pelvis aligned in a posterior tilt which is required.

If the patient is unable to shift the weight well enough on the affected lower limb, then activities which train the same are started as shown in Figures 12.5A to D.

Sound lower limb of the patient is crossed on the affected limb as shown in Figure 12.5A. Both the upper limbs can be clasped and held in front of the body. The therapist assists the shift of the weight on the affected side. The patient bends little forwards and with the assistance from the therapist, tries to lift up the pelvis off the chair. This is a difficult activity for most of the patients and hence, is carried out with utmost care; safety of the patient should never be compromised. Note that the optimum height of the chair is mandatory for getting up easily. Maintaining the posture midway will help develop the eccentric control of the muscles of the lower limbs. Note the contraction of the abdominal muscles in Figures 12.5A to D. Once the control of the lower limb is developed, the patient may be asked to stand fully although with guarded knee extension. (In above mentioned activities, note the position of the therapist on sound side as the patient may hold on to the therapist with sound upper limb in case of imbalance).

PELVIC ALIGNMENT IN STANDING

Equal weight bearing on both the lower limbs is one of the most important activities in the entire rehabilitation program of the hemiplegic patient. It should be started as early as possible as, in advanced and chronic stages, it becomes extremely difficult to train weight transference. As it can be assumed, weight transference on the affected lower limb cannot be achieved without the adequate shift from the pelvis, participation from the lumbar region and alignment of the upper segments of the spine, in addition to the distal control of the lower limb.

The therapist sits in front of the patient in level of the pelvis as shown in the Figure 12.6. The therapist puts his feet in between patient's feet for spacing. Patient keeps both the hips slightly externally rotated and knees slightly flexed. The therapist facilitates the gluteal contractions on both the sides by tapping gently and then asking the patient to maintain the contraction. One hand of the therapist facilitates the contraction of abdominals and hence, posterior pelvic tilt is maintained. The therapist shifts the pelvis on the affected side if need be, without allowing the patient to side flex the trunk on the affected side.

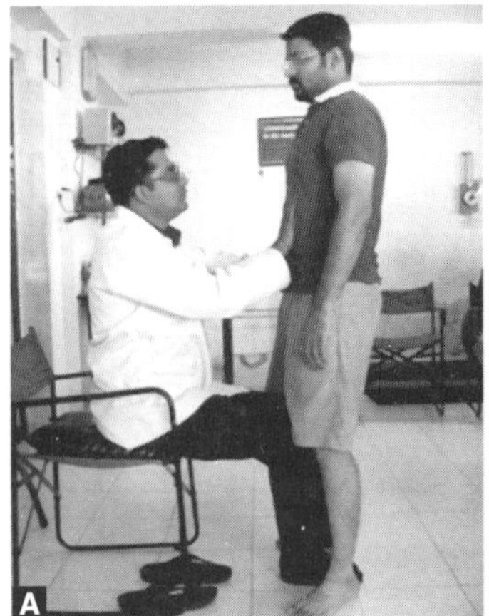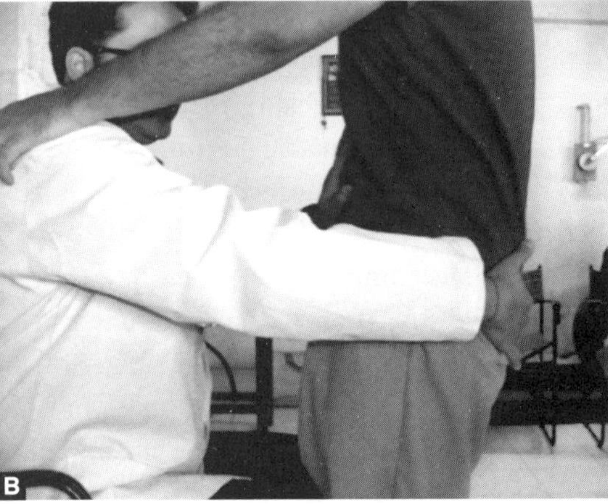

FIGURES 12.6A and B: Maintaining posterior pelvic tilt in standing with knees unlocked, left hemiplegia

Figure 12.7 shows exaggerated anterior pelvic tilt. This is caused by inadequate abdominal and hip extensor activity. Also note the hyperextension of the knee and shifting of the lower end of tibia posteriorly on talus resulting into close chain planter flexion. Though this is a weight bearing position, it will not give any advantages of the same as it is mechanically at fault. Apparent length of the affected side increases due to planter flexion and hence, the weight bearing on affected side is reduced to a minimum. In chronic cases, this position leads to damage of the ligaments of the knee, which are irreversible. No amount of splintage can tackle this issue and hence, it should be avoided from initial stages.

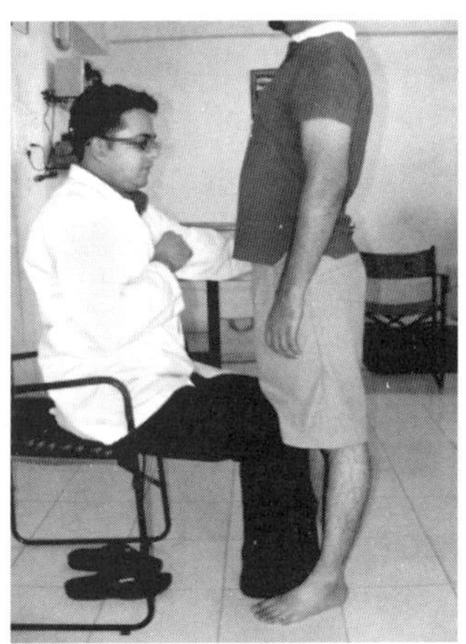

FIGURE 12.7: Incorrect method of standing with anterior pelvic tilting and increased lumbar lordisis, left hemiplegia

UNILATERAL WEIGHT BEARING

As the patient can maintain some balance independently in standing, unilateral weight bearing i.e., standing on one leg can be started. To take the entire weight on the affected side, the therapist assists the patient by sitting on the affected side. With one knee of the therapist behind the patient's knee and one hand in front of the knee, the therapist controls the amount of knee flexion. Other hand of the therapist is encircled around the patient's waist to maintain

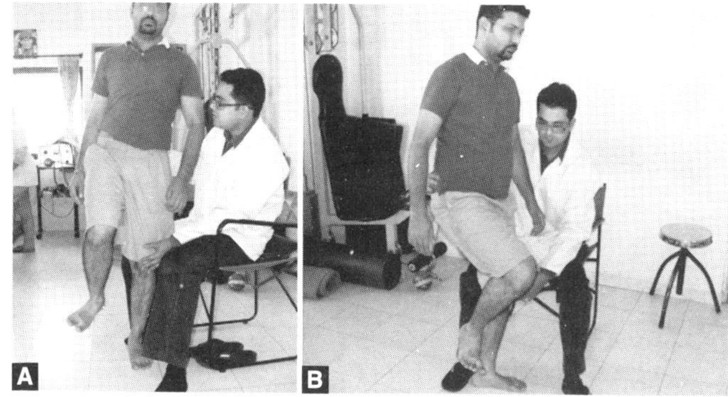

FIGURES 12.8A and B: Unilateral weight-bearing on affected side, assisted, left hemiplegia

the lateral tilt of the pelvis and overall balance. Then the patient is asked to gradually take the sound leg off the floor, shifting the entire weight on the affected lower limb (Figure 12.8). This movement is carried out gently and balance is maintained throughout.

Patient can practice selective knee flexion and extension in weight bearing position in a guarded manner. The therapist controls the motion of the lower limb unless the patient is in a position to maintain the position himself. Throughout the movement, patient is asked to maintain posterior pelvic tilt as shown in

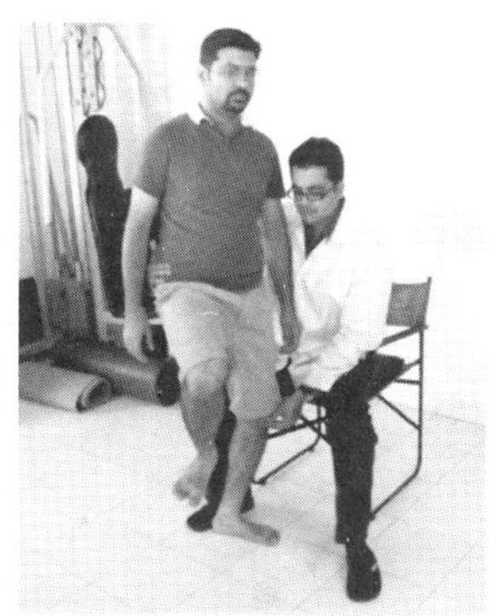

FIGURE 12.9: Moving sound limb while weight-bearing on affected side with knees semiflexed, left hemiplegia

Figure 12.9. In the same position, the sound lower limb of the patient can be moved in various directions as a progression.

ASSISTED ACTIVITIES WITH THE HELP OF A TABLE

Modified plantigrade is an ideal early standing posture to develop control. The affected arm is extended and weight is shifted on to it. In addition, the posture has a wide base support and is very stable. Progression to upright standing activities can then occur, first with arm support, and then without arm support.

Patient is made to stand in front of a table in a manner as shown in Figure 12.11A. This position gives adequate support to the patient's thighs and hence, fear of falling decreases. This reduction of fear reduces the hypertonicity throughout the affected side. The patient is assisted to stand erect taking equal weight on both the lower limbs while the thighs of the patient are supported by a table in front. Similarly, patient can take weight on both the upper limbs by keeping them on the table top as shown in Figure 12.10. The therapist aligns the spine of the patient as required. The patient is then asked to lift the sound leg off the ground and take entire weight on affected lower limb only. Abdominal muscles and gluteal muscles contractions tilt the pelvis posteriorly and align the femur so that knee joint remains neutral and does not fall into hyperextension. Note Figures 12.11A and B and difference in position of pelvis and knee in both of them.

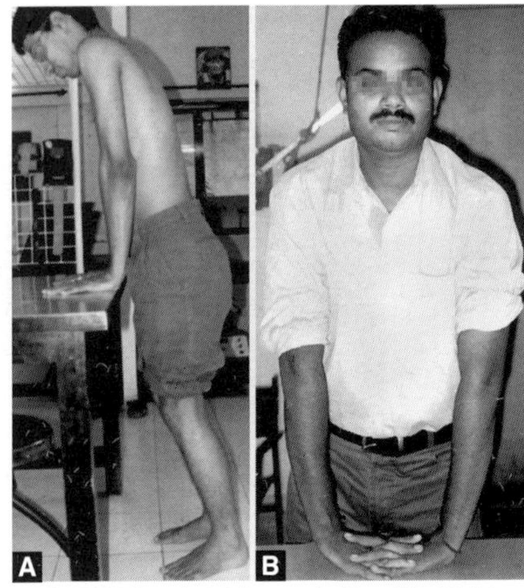

FIGURES 12.10A and B: (A) Taking weight on upper limbs in standing, right hemiplegia, (B) taking weight on clasped hands with wrist in extension

The patient is made to stand on a foam wedge in a stride position with the affected leg in front as shown in Figure 12.12A. The front thigh of the patient is supported by the table. Both the upper limbs are clasped and taken in front of the body. The therapist guides the pelvis in a posterior tilt and assists the weight transference on the affected front leg. Note the knee joint which is in few degrees of flexion. The patient is then asked to flex the trunk and put the weight on both the elbows on table top. Note the weight on the heel as the ankle dorsiflexes. The use of a foam wedge trains the proprioception and balance. The same

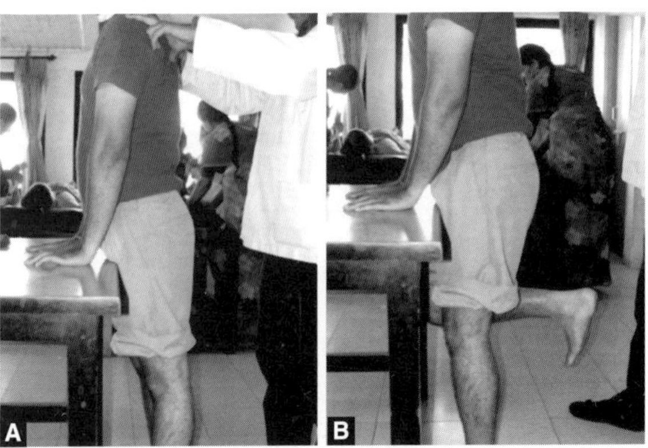

FIGURES 12.11A and B: (A) Standing straight with thigh supported by a table, left hemiplegia, note anterior pelvic tilt which can be corrected and (B) weight-bearing on affected side with knee in neutral or slight flexion in standing, left hemiplegia, pelvis posteriorly tilted

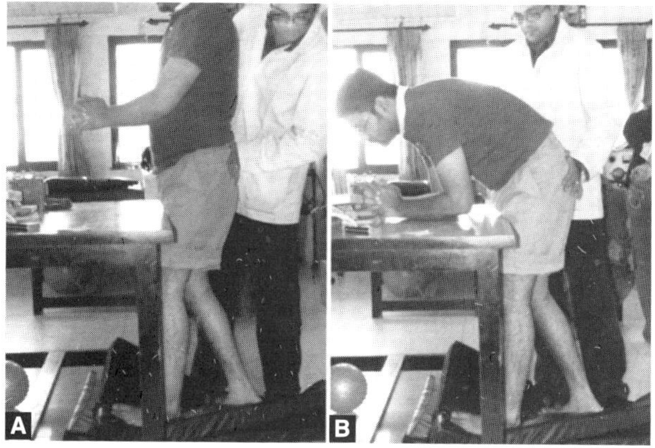

FIGURES 12.12A and B: (A) Stride standing on a foam wedge and (B) stride standing on a foam wedge with flexion of trunk, left hemiplegia

activity can be done with the sound (right) leg in front and training of affected side ankle plantar flexors can be carried out. A contraction of abdominal muscles is maintained throughout along with relaxed breathing.

Weight bearing on Extended Arm

Practice of weight bearing through the extended arm in standing is carried out by placing both the upper limbs in external rotation position from shoulder, extension from elbow, supination of forearm, wrist and fingers extension, and thumb abducted and extended (Figure 12.13). As a part of progression, only the affected side can be used for weight bearing. Elbows can be flexed and extended in the weight bearing position to train activities of triceps in close chain position.

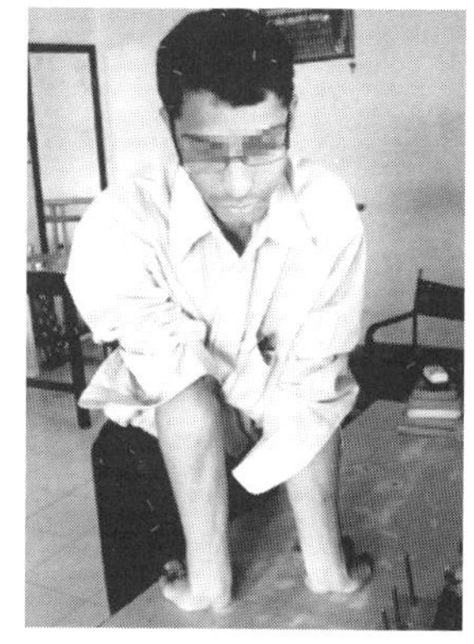

FIGURE 12.13: Weight-bearing on both upper limbs in external rotation of shoulder, right hemiplegia

The patient can flex the lower limbs while the upper limbs are still on the table either in front or behind as shown in Figures 12.14A and B. While flexing the trunk, both the hands are kept on table as shown. If affected hand slides off the table, it can be secured by putting sound hand on top of it. This activity trains close chain upper limb function of shoulder flexion primarily with flexion pattern of trunk. Both the upper limbs can be placed on a table which is kept behind and weight bearing posteriorly can be carried out. In this position, external rotation of the shoulder is easily maintained. As a progression, therapist can ask the patient to flex the lower limbs and squat as far as possible. If the patient is unable

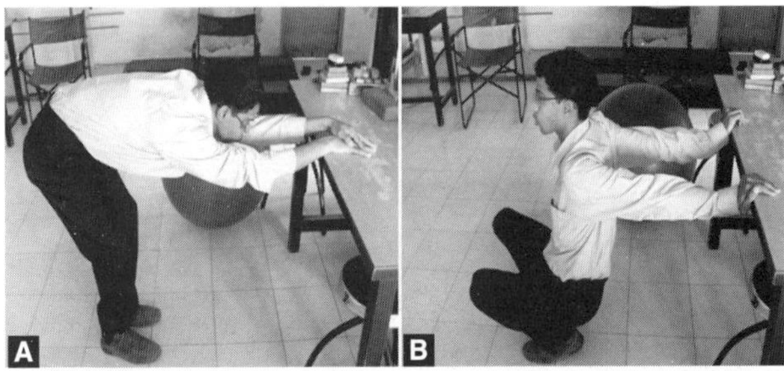

FIGURES 12.14A and B: (A) Weight bearing on upper limbs with trunk flexion, right hemiplegia and (B) weight bearing on upper limbs with shoulder extension and knee flexion, right hemiplegia

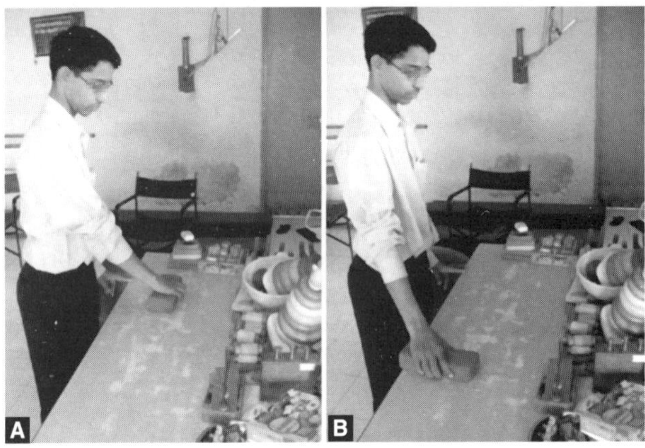

FIGURES 12.15A and B: Table mopping, right hemiplegia

to maintain position of affected hand on table then, the therapist can assist in doing so.

Patient can carry out mopping activities, once the weight bearing on the upper limb in standing improves. If motor control of the affected side is not sufficient enough, sound hand is placed over the affected hand and assisted mopping can be carried out in full range of motion; forward backwards and side to side (Figure 12.15). This activity trains functional movements of upper limb. It also helps in normalizing muscle tone of affected upper limb. Partial weight given through affected upper limb facilitates proprioception and helps in awareness of position of that part in space.

STEP-UP ACTIVITIES

While standing on patient's affected side, the therapist draws his weight towards himself, giving as much support as required. The therapist then asks the patient to take steps on the bolster with the sound leg, preventing the knee from snapping back into extension by keeping the hip well forward.

A bolster is placed in front and the patient is asked to keep one leg on it (Figure 12.16). The bolster being a movable surface, the patient may have to control the lower limb and if not, the extensor thrust of the lower limb will slide the bolster forwards. Adequate support by the therapist may be required initially. So as explained before, support from the pelvis is given. If need be, patient may hold on to a stable object by the sound limb but care must be taken not to allow the patient to lean on the object of support. Training is done for both the lower limbs. Affected side raises will train the hip flexion and knee flexion with dorsiflexion of ankle in a controlled manner. The sound leg raises will train the affected side weight bearing and balance. Bolster can be moved back and forth in a controlled fashion to train selective motor movement in standing (Figure 12.17).

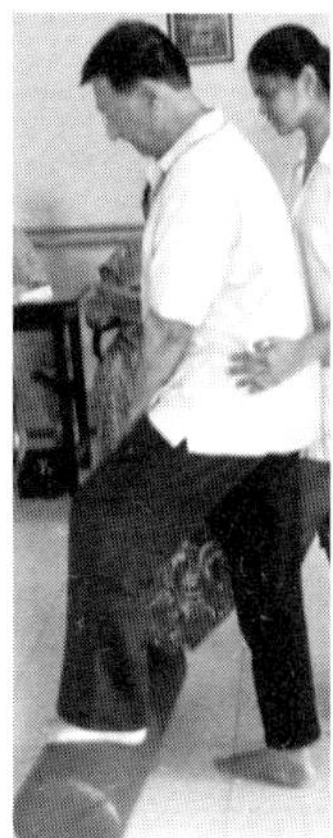

FIGURE 12.16: Stepping up on a bolster with affected lower limb, left hemiplegia

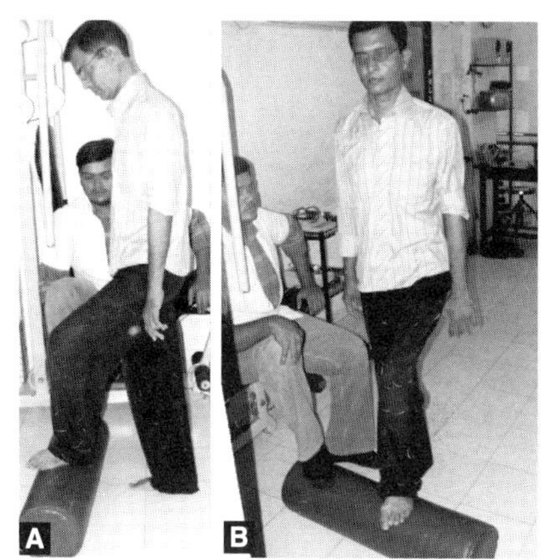

FIGURES 12.17A and B: Dynamic activities on a bolster, sensory stroke, left hemiparesis

WEIGHT BEARING ON THE AFFECTED LEG

In standing position, ask the patient to place his sound foot lightly on and off a step in front of him. Repeat the activity with the step placed well, out to the side. Encourage the patient to keep his affected hip against your hip. Prevent the patient's knee from locking back, and ask the patient to draw large letter on the floor with the sound foot, ensuring weight bearing on a mobile leg. Make the patient stand on the affected leg and lightly place the sound foot at a right angle in front or behind the other foot, without transferring the weight onto it. If the activity is performed accurately, it helps the patient to gain control of the hip abductors and extensors. Place the patient's affected leg on a 15 cm (6 inches) step in front of him. With your hand pushing down on the knee and keeping the weight well forward, the patient steps up onto the step. Practice stepping down with his sound leg placing further and further back, and tapping it on the floor behind, keeping the weight forwards on the affected leg. Put the affected leg on the step and help the patient to push up and step right over and back again (Figures 12.18A and B).

Patient is trained for side lifts of affected and sound lower limb as shown in Figures 12.19A to C. Here, the affected side is left. The therapist stands behind the patient with the pelvis fully supported and maintaining the balance of the body. The affected upper limb is held in a reflex inhibiting position (shoulder extension, external rotation, elbow extension, forearm supinated and wrist and fingers extended and thumb extended and abducted) as shown in Figures 12.19A and B. A small stool of optimum height is kept at the affected side first. The patient is asked to take the affected lower limb sideways, upwards and to put the foot on the stool. The therapist guides the pelvis so that it

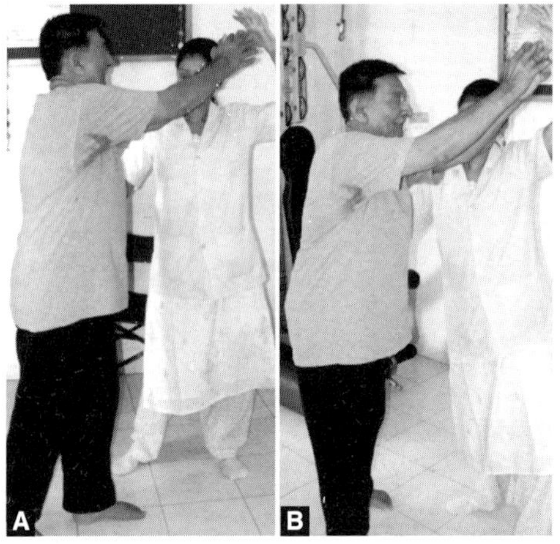

FIGURES 12.18A and B: (A) Reaching outs with affected lower limb in front, left hemiplegia, and (B) reaching outs with sound lower limb in front, left hemiplegia

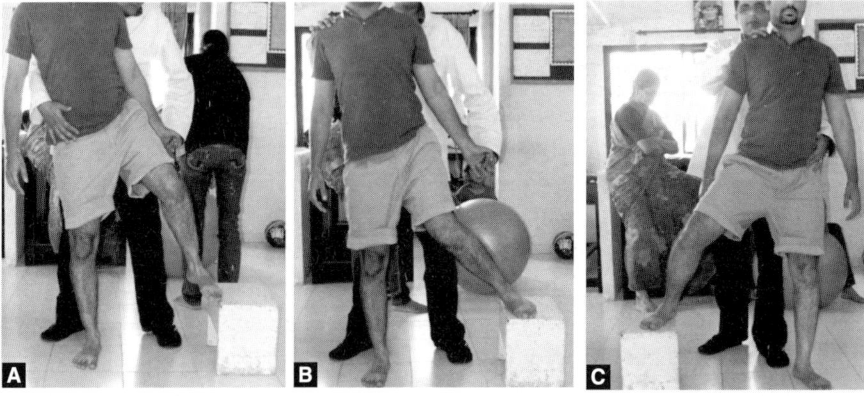

FIGURES 12.19A to C: (A) Putting affected foot on a step sideways, left hemiplegia, (B) note hip internal rotation with adduction on left side, and (C) putting sound foot on a step sideways, left hemiplegia

does not fall into gravity and asks the patient to maintain the position. Gradually, the assistance given by the therapist is reduced and the activity is carried out more and more independently. Similar side lifts can be carried out by the sound lower limb also. Note the difference in position of pelvis in Figures 12.19A to C when the sound limb is lifted and when the affected limb is lifted.

Posterior Pelvic Tilts against the Wall

Symmetrical weight bearing on both lower extremities and knee control can be trained along with contraction of abdominal muscles in standing position. Patient is made to stand with the back totally supported by a wall. Both the feet are kept apart in the line of pelvis. Both the hips are kept slightly externally rotated and knees are flexed to about 15 to 20 degrees. Both the feet are kept firmly on the ground. The patient is then asked to posteriorly rotate pelvis by contraction of abdominal muscles in front and gluteal muscles at the back so that lumbar lordosis is obliterated (Figure 12.20). A small ball can also be kept at the lumbar region to "feel" flattening of the lumbar spine. This activity helps in maintaining a symmetrical and correct posture which eventually helps in all functional tasks.

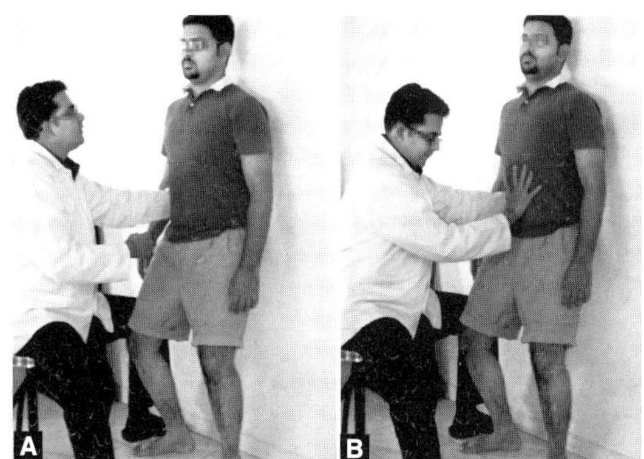

FIGURES 12.20A and B: Practicing posterior pelvic tilts, supported by wall, left hemiplegia

TRAINING PLANTAR FLEXION

Selective motor activity of plantar flexion in standing position is essential for terminal stance phase and push-off of gait cycle. Contraction relaxation coupling of dorsi and plantar flexors is required for aligning tibia in relation to talus and femur, thus providing stability at ankle and knee joints, respectively. Use of the gait cycle in training plantar flexors is usually incorporated. The patient is made to stand in a stride standing position with the sound limb

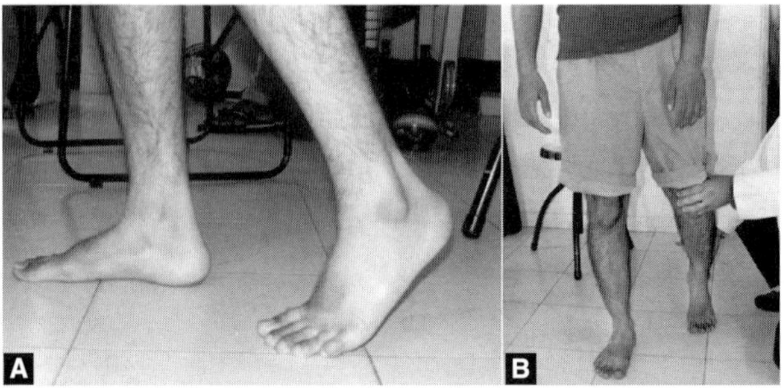

FIGURES 12.21A and B: Plantar flexion in stride standing position, left hemiplegia

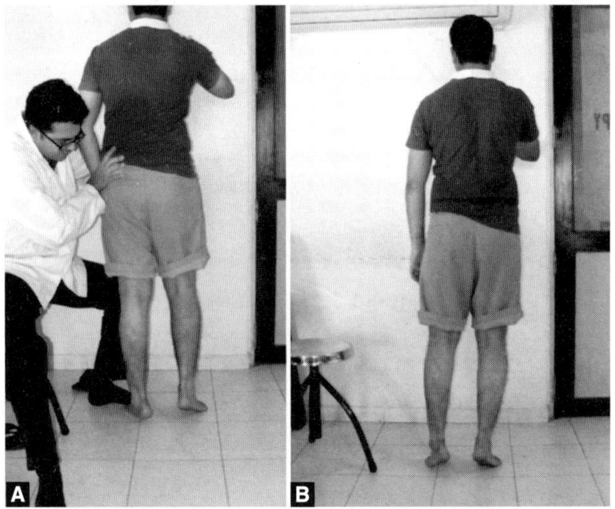

FIGURES 12.22A and B: (A) Toe standing, assisted but still asymmetrical, left hemiplegia, and (B) toe standing, symmetrical, left hemiplegia

in front and affected limb behind. The patient is then assisted to shift the weight onto the sound limb while concentrating on plantar flexion of the affected limb which is behind. Few degrees of knee flexion may be associated to unlock the knee while doing so. Please note Figures 12.21A and B.

If the patient fails to plantar flex the ankle actively, the therapist assists by lifting the heel off the ground as shown in Figure 12.21B. Standing up on the toes with the support of the wall can also be carried out as it would become a bilaterally symmetrical pattern of activity (Figures 12.22A and B).

TRAINING SELECTIVE KNEE FLEXION IN STANDING

To counteract exaggerated extensor thrust response in standing, selective knee flexion is started as soon as possible. The patient is asked to flex the affected

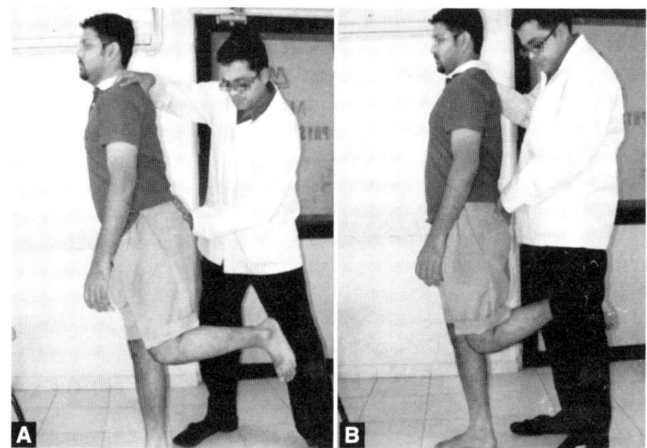

FIGURES 12.23A and B: (A) Active knee flexion in standing, left hemiplegia, note reactions of trunk, and (B) assisted knee flexion in standing with stable trunk, left hemiplegia

knee in standing while the therapist prevents the associated unwanted contraction in trunk and hip region by stabilizing upper trunk with one hand and pelvic region with the other. The therapist can hold the patient's ankle (while the knee is flexed), in between his both lower limbs. Eccentric contraction of hamstring can be trained when the patient is asked to lower the leg which is flexed from the knee assisted by the therapist. Please note Figures 12.23A and B. Eccentric contraction of hamstring is useful in deceleration of the leg in terminal swing phase of the gait.

DYNAMIC ACTIVITIES FOR LOWER LIMB CONTROL AND GAIT

Releasing the Knee and Moving the Hemiplegic Leg (Preparation for the Swing Phase of Gait)

The patient stands with his feet close together. Guide the pelvis forward and down to release the knee on the affected side. Instruct the patient to straighten it again, without pushing the whole side back. The patient must remain in contact with the floor; this is only possible if the pelvis drops forward. The same activity is practiced in step standing with the affected leg behind, and the weight forwarded over the extended sound leg. The patient stands with the weight on his sound leg. Facilitate small steps backward with the other foot by holding the toes dorsiflexed and instructing not to push down. Do not allow to hitch the hip back. The patient walks sideways along a line crossing one foot in front of the other. When the sound leg takes a step, the affected limb must be kept well forward so that his knee does not snap

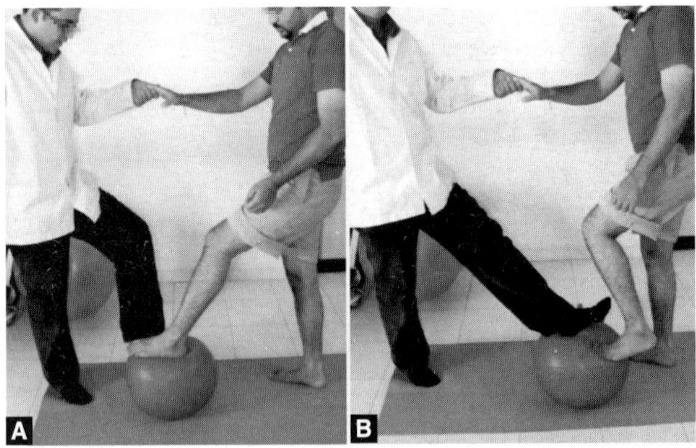

FIGURES 12.24A and B: Movements of affected lower limb in standing using a ball, left hemiplegia

back into extension.

Patient is trained to move the affected lower limb in a controlled fashion in standing position by using a vestibular ball of optimum size as shown in Figures 12.24A and B. The patient puts the affected foot on the ball, while taking majority of the weight on the sound lower limb. The patient then moves the ball in various directions starting from single plane activity progressing to multiplanar activities. The therapist may guide or control the movements by putting his own foot on the ball. This way, all the functional movements of the lower limb can be trained for direction of the movement, range of movement and velocity of movement. During this activity, the basic correction of the posture as explained before is strongly advocated. Similar activity can be carried out by putting the sound foot on the ball while the affected lower limb maintains the balance of the body in a weight bearing position.

Training for Taking Steps

Figures 12.25A and B show the correct method for avoiding hyperextension of knee and exaggerated extensor thrust while walking. The therapist stabilizes the patient's affected knee joint in a few degrees of flexion in the stride position as shown in the above Figure. The knee joint is held in partially unlocked position and the hip is held in extension while the foot rests completely on the ground. The patient is asked to take a step forward with the sound lower limb. Any exaggerated movement on either side should not be allowed at all. As this movement happens, the therapist guides the affected knee into few degrees of flexion and ankle in few degrees of planter flexion, simultaneously maintaining adequate extension at the hip by asking the patient to contract gluteal muscles. This activity is of paramount importance in training various phases of gait cycle. In initial stages, adequate support for maintainance of

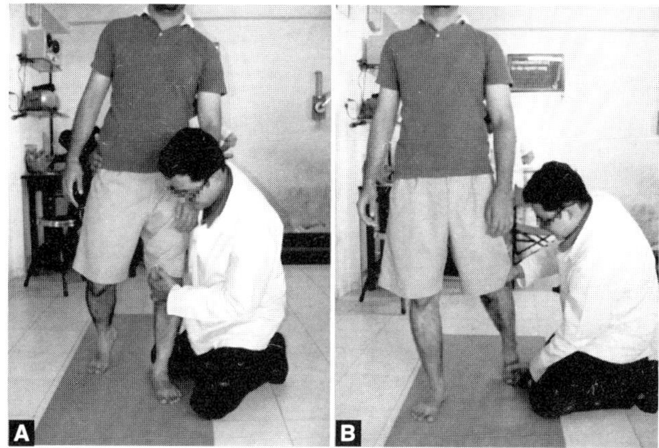

FIGURES 12.25A and B: Taking step with sound lower limb, guiding done for affected limb, left hemiplegia

the balance is usually required and hence promptly provided.

The affected limb swing phase can also be trained with the therapist guiding and controlling the active motion throughout the range.

Abnormal Gait Pattern

To walk upright on a narrow base has played a key role in our life style for over two and half million years. This ability has enabled us to acquire numerous challenging skills like running, jumping, dancing, rope walking, etc. To support the upright posture on a narrow base on either both the legs or one leg support demands a highly complex postural reaction to maintain balance and postural adjustments throughout the ongoing gait sequence. In walking, the shift in position of torso and hips over the feet initiate the movements in each foot. The ability to stand up and sit down symmetrically and safely plays an integral role in normal functional walking. Normal gait pattern is automatic and symmetrical; there is continuous shift of center of gravity in posterior, lateral and forward directions. The femoral trochanters face anteriorly and the hips move forwards in a smooth wave-like pattern. The rhythm, the step length and support time on each leg are equal.

Factors responsible for abnormal gait pattern

- **Primary neurogenic**

  Sensory motor impairments as a result of the lesion in the CNS
  - Alteration in muscle tone, spastic extensor tone
  - Inadequate or distorted tactile-kinesthetic information from within and from the environment
  - Depression of motor activity, weakness or paralysis of the muscle
  - Loss of selective motor activity, reciprocal inhibition and movement dexterity

- Abnormal coactivation of the weak muscles emerge as patient attempts to load the affected limb resulting in altered normal biomechanics in the leg
- Insecurity and fear of fall due to inadequate balance and equilibrium reactions affecting the normal postural adjustments during the gait sequence.

■ **Adaptive patterns**

Adaptive patterns occur as a result of faulty habits

- The patient attempts to walk in his best possible manner irrespective of proper balance and movement sequence
- Improper inputs and facilitation given by the team members and family
- Adverse neural tissues result in shortening of soft tissues, muscles and musculoskeletal contractures and joint stiffness. Muscle length shortening or contractures are observed in truncal muscles, low back extensors, hip flexors specially rectus femoris, hip external rotators and iliotibial band, adductors, knee flexors, calf muscles and occasionally in tibialis anterior and extensor hallusis longus. The adverse tissue tensions alter the biomechanics in the leg restricting forward weight shift of the body mass over the stance leg.

Main difficulty is a short stance phase on the hemiplegic leg with a quick active swing phase and long stride length. This results into prolonged stance phase and abruptly ending swing phase of the normal leg.

Stance Phase

Stance phase sets up the most favorable condition for the swing phase. Many problems observed in the swing phase are related to stance phase. An asymmetrical flexed posture with the center of gravity well behind the normal line make it difficult for the patient to extend the trunk on his hips and to shift body weight forward over to supporting leg. The extensor spasticity, the hyperextension in the knee, weakness in the extensors and truncal muscles and inadequate postural adjustments result in flexion of the trunk on hips (flexion attitude). Shortened and inactive plantar flexor reduces the force for the push off.

Swing Phase

The problems observed in the stance phase cause difficulty in achieving a low energy swing phase following a forward step with the unaffected leg. The swing phase of the sound leg too is affected, the foot falls flat on the ground without heel strike and the knee remains 15–20 degrees flexion on floor-foot contact. The patient actively extends the supporting leg to raise his center of gravity in an effort to shorten the hemiplegic leg for the swing phase. The swing phase of the hemiplegic leg is a high-energy active movement. The patient hitches the pelvis up and with circumduction brings the leg forward in total extension pattern. The floor-foot contact is either on the toes, ball of the foot or in supination due to spastic pull of tibialis anterior and tibialis posterior and loss of their inhibition. There is an inability to transfer the weight adequate over the sound leg to free the affected leg for swing phase. The foot continues to push against the floor for clearance, the patient translates the weight sideways to the hitching the pelvis. The patient literally walks sideways.

Typical Characteristic Features

- Loss of automatic gait pattern
- Significantly reduced speed and stride length
- Alteration in cadence and rhythm
- Short stance phase on hemiplegic leg and active high energy swing phase
- Long step length with the hemiplegic leg
- Increased double leg support
- Abnormal coactivation of truncal and leg muscles alter the biomechanics of the leg
- Inadequate balance, postural adjustments and weight transfers.

Re-education and Gait Facilitation

Restoration of functional walking plays a major role in the rehabilitation of the CNS lesions. A hemiplegic patient, who stands up asymmetrically, experiences difficulty to bear weight on his hemiplegic leg and maintain an upright posture. The asymmetrical posture affects the gait sequence from very first step. To facilitate gait, the therapist uses the skill in his hands to prevent all the observed difficulties. The hands either assist the selective movement pattern or inhibit and prevent unwanted activity. Quoting Ms. Bobath (1976), *"All the various phases of walking can be prepared for in standing."* To prepare the patient for a reasonably good gait pattern balance, stance and weight transfer should be practiced in standing for the stance phase. The patient requires to release his spastic muscles at hip, knee and ankle for push off and to swing the leg forward. In the mid swing phase, patient must control his extending knee for a well-timed heel strike or floor-foot muscle. These preparatory exercises assist the patient to develop a better and stable walking pattern.

The treatment goal aims at:

- Bearing equal weight and balance on both the legs and on each individual leg
- Shifting the weight laterally and forward
- Walking without aids and with good speed and rhythm
- Ability to regain balance
- Learning to walk sideways and backwards to cross the steps and to walk on uneven surfaces
- Ability to go up and down the stairs
- Walking with confidence and stability on the streets.

Gait Training

Walking is usually initiated early on, before selective movement and balanced control are achieved. It can be used to motivate patients and minimize deconditioning but increases the risk of developing persistent and faulty habits. While ambulation, aids such as quadripod canes assist early mobilization; they can also distort balance, promoting an excessive weight shift on to the unaffected side. Gait training should focus on the attainment of control in the selective movements necessary for gait with appropriate timing. Specific movement deficiencies should be identified and corrected. Initially, this may require focusing on the specific muscle actions or combinations in other less demanding postures and then practicing them in an upright position (e.g. lower trunk rotation is practiced first side-lying, then kneeling, plantigrade, and finally standing and walking). Performance is context specific. The therapist cannot assume carrying over from practice in one position to another. Persistent posturing of the upper extremity in flexion adduction during gait can be controlled through positioning the hemiplegic arm in extension and abduction with the hand open.

Orthosis in Gait Training

An orthosis may be required when persistent problems prevent safe ambulation. Prescription will depend upon the unique problems each patient presents. The pattern of mediolateral instability and weakness at the ankle and knee, and the extent and severity of spasticity and sensory deficits of the limb are the major factors to be considered when prescribing an orthosis. Temporary devices (e.g. dorsiflexion assists) may be used during the early stages while recovery is proceeding, to allow the patient to practice standing and early walking. Permanent devices are prescribed once the patient's status is relatively stable. Extensive bracing using a knee-ankle-foot orthosis (KAFO) is rarely indicated or successful.

An ankle-foot orthosis (AFO) is commonly prescribed to control deficient knee and ankle and/or foot function (Figure 12.26). These may include a molded AFO (polypropylene AFO, plastic spiral AFO, plastic solid ankle AFO), or conventional double upright/dual channel AFO. In this latter device, a posterior stop can be added to limit plantar flexion while a spring assist can be added to assist dorsiflexion. An air-stirrup ankle brace can be used to provide

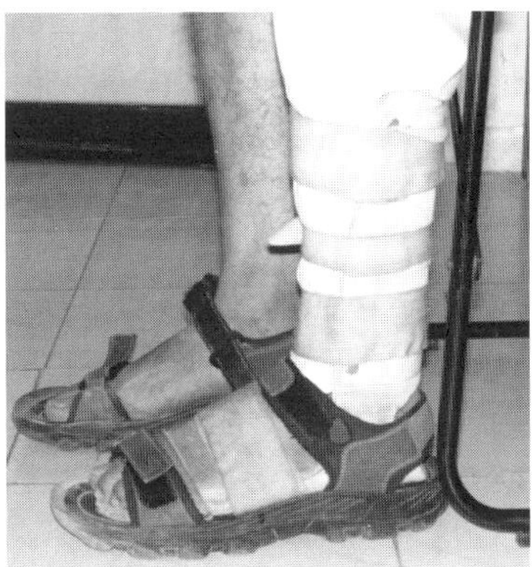

FIGURE 12.26: Ankle-foot orthosis, left hemiplegia

mediolateral stability at the subtalar joint while allowing dorsiflexion and plantar flexion. Knee problems in hemiplegia can usually be controlled by adjusting the position of the ankle. An ankle set in 5 degrees plantar flexion stabilizes the knee during mid stance. A patient with mild knee hyperextension without foot and/or ankle instability may benefit from the application of a Swedish knee cage to protect the knee. The therapist must frequently reassess the patient's motor function and the need for an orthosis, since continuing recovery may warrant a prescriptive change or discontinuing the use of a device.

Various Activities During Gait Cycle

Each phase of gait cycle is trained individually on both sides before actual walking is begun to avoid abnormal reflex activity paterns to takeover. During walking, to counteract the flexor synergy of the affected upper limb, one of the method can be used is explained below. The patient is given a large ball to hold with both the upper limb while walking a shown in Figure 12.27. This activity also facilitates movement of thoracic and lumbar region. Mass synergistic pattterns of activities are reduced as the patient voluntarily tries to hold the ball with both the upper limbs.

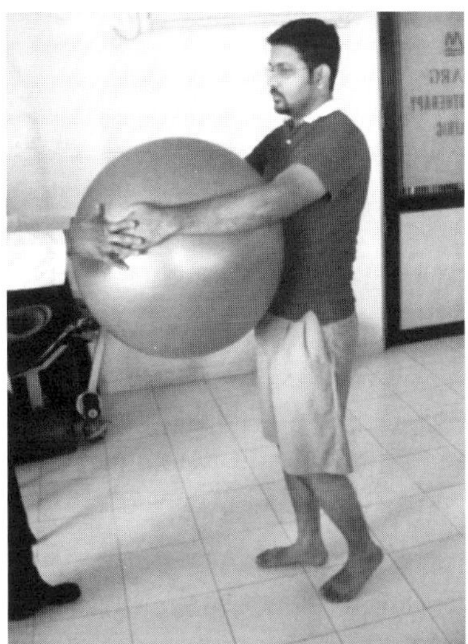

FIGURE 12.27: Walking with a large ball held in front, assisted, left hemiplegia

The patient can also walk with both the hands clapsed together in front in initial stages. Furthermore, the therapist may hold the affected upper limb in reflex inhibiting posture (shoulder extension; abduction and external rotation; elbow extension; forearm supinated; wrist and fingers extension; thumb extension and abduction). The rotation of upper trunk in either direction is essential for normal arm swing during walking. This can be trained by the therapist by holding both the upper limbs from either behind or front and assisting

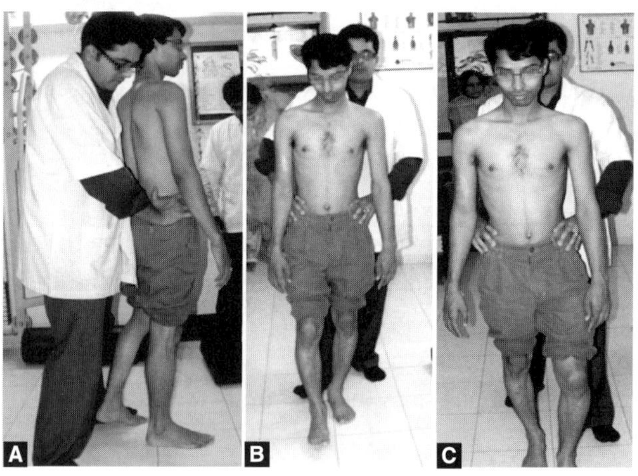

FIGURES 12.28A to C: Gait facilitation by guiding the pelvis, right hemiplegia

rotation of the upper trunk (Figure 12.28).

The therapist can assist the pelvic movement of the patient while walking from behind. The therapist holds the pelvic rim of the patient on both the sides and assists the pelvic motion in the following manner.

- Swing phase: Pelvic movements upwards and forwards progressing to forwards and downwards during heel strike
- Heel strike: Downward pressure
- Stance phase: Downwards and backwards.

The above movements are done in a cyclic fashion without changing the hold and continuity is maintained throughout the movement.

For training dorsiflexion during walking, the therapist tips the patient backwards from pelvis. This movement elicits the response of dorsiflexion of ankle. The patient is then asked to carry out the dorsiflexion actively in standing position. As shown in Figure 12.29, the therapist holds the

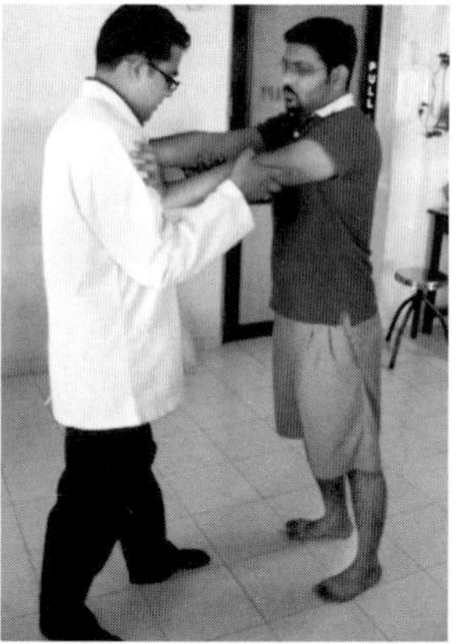

FIGURE 12.29: Tipping backwards for dorsiflexor activity, left hemiplegia

patient from the arms on both the sides while the patient places both the hands on the therapist's chest in front (Figure 12.30). The therapist in this position can resist the forward motion of the patient's body, thus training the abdominals dynamically. The activity should be smooth in nature and no amount of jerky activity is allowed. This activity also trains the affected upper

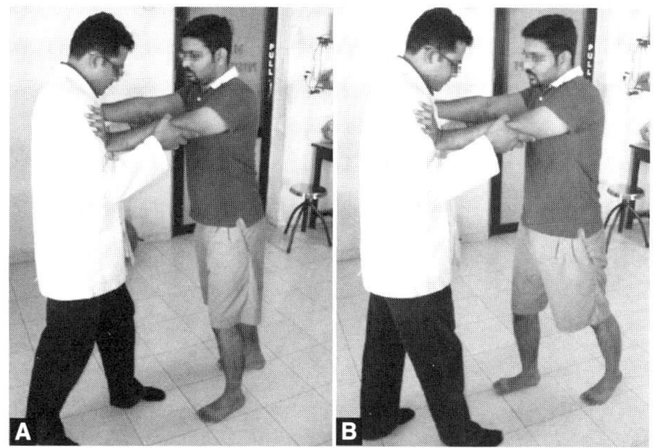

FIGURES 12.30A and B: Resisted gait training, left hemiplegia

limb in weight bearing in front and hence, decreases the chances of flexor synergy while walking.

The same position can be easily utilized for resisting the action of walking. It is very useful in training functional walking in normal environment. Resisted walking facilitates normal gait pattern.

Gradually, as the patient progresses, the upper limbs can be removed from the therapist's chest and the therapist can provide resistance to the movement by applying pressure over sternum. This activity trains the appropriate alignment of the of the body parts while walking so that the center of gravity is maintained insde the base of support. Rather than holding the patient for giving support, the therapist can use this activity as the patient feels supported and hence fear of fall decreases. As it can be noted from the Figures 12.31A and B, reisted walking will elicit dorsiflexion of the affected side and hence, heel strike is facilitated. A combination of many such techniques may be required to train individual phases of the gait.

Advanced gait training should continue to emphasize selective movement control and normal timing. Gait can be practiced forwards, backwards, sideways, and in crossed pattern (braiding) (Figure 12.32). Elevation activities (stair climbing, step over step; over and around obstacles) and community activities (on different terrains) should also be practiced. Timings can be improved through the use of resisted progression technique, stimulating music, or a treadmill. At this point

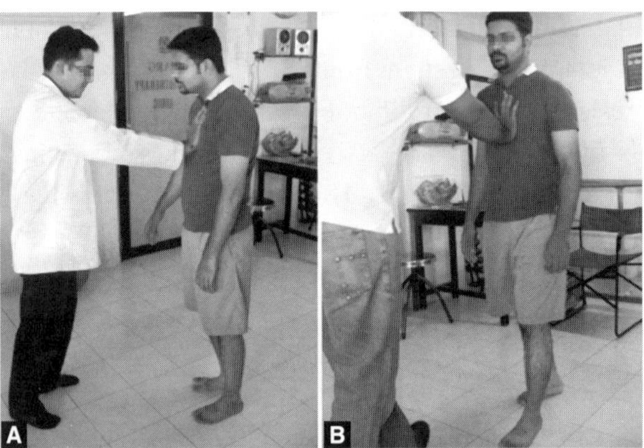

FIGURES 12.31A and B: Reisisted walking with one hand, left hemiplegia, note facilitation of dorsiflexion of ankle on affected side in Figure B

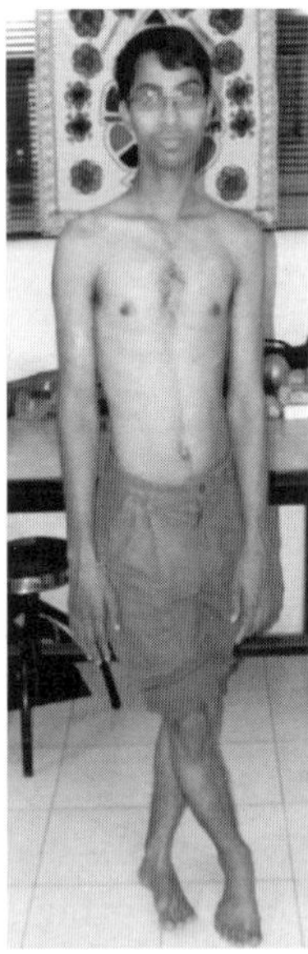

FIGURE 32: Braiding, crossing one leg in front of other leg while walking, right hemiplegia

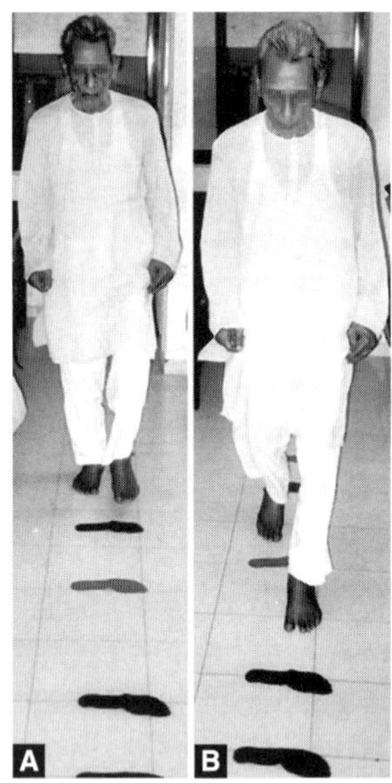

FIGURES 12.33A and B: Pattern walks for training coordination of step length

in recovery, the patient should be able to monitor his or her own performance and reorganize and initiate corrective actions. The patient should be able to vary speed of walking and maintain performance while confident walking in all types of situations likely to be encountered in daily life. For training steps length, various marks on the floor can be made and the patient is asked to walk according to them. For an example, foot marks are placed which are at an appropriate distance with each other and the patient is asked to place the foot right on them. This activity can be made more challenging by altering the distance between the marks frequently (Figure 12.33).

In many cases, the basic structure of the patient's lower limbs are not stable to carry out complete weight bearing on the lower limbs. Orthopedic injuries or previous surgeries to the back or lower limbs may cause instability of the lower limbs. Neurological involvement like stroke decrease the motor control of the muscles and hence, more strain occurs on the ligaments. Thus, modification

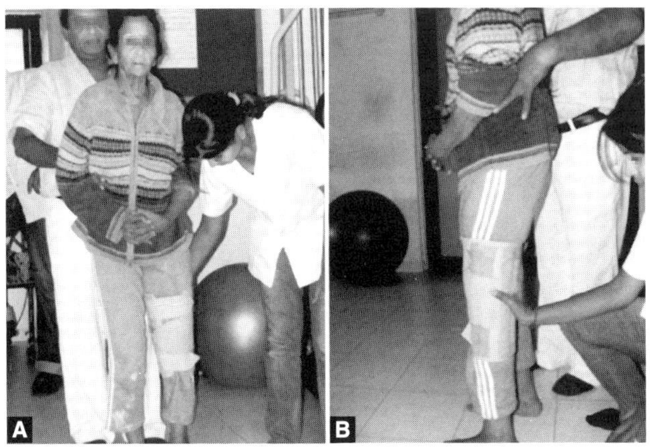

FIGURES 12.34A and B: Use of an AKBK splint in a patient with TKR, left hemiplegia

of activities has to be carried out and a patient specific customized approach is carried out.

Figures 12.34A and B show an elderly female patient with left-sided hemiplegia. She had undergone total knee replacement surgery before two years of the onset of stroke. Due to these events, there was gross instability of the knee joint and hence, all the weight bearing activites were carried out using an AKBK (above knee below knee) splint which can be seen in Figures 12.34A and B. Apart from the splint, adequate manual support was also provided by the therapist.

The lunges as shown in the Figure 12.35 are a helpful tool in gaining dynamic weight bearing on the lower limbs. The patient is asked to keep the trunk stable and erect throughout the movement and weight is shifted on lower limb on one side. The patient stands with both the feet apart and is firstly asked to shift the weight on sound side as it is easier to learn. Once a correct pattern of the lunges is learnt, the therapist asks the patient to lunge on the affected side. Lunges are carried out as low as the patient can maintain. Forward lunges can also be practiced by keeping one leg in front. The forward limb is bent while the back limb is kept extended form the knee. Along with the weight shift forwards on the lower limb, the patient can be asked to reach

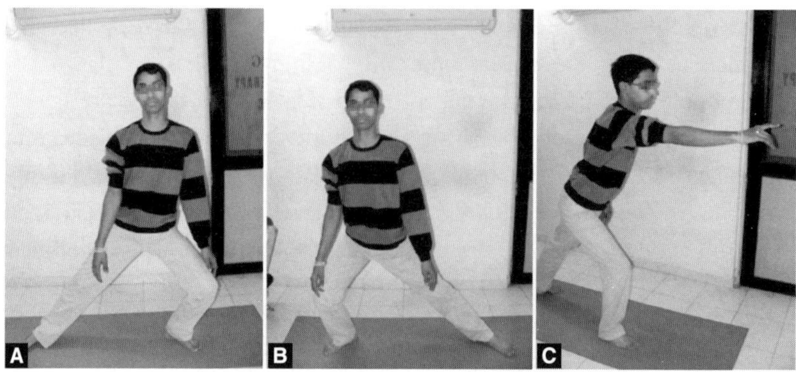

FIGURES 12.35A to C: (A) Lunge to left, right hemiplegia, (B) lunge to right, right hemiplegia, and (C) forward lunge with right leg in front, right hemiplegia

out with the affected upper limb in front which will elicit the response of wrist and fingers extension. Please note the Figure 12.35C.

STAIRS

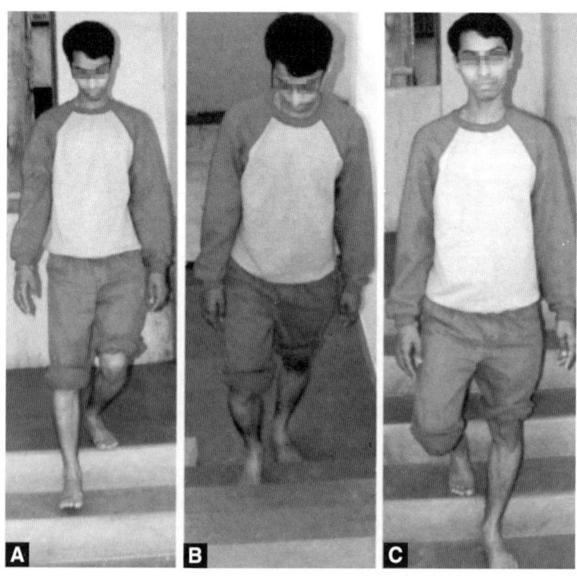

FIGURES 12.36A to C: Stair climbing, unsupported, right hemiplegia

Climbing stairs at an early stage, even before independent gait is achieved, is both therapeutic and functional. The patient is taught to perform the activity in a normal manner, i.e. one foot on each step and without the support of the hand-rail (Figures 12.36A to C).

Ascending

In the early stage, it may be necessary for the therapist to lift the affected leg on to the step rather than allowing the patient to struggle. Support the affected knee as steps are taken with the sound leg and keep the weight forward. The therapist can hold the patient from pelvis by remaining on the affected side by one hand and by the other hand can control the affected lower limb from the knee joint. As said earlier, the therapist can assist the patient in keeping the affected lower limb on the step. By guiding the pelvis well forwards and at the same time, keeping the affected side knee joint stabilized, the therapist asks the patient to climb up. Snapping of the affected knee joint is prevented by proper stabilization. Rail on unaffected side can be used for support but the patient is not allowed to transfer the weight on sound side completely. The patient can also be taught to climb the step by putting the sound lower limb first. In this activity, the therapist stabilizes the affected lower limb which is supporting the body weight while the sound lower limb is kept on the step. Along with providing adequate support for balance, the patient is asked to keep the sound lower limb very slowly and in a controlled fashion to achieve smooth weight transference on to the affected side. During this activity, the therapist can stabilize the patient's affected side knee joint in few degrees of flexion to prevent hyperextension.

Descending

Guide the pelvis well forward on the affected side as the patient puts the foot down preventing the leg pulling into adduction. The therapist's hand on the patient's knee will give support as steps are taken down with the sound leg. The grip of the therapist on the patient is similar to that during the stair case ascending. While putting the affected lower limb down on the step first, the therapist has to control the hip adduction in addition to the knee control. Care should be taken that the foot lands completely in the middle of the step, as half foot on the step can trigger fear of fall or ankle clonus. While putting the sound lower limb first, the therapist controls the knee, hip and pelvis movements on the affected side till the active eccentric control develops.

DYNAMIC BALANCE ACTIVITIES

Postural reactions are organized in to a limited number of motor strategies or synergies. Patients with stroke typically exhibit delayed, varied, or absent responses. Latency, amplitude, and timing of muscle activity are all characteristically disturbed. It is, therefore, important to proceed slowly in training and to select challenges appropriate for the patient's level of control. The patient's attention should be directed to the appropriate muscle activity and strategies needed to maintain balance. Postural biofeedback provided from standing on a force plate system has been effective in improving balance responses in patients. There are a number of different balance devices currently on the market that can be utilized in training. Finally, safety education on the prevention of falls is a critical factor in ensuring maintenance of the patient's hard-won functional independence.

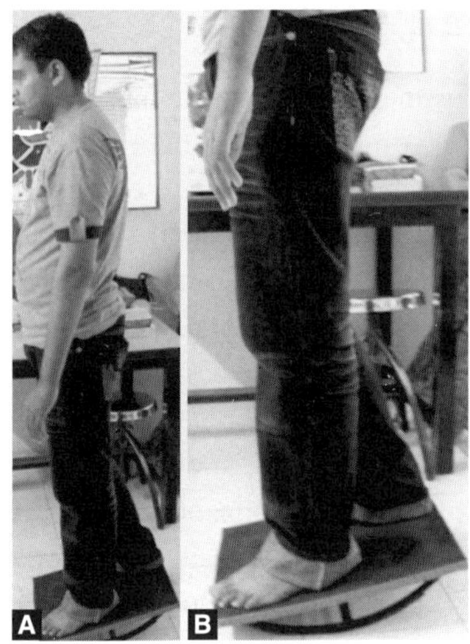

FIGURES 12.37A and B: Forward weight shifts on affected side on tilt board, left hemiplegia

The tilt board is not only essential for treatment but is also most helpful when re-educating correct transference of weight.

The therapist stands on the floor behind the patient and helps to step on to the tilt board with one foot on either side. The patient's feet should be parallel to one another throughout the exercise (Figure 12.37A). Tilt the board slowly from side, pausing at each extreme to correct the patient's position and make sure that the hip comes right above the foot, that the side lengthens and that the pelvis does not rotate (Figure 12.37B).

The therapist should take care that the patient takes full weight on the affected lower limb as this is not possible actively during the acute stage. The therapist assists the pelvis from behind and ensures that hip is extended on the affected side. The back leg which is unaffected will bend from the knee, while the affected front leg remains extended at the knee.

When taking the sound limb in front, the back sided affected leg has to flex from the knee and hence, there is closed chain dorsiflexion at the ankle joint and close chain flexion at the knee which are desired movements.

When doing side to side movements, there is alternate flexion and extension at the knee with alternating weight bearing on each leg. The trunk should follow the limb which has the weight. If this movement is not possible actively, assistance is given by the therapist (Figure 12.38).

When adequate balance is achieved and the patient is able to maintain balance while maintaining posterior pelvic tilt, more dynamic activities like

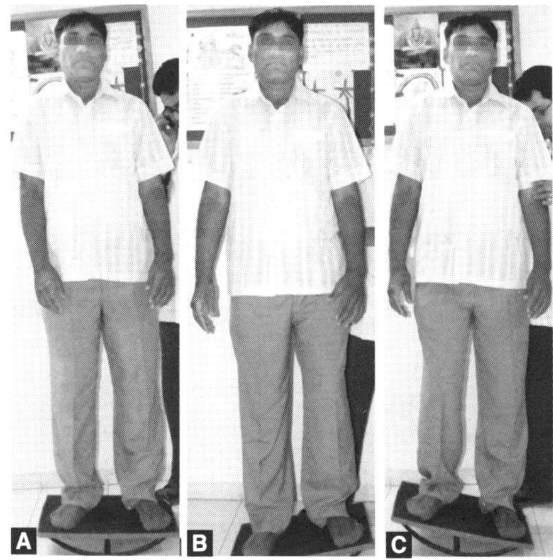

FIGURES 12.38A to C: Weight shifts sideways on both sides on tilt board, left hemiplegia

reaching outs while on the vestibular board can be started. Ball catching and throwing, while on the board will test the skill of the patient tremendously. Care should be taken for the safety of the patient.

Proprioception can be furthermore attenuated by taking the patient on

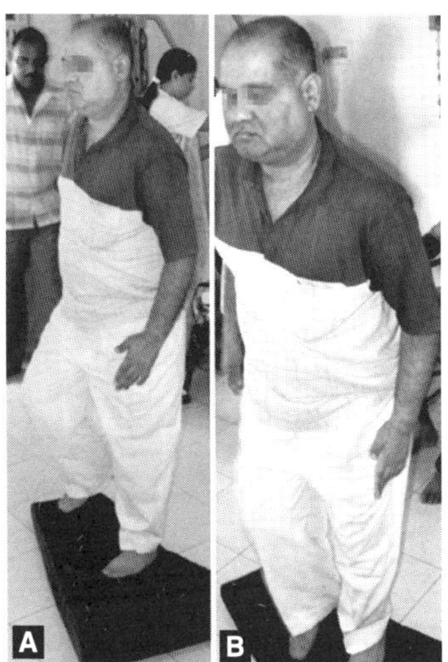

FIGURES 12.39A and B: Marching on a foam wedge with eyes closed, left hemiplegia

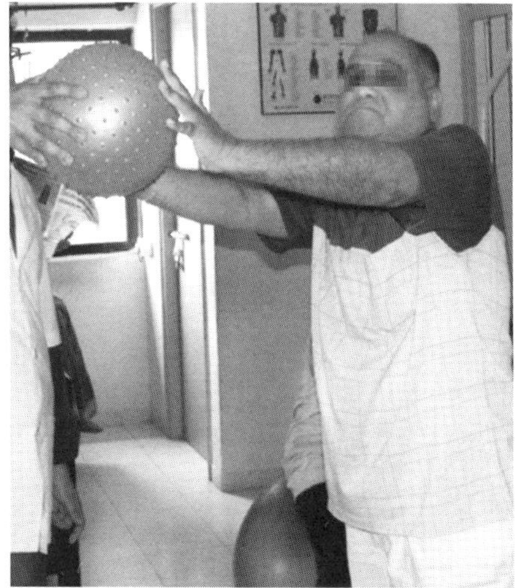

FIGURE 12.40: Reach outs with a ball, on a foam wedge, left hemiplegia

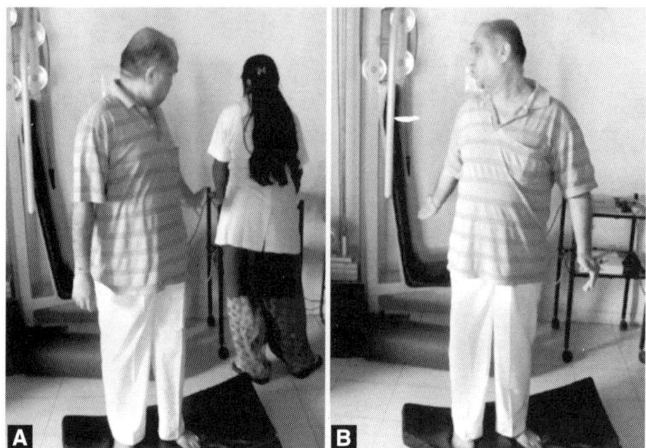

FIGURES 12.41A and B: Trunk rotation with supination of forearm, on foam wedge, left hemiplegia

the foam wedge. The patient is asked to first maintain the balance. Secondly, the patient is asked to do marching on the wedge first with the eyes open and then with the closed eyes. The progression can be made by reaching out activities while the patient is on the foam wedge (Figures 12.39 and 12.40).

While the patient stands on the foam wedge, active rotation of the trunk can be used in eliciting external rotation at shoulder and supination at forearm. The patient is asked to carry out the above mentioned, actively on both the sides (Figure 12.41). Assistance by the therapist in the movements of trunk and upper limb can be given if needed. These activities are carried out in rhythmic fashion.

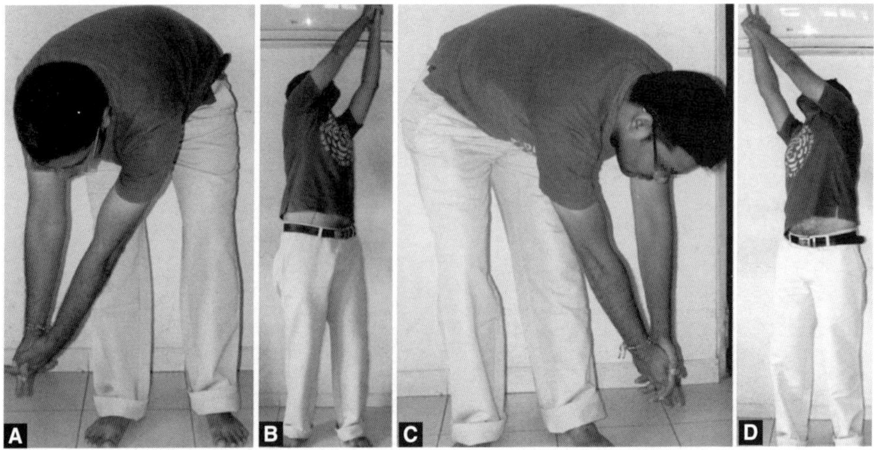

FIGURES 12.42A to D: Wood chopping: (A) Down and to the right, (B) up and to the left, (C) down and to the left and (D) wood copping, up and to the right, left hemiplegia

PNF WOOD CHOPPING

Diagonal patterns of trunk with upper limbs clasped together can be carried out easily in standing. Patient stands erect with equal weight bearing on both the lower limbs with the hands clasped together. The patient is then asked to take both the hands down towards right foot by bending and rotating the trunk towards right side (Figure 12.42A). From this position, the upper limbs are taken up and towards left by extending and rotating the trunk towards left side (Figures 12.42B and C). Similar activity can be performed on other side also (Figure 12.42D). Throughout the movement, patient's head and neck moves in the direction of the motion and the eyes follow the moving upper limbs. If the patient is unable to flex the trunk completely with knee in extension due to soft tissue tightness, flexion of the knee can be allowed. This activity strengthens the trunk musculature as well as stretching of tight structures of the trunk is duly carried out. The affected upper limb moves in a reflex inhibiting posture and hence, spasticity is reduced. As a progression of this exercise, the patient may hold a ball in both the hands rather then clasping. All these movements can be resisted manually by the therapist by either applying pressure over the moving clasped hands or on the moving trunk. This activity is also used in strengthening the stabilizers of scapula like serratus anterior and also helps in improving dynamic balance reactions. It should be noted by keeping both the knee slightly flexed, eccentric contraction of the stabilizers of the lower limb are carried out.

UPPER LIMB ACTIVATION

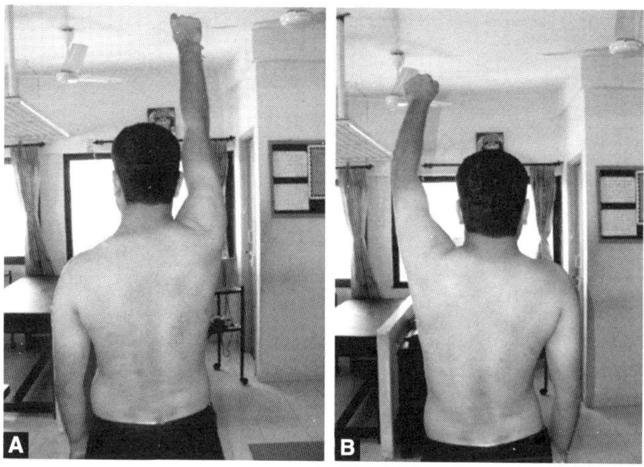

FIGURES 12.43A and B: (A) Raising sound upper limb and (B) raising affected upper limb, left hemiplegia

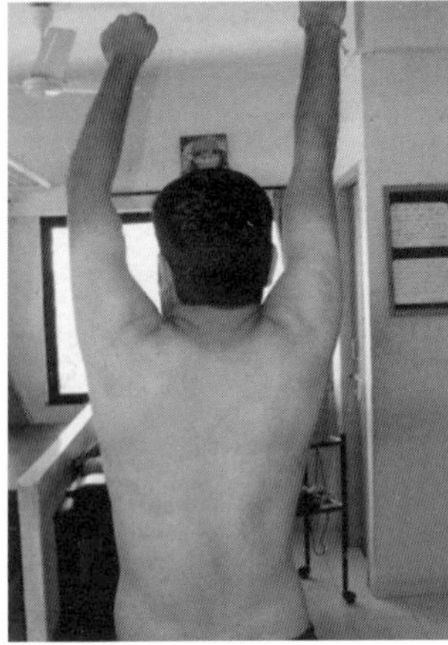

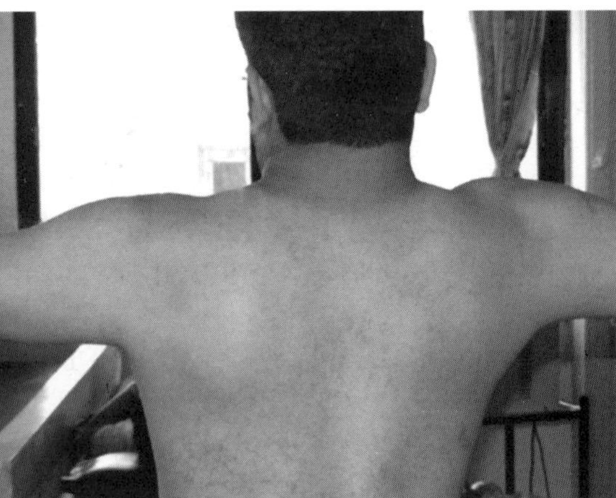

FIGURE 12.44: Bilateral elevation of both the upper limbs, note movement of scapula on both sides, left hemiplegia

FIGURE 12.45: Bilateral abduction of both upper limbs, note the movements of scapula on both sides, left hemiplegia

All the movements of the upper limb, especially that of scapula and shoulder can be checked and treated in standing position for the ease of application. Any assessment which needs to be carried out is done by proper exposure of the part. As shown in Figures 12.43A and B, the left side of the patient is affected side and proper observation alone can show the abnormality of the motion if any. Figure 12.43B shows the exaggerated outward rotation of scapula with protraction on the affected left side. Due to this reason, the head of the humerus fails to align with the glenoid cavity at optimum level and hence, full range of shoulder flexion and abduction is not gained. Figure 12.44 shows the dynamic alignment fault while attempting to raise both the upper limbs.

Winging of the scapula on the left side can easily be seen when the patient attempts active abduction of both shoulders. On the right side, proper alignment of the scapula can be noted.

After studying the abnormal motion on the affected side, the therapist can treat the disorder by fixing the scapula and aligning it to the thoracic cage. This can be done passively in the initial stage of treatment and later on, active fixation can be achieved by contraction of the muscles which stabilize the scapula. The therapist should not fix the scapula in a specific position while the arm is in motion , but rather the therapist assists the normal biomechanical scapular motion dynamically (Figure 12.45). As seen in the above case, if the motion of the scapula on the affected side is exaggerated at two levels, i.e. outward rotation and protraction, then the therapist fixes the scapula from start of the movement and asks the patient to raise the arm. All throughout the movement, the therapist stabilizes the scapula so that the outward rotation and protraction doesnot occur more than that of the normal side, and allowing the scapula to move normally in the entire range of motion. The therapist can also assist the movements if active contraction of the scapular muscles fails to produce desired movements.

The above explained activity can be done in any part of the body with proper understanding of the biomechanics and kinesiology. Comparing the movement to that of the normal side is the best guide for the therapist. To

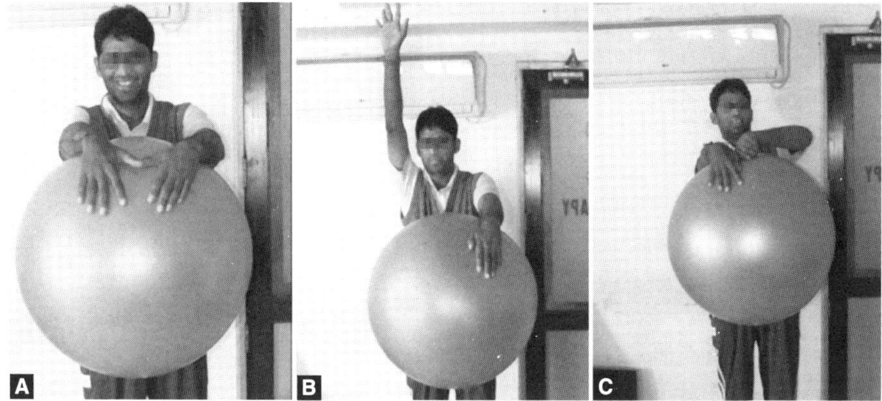

FIGURES 12.46A to C: (A) Holding a ball in front with both upper limbs, (B) holding the ball with affected upper limb, and (C) holding the ball with sound upper limb while the affected upper limb is tried to elevate, left hemiplegia

maintain the corrected position, scapula can be taped adequately.

The patient stands erect with a ball of optimum size held in front of the body with both the upper limbs as shown in Figure 12.46A. This activity decreases the tone of the spastic muscles on the affected side. This activity is a bilaterally symmetrical pattern of activity and hence, activity on the affeccted side will be enhanced in accordance with the movement on the sound side.

As the patient becomes comfortable in this position, the sound upper limb can be raised upwards while the affected upper limb holds the ball against the body as shown in Figure 12.46B. The patient is then asked to lift the affected upper limb upwards while the sound limb holds the ball. Note that the affected side is left in Figures 12.46A to C. Also note that even though motor control on the affected left side is inadequate to produce sufficient movement, the same affected limb can hold the ball alone without the support

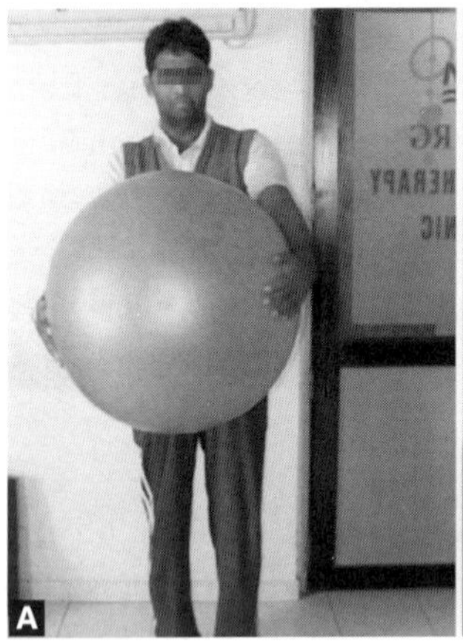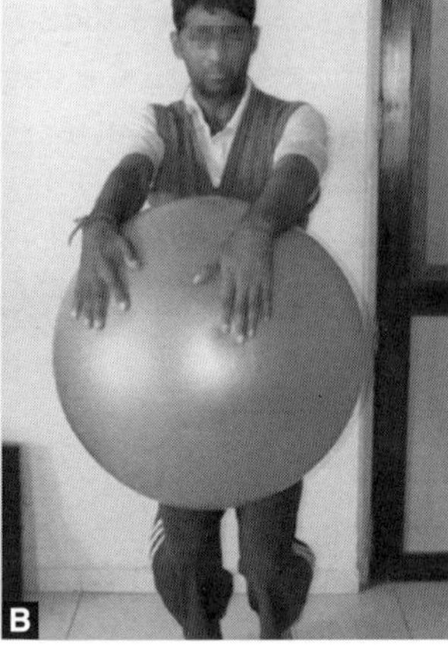

FIGURES 12.47A and B: (A) Holding a ball with upper limbs on side, left hemiplegia, and, (B) squats while holding a ball, left hemiplegia

of the sound upper limb. As the motor control of the upper limb develops, the ball can be held with the upper limbs kept sideways on the ball as shown in Figure 12.47A. This requires supination of forearm and external rotation of the shoulder. Ball can be moved sideways to the right and to the left with the rotation of the trunk. It should be noted that during all these activities, head and neck should be straight, shoulders should be in line, abdominal and gluteal muscles contracted for posterior pelvic tilts, and weight bearing should be equal on both the lower limbs (Figure 12.47B). Mini or half squats can be performed with the ball in the hand which improves the muscle control of the entire body.

Dynamic tasks such as catching or kicking a ball challenge balance and include the added challenge of anticipatory timing. These tasks also redirect the patient's attention to a task at hand rather than on balance itself, thus testing the automaticity of postural responses. The patient can bounce the ball on the ground and catch it with both the hands which elicits a response of wrist and fingers extension. If during initial stages or due to spasticity, patient is unable to open up the fingers, the therapist assists the affected side wrist and fingers extension.

It can be noted from Figures 12.48A and B that the affected side is the right side. Even with partial amount of motor control, the patient can perform this task with concentration.

Ball catching activity in standing is an enjoyable activity for the patient, which trains eye-hand coordination, upper limb motor control, bilateral activities of upper limbs, and dynamic balance reactions in functional manner. The therapist can make this activity challenging by throwing the ball at different speeds and in different directions and asking the patient to catch it (Figure 12.49).

Standing position provides dynamic posture for many of the upper limb

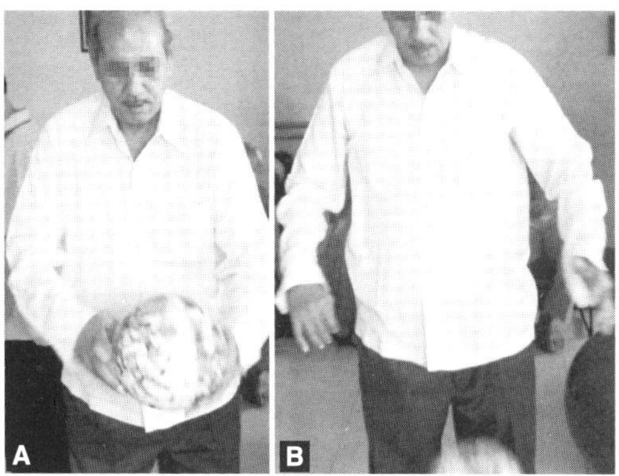

FIGURES 12.48A and B: Bouncing a ball and catching it, right hemiplegia

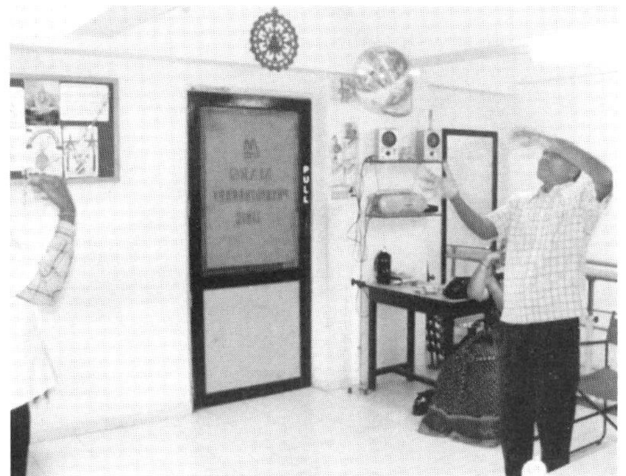

FIGURE 12.49: Catching a ball, left hemiplegia

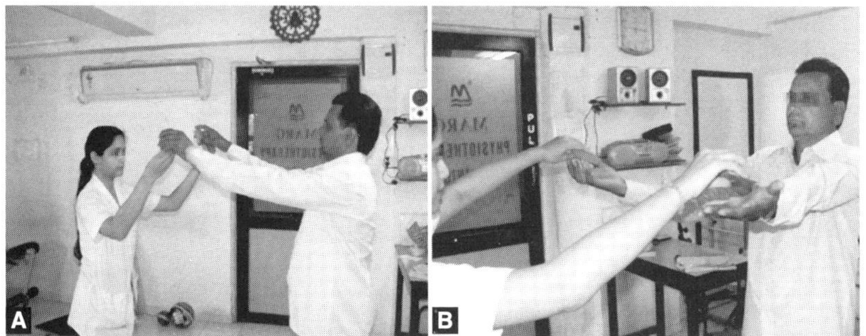

FIGURES 12.50A and B: Grasping objects with both hands at various angles, right hemiplegia

tasks. Figures 12.50A and B shows the training of bilaterally symmetrical upper limb activities which involve holding of objects at various levels of upper limbs. Note the difference between the two Figures, where in one, the hands of the patient are pronated while in other, they are supinated. These activities can also be carried out while the patient is walking, which adds

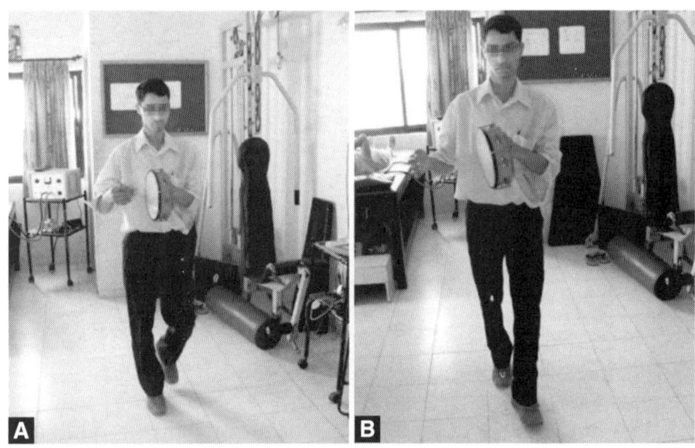

FIGURES 12.51A and B: (A) Walking forwards while beating a drum and (B) walking backwards while beating a drum, right hemiplegia

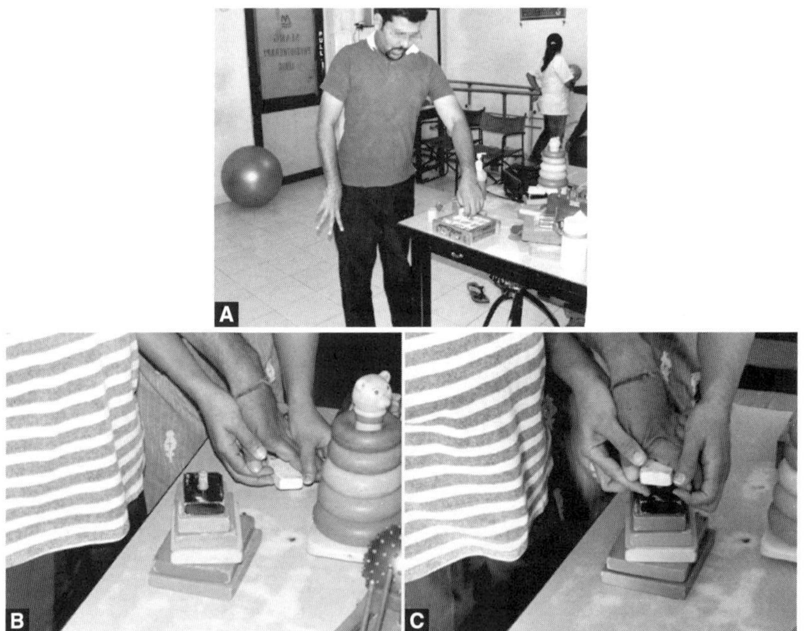

FIGURES 12.52A to C: Various hand functions in standing position

a dynamic component to the task and makes it difficult. Catching the ball, tapping the ball on the ground and catching it, beating a drum (Figure 12.51), or clapping while walking are all highly interesting tasks for the patient to perform and increase the skill of movement.

Hand functions to improve dexterity of the fingers can be performed while the patient is in standing position. Figures 12.52A to C show the patient performing hand functions with the affected left hand. Note the associated reaction which can be seen in the sound right upper limb.

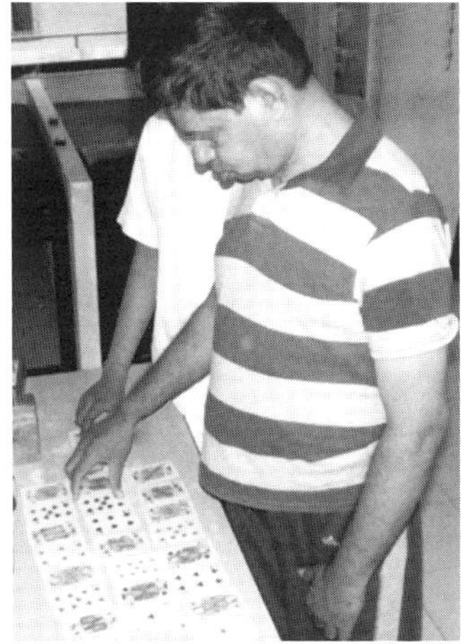

FIGURE 12.53: Arranging playing cards, left hemiplegia

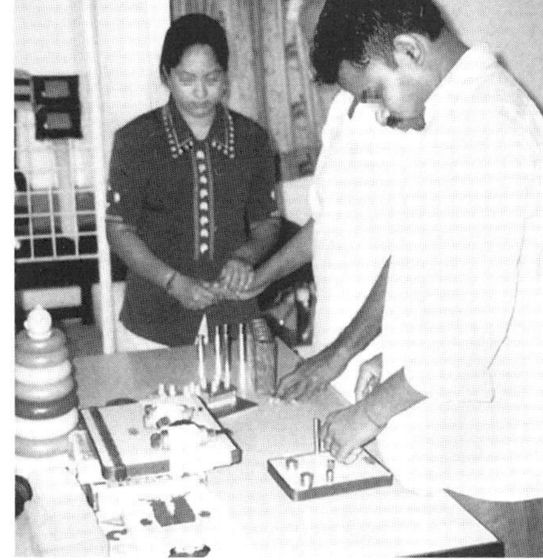

FIGURE 12.54: Hand functions in a group

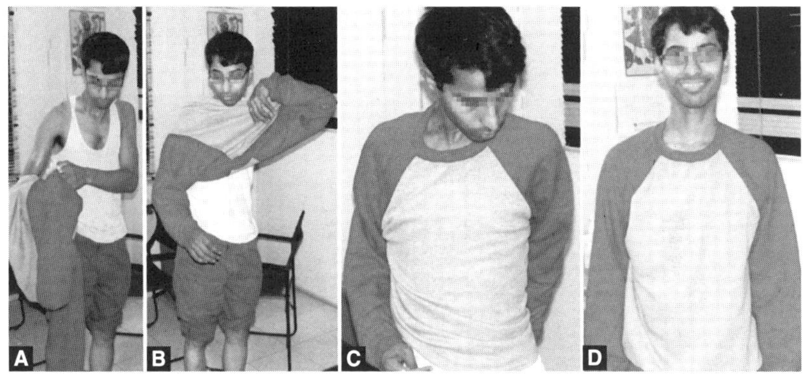

FIGURES 12.55A to D: Dressing up independently, right hemiplegia

Figure 12.53 shows the left-sided hemiplegic patient, arranging playing cards with right hand in standing position. Arranging playing cards numberwise, colorwise or patternwise will train sensory perception. Doing various activities in standing position takes the attention away from the act of standing and yet the patient has to maintain the postural balance in a subconscious way. This activity thus prepares the patient to face the normal environment where standing and walking is a basic need for carrying out various functional activities.

As shown above, guiding may be required in carrying out complex activities of the hand in absence of adequate motor control. Usually, patient may be able to pick up an object actively, while during release of the object, the therapist guides by either opening up the fingers or adjusting the position of the wrist passively (Figures 12.53 and 12.54).

As the recovery progresses, the patient is taught to do the day-to-day tasks independently like the one showed above, dressing up (Figures 12.55A to

D). Other functional activities are practiced till the efficiency of the same is increased. The time taken up for the functional activity is calculated and patient tries to minimize the time consumed for the activity with the higher precision level.

OBSTACLE WALKING

Walking in the normal environmental circumstances require negotiating various hurdles and obstacles, especially in our country. Training of obstacle walking in a clinical set up requires simple tools like a small board to cross over, some stools to go around, a mat to train walking on a soft surface, low height stool to climb on and get down, marked tiles for coordinated steps, etc. Adequate support to the patient is given before the patient can actively negotiate the obstacles. Figures 12.56A and B shows the cross over activity done by a child.

Figure 12.57 shows a young boy with left-sided hemiplegia playing cricket in the clinical set up. On carrying out the activity of choice, motor response

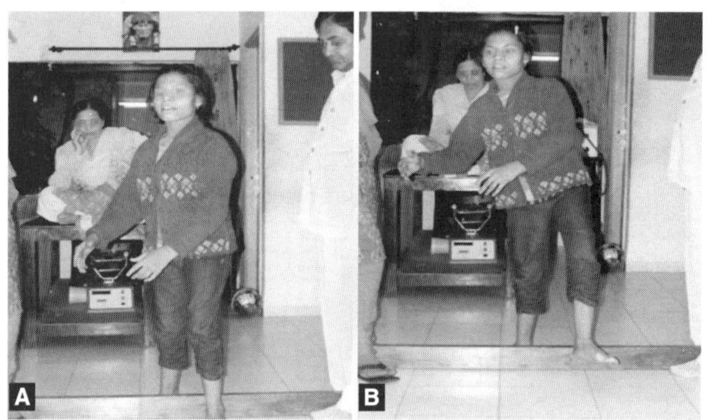

FIGURES 12.56A and B: Crossover walking independently

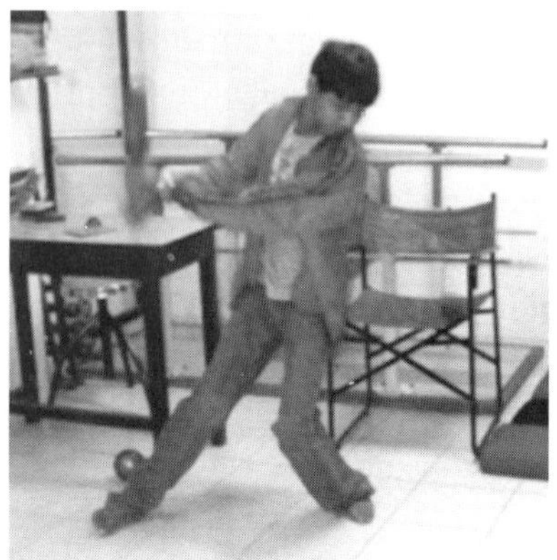

FIGURE 12.57: Playing cricket, left hemiplegia

throughout the body is of the best quality. It also promotes sensory awareness, sequencing of the movements and problem solving. All the patients of various age groups are encouraged to play or carry out activity of their choice, as soon as the physical condition allows.

STRENGTHENING EXERCISES USING RESISTIVE TUBING

Use of a tubing of various resistance levels can be useful for strengthening of the muscles. Although manual resistance provided by the therapist is best in cases of hemiplegia, the tubing or the elastic bands give an ease of application and the patient can perform these activities as a part of home program also once they have mastered it.

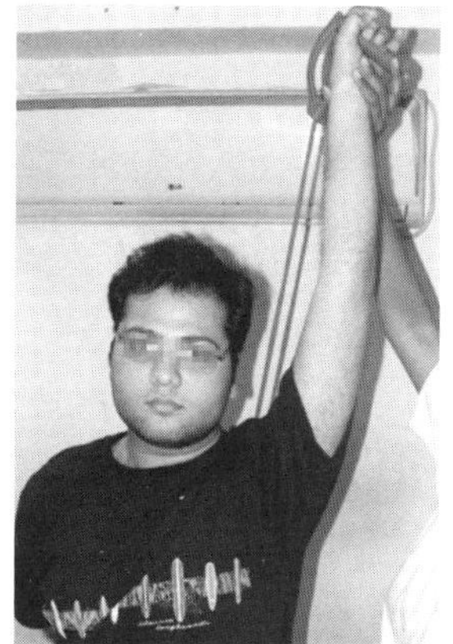

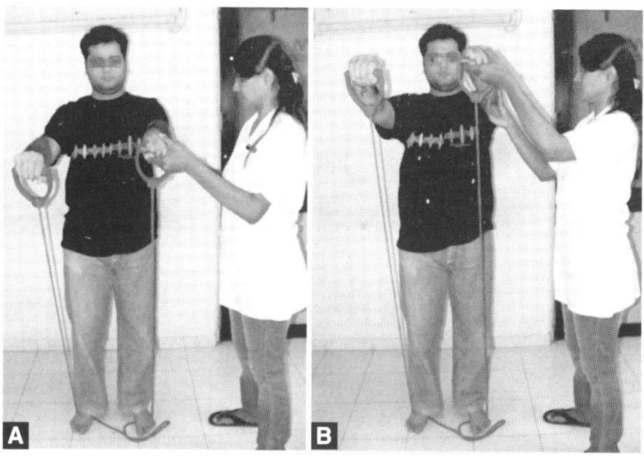

FIGURE 12.58: Resisted triceps workout using a tubing, left hemiplegia

FIGURES 12.59A and B: Bilateral shoulder flexion strengthening using tubing, left hemiplegia

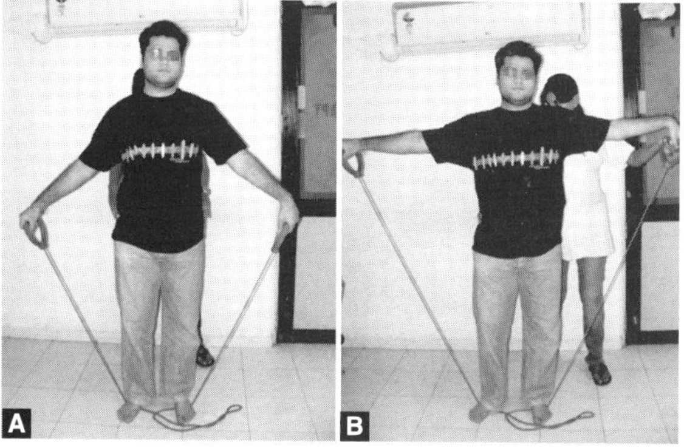

FIGURES 12.60A and B: Bilateral shoulder abduction strengthening using tubing, left hemiplegia

Figure 12.58 shows the resisted workout for triceps muscle on affected left side.

Figures 12.59A and B show the resisted workout of shoulder flexors on both the sides.

Figures 12.60A and B show the resisted workout of shoulder abductors on both the sides.

Figure 12.61 shows resisted workout for a combination of the movements of shoulder flexion, abduction and horizontal abduction on both sides.

In all the above Figures, note that the therapist guides and supports the movements wherever needed. Similarly, resisted activities of many other movements of upper limb, lower limb and the trunk can be performed using an exercise

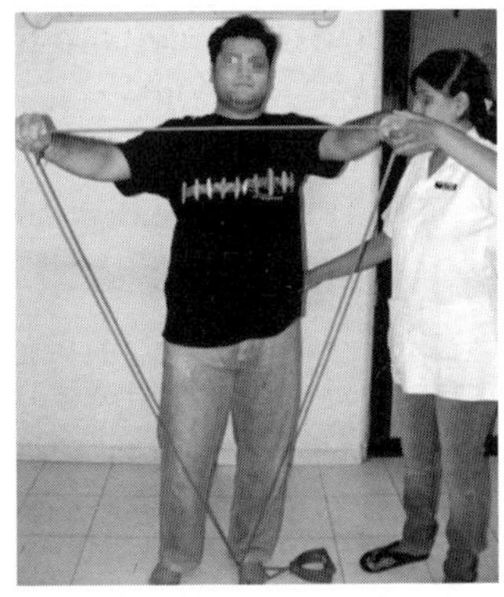

FIGURE 12.61: Strengthening shoulder flexion and abduction, with the use of tubing, left hemiplegia

tubing or an elastic band. All these bands and tubings are available in different resistance levels, and an adequate and optimum one is selected for the patient. Recoil of the elastic material is faster and harder as the resistance level increases and hence, the patient is asked to carry out the exercise smoothly and while returning to the starting position, enough control is maintained.

List of the Muscles which can be Strengthened by Tubing or Elastic Bands Easily

The following is the list of the muscles which can be easily strengthened by the use of elastic bands and tubings. The best position in which this can be achieved is also listed. It is understood that the practicing therapist can modify the position according to the circumstances and needs of the patient.

- Serratus anterior
  - Sitting, standing
- Trapezius upper, middle, lower
  - Prone-lying, sitting, standing
- Latissimus dorsi
  - Prone-lying, sitting, standing
- Subscapularis
  - Side-lying, sitting, standing
- Infraspinatus
  - Side-lying, sitting, standing
- Supraspinatus
  - Standing
- Teres major and minor

- Side-lying, sitting, standing
- Rhomboids major and minor
  - Sitting, standing
- Pectoralis major and minor
  - Supine-lying, sitting, standing
- Deltoid—all fibers
  - Supine-lying, side-lying, sitting, standing
- Biceps, brachialis, brachioradialis
  - Supine-lying, sitting, standing
- Triceps
  - Sitting, standing
- Long flexors of wrist and fingers
  - Sitting
- Long extensor of wrist and fingers
  - Sitting
- Abdominals including the obliques
  - Sitting, standing
- Iliacus and psoas major
  - Supine-lying, sitting, standing
- Gluteus maximus
  - Prone-lying, supine lying, standing
- Gluteus medius
  - Supine-lying, standing
- Adductor magnus, longus and brevis
  - Supine-lying, standing
- Hamstrings
  - Prone-lying, sitting, standing
- Quadriceps
  - Supine-lying, sitting, standing
- Gastrocnemius and soleus
  - Half-lying, long sitting, sitting
- Peroneus longus and brevis
  - Half-lying, long sitting
- Tibialis anterior and posterior
  - Half-lying, long sitting.

ADVANCED FUNCTIONAL TRAINING

Functional walking in the external environment effectively boosts up the confidence of the patient. The patient can be taught to drive the vehicle which is feasible. Gradually, all the activities are trained by the therapist and should be practiced well by the patient to achieve functional independence.

To increase the muscle strength after the spasticity has significantly reduced and motor function has improved, gymnasium activities can be started (Figures 12.62 and 12.63). Care should be taken not to overdo the exercises as they can increase spasticity and can produce injury. These activities are always carried out under strict supervision of a physiotherapist. Swimming can be started as it is a wholesome exercise. It is easier if the patient had already learned swimming in premorbid state. Learning swimming after hemiplegia can be a challenging task. Nevertheless, it can be learned and practiced safely in a controlled environment like shallow water.

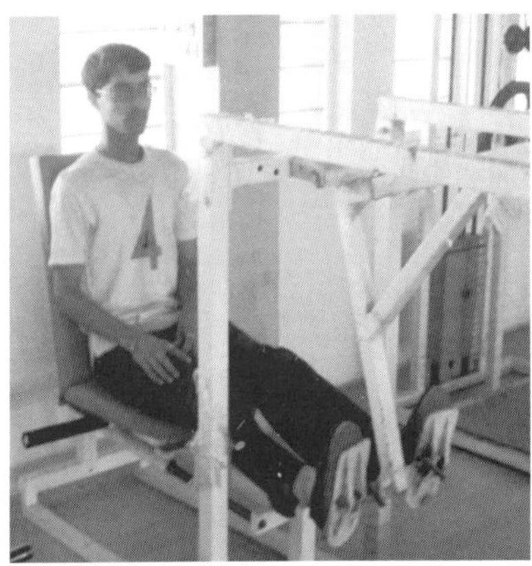

FIGURE 12.62: Gym activities, right hemiplegia

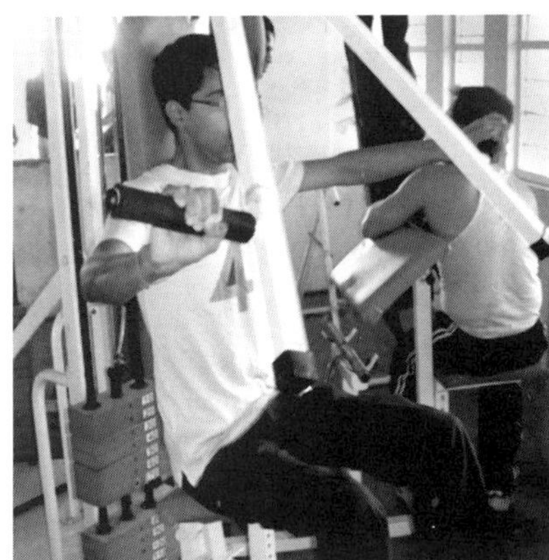

FIGURE 12.63: Gym activity for increasing strength, right hemiplegia

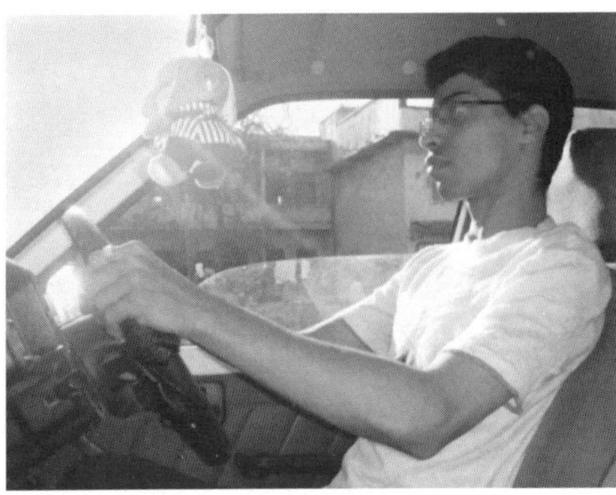

FIGURE 12.64: Driving a car, right hemiplegia

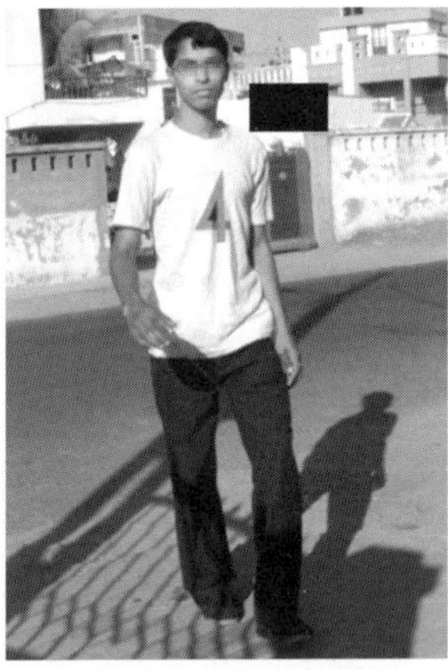

FIGURE 12.65: The normal walk, at last!!!

Advanced functional activities like walking on the road and driving (Figures 12.64 and 12.65) can make the patient totally independent and confident for facing the newer challenges posed by the life.

GROUP THERAPY

Hemiplegic patients require prolonged rehabilitation program in most of the cases. Patients go to the physiotherapy and rehabilitation clinics for a long period of time, daily. The exercise sessions may become routine and boring, especially in the chronic phase because of the time taken for the recovery. Many a times, a small amount of improvement will take as long as few months. In such a case, the patients need to interact with other patients to boost the morale and prepare for the time ahead. If the patients of similar recovery are arranged in a group therapy session, all the patients will enjoy the therapy session and the interaction with each other will make the patient fell that they are not alone. In the group, there will be a sense of healthy competition amongst the patients and the patients will try to do their best.

Functional activities and the activities of daily living are best done in a group. The physiotherapist's time will be saved as the patients will monitor each other's progress with zeal and enthusiasm. Patients may play a game or a two during such a session, which will ease out the stress and improve the interpersonal relationships. They make newer friends and the sense of isolation and the fear of nonacceptance in the society will decrease tremendously. The patient will become punctual as the group has to meet at a fixed time and this will stress the importance of time and scheduling in the patient who is physically differently-abled for a long time. The more disabled patients will get help from the more active members and thus, the activities which are designed become easy for each member.

Therefore, the group has a very positive effect on the psyche of the patient and is proved long before that such patients recover faster than the conventionally treated patients in isolation. The group can be formed by the physiotherapist and for forming the group, help from the patients who are coming for a longer duration can be taken. The group can meet in the clinic once a week or as designed by the physiotherapist. Group therapy is valuable tool in the treatment of the patient and should be used extensively but, judiciously for each patient attending the clinic. Even the home visit patients can be called for the group session once a week, as it may not be difficult to bring in the immobile patient in the wheelchair. The patients, who may not be fit for the group, may be the patients who are very old and severely osteoporotic, patients with severe psychiatric problems and patients with active infective disease.

Proprioceptive Neuromuscular Facilitation (PNF) Activities

Proprioceptive neuromuscular facilitation (PNF) activities are extremely useful in treatment of hemiplegia. There are many methods of application by which desired results can be achieved. Some of the very useful techniques are described here.

FLEXION—ABDUCTION—EXTERNAL ROTATION

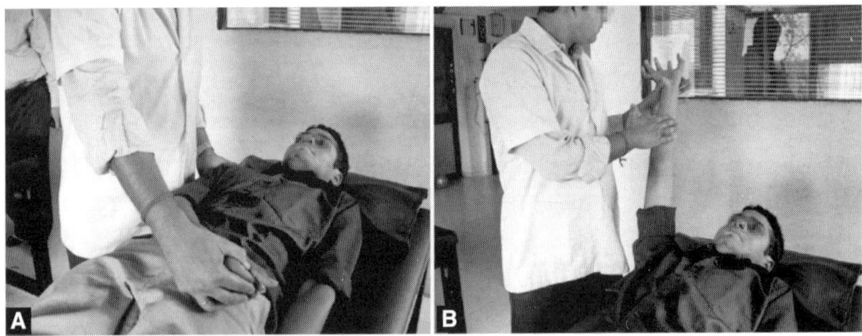

FIGURES 13.1A and B

Joint	Movement	Muscles: Principal components
Scapula	Posterior elevation	Trapezius, levator scapulae, serratus anterior
Shoulder	Flexion, abduction, external rotation	Anterior deltoid, long head of biceps, coracobrachialis, supraspinatus, infraspinatus, teres minor
Elbow	Extended—position unchanged	Triceps, anconeus

Forearm	Supination	Biceps, brachioradialis, supinator
Wrist	Radial extension	Extensor carpi radialis—longus and bravis
Fingers	Extension, radial deviation	Extensor digitorum longus, interossei
Thumb	Extension, abduction	Extensor pollicis—longus and brevis, abductor pollicis longus

FLEXION—ABDUCTION—EXTERNAL ROTATION WITH ELBOW EXTENSION

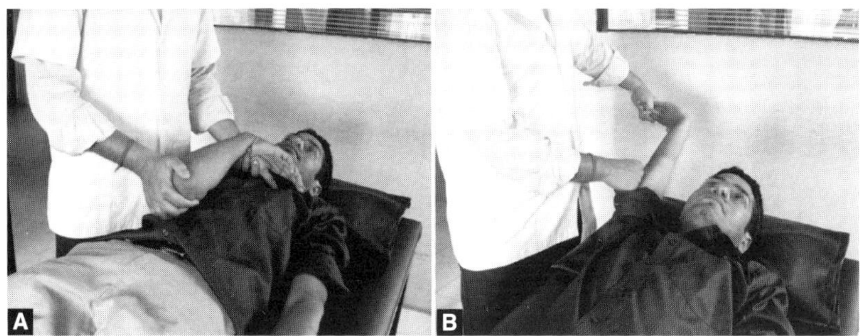

FIGURES 13.2A and B

Joint	Movement	Muscles : Principal components
Scapula	Posterior elevation	Trapezius, levator scapulae, serratus anterior
Shoulder	Flexion, abduction, external rotation	Anterior deltoid, long head biceps, coracobrachialis, supraspinatus, infraspinatus, teres minor
Elbow	Extension	Triceps, anconeus
Forearm	Supination	Biceps, brachioradialis, supinator
Wrist	Radial extension	Extensor digirorum longus, interossei
Fingers	Extension, radial deviation	Extensor digitorum longus, interossei
Thumb	Extension, abduction	Extensor pollicis—longus and brevis, abductor pollicis longus

FLEXION—ADDUCTION—EXTERNAL ROTATION WITH ELBOW FLEXION

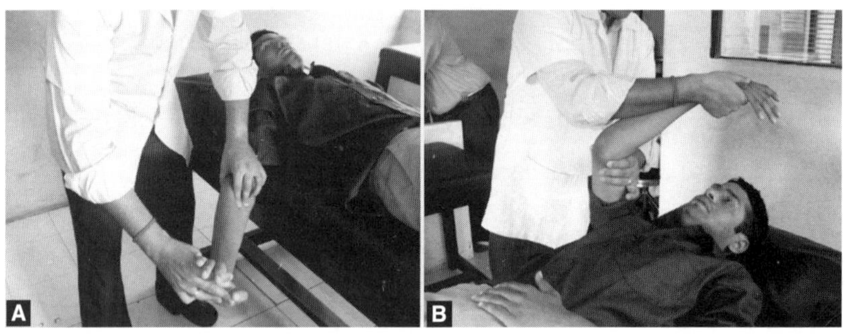

FIGURES 13.3A and B

Joint	Movement	Muscles : Principal components
Scapula	Anterior elevation	Upper Serratus anterior, trapezius
Shoulder	Flexion, adduction, external rotation	Upper pectoralis major, anterior deltoid, biceps, coracobrachialis
Elbow	Flexion	Biceps, brachialis
Forearm	Supination	Brachioradialis, supinator
Wrist	Radial flexion	Flexor carpi radialis
Fingers	Flexion, radial deviation	Flexor digitorum superficialis and profundus, lumbricales, interossei
Thumb	Flexion, adduction	Flexor pollicis longus and brevis, adductor pollicis

FLEXION—ADDUCTION—EXTERNAL ROTATION WITH ELBOW EXTENSION

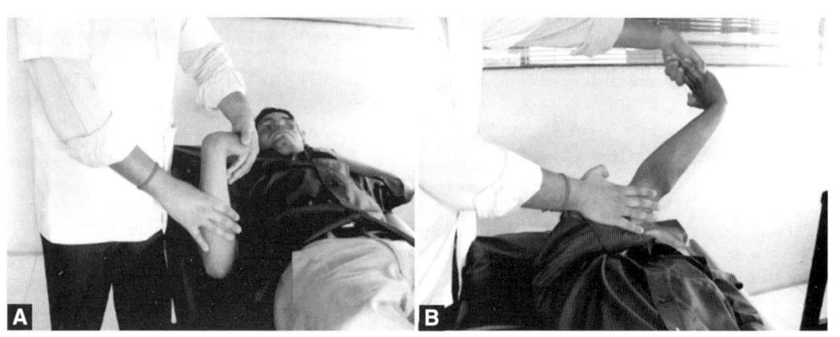

FIGURES 13.4A and B

Joint	Movement	Muscles : Principal components
Scapula	Anterior elevation	Upper serratus anterior, trapezius
Shoulder	Flexion, adduction, external rotation	Upper pectoralis major, anterior deltoid, biceps, coracobrachialis
Elbow	Extension	Triceps, acnoneus
Forearm	Supination	Brachioradialis, supinator
Wrist	Radial flexion	Flexor carpi radialis
Fingers	Flexion, radial deviation	Flexor digitorum superficialis and profundus, lumbricales, interossei
Thumb	Flexion, adduction	Flexor pollicis longus and brevis, adductor pollicis

EXTENSION—ABDUCTION—INTERNAL ROTATION WITH ELBOW EXTENSION

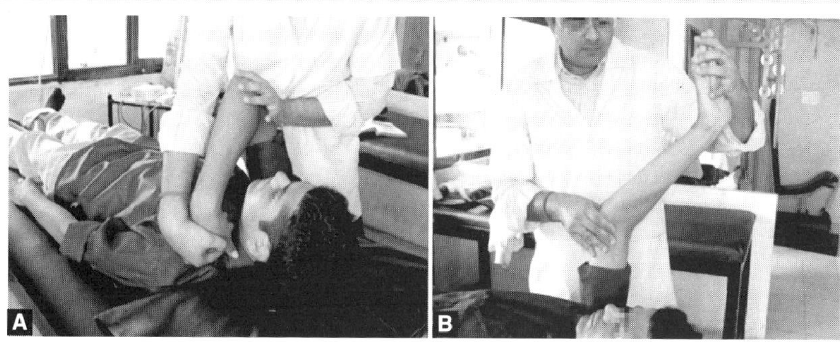

FIGURES 13.5A and B

Joint	Movement	Muscles : Principal components
Scapula	Posterior depression	Rhomboids
Shoulder	Extension, abduction, internal rotation	Latissimus dorsi, deltoid— middle and posterior, triceps, teres major, subscapularis
Elbow	Extension	Triceps, acnoneus
Forearm	Pronation	Brachioradialis, pronator teres and quadratus
Wrist	Ulnar extension	Extensor carpi ulnaris
Fingers	Extension, ulnar deviation	Extensor digitorum longus, lumbricales, interossei
Thumb	Palmar abduction, extension	Abductor pollicis brevis, extensor pollicis

BILATERAL SYMMETRICAL: FLEXION—ABDUCTION—EXTERNAL ROTATION

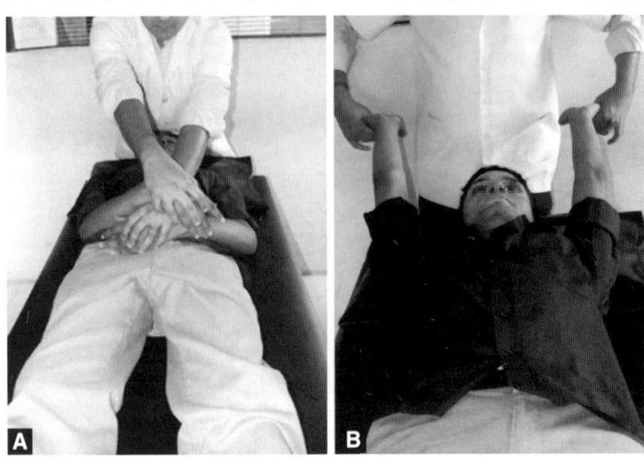

FIGURES 13.6A and B

These movements train upper limbs in a bilaterally symmetrical pattern. The sound upper limb movements reinforce the movements on affected side. These activities are useful in initial stages when motor control is developing.

BILATERAL ASYMMETRICAL: FLEXION—ABDUCTION—EXTERNAL ROTATION WITH THE RIGHT ARM; FLEXION—ADDUCTION—EXTERNAL ROTATION WITH THE LEFT ARM

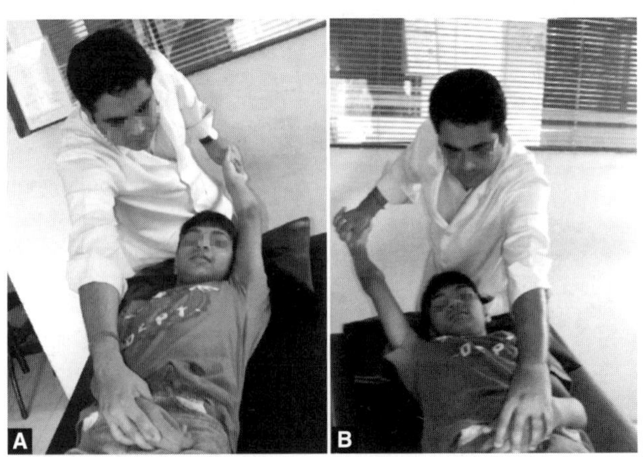

FIGURES 13.7A and B

These movements train upper limbs in bilaterally asymmetrical pattern. They are useful in later stages of recovery to dissociate one limb movements from other.

FLEXION—ABDUCTION—EXTERNAL ROTATION AT END RANGES, LYING PRONE ON ELBOWS

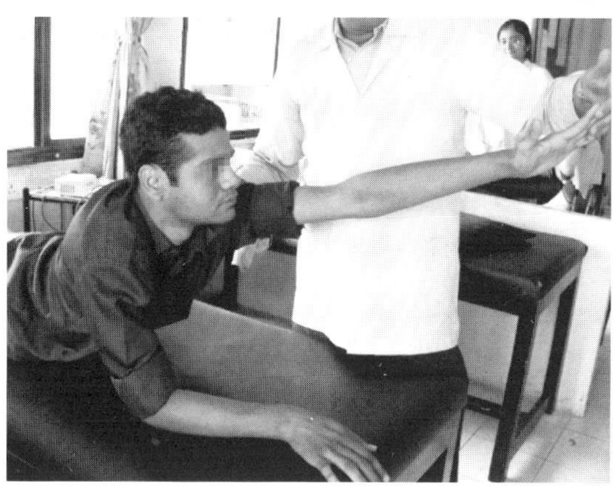

FIGURE 13.8

These activities train weight-bearing on affected side in prone, movements of upper extremity in prone and end range shoulder and scapular motion.

FLEXION—ABDUCTION—INTERNAL ROTATION

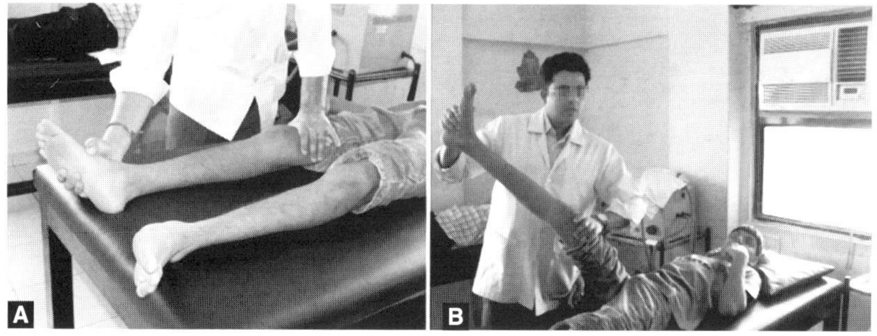

FIGURES 13.9A and B

Joint	Movement	Muscles : Principal components
Hip	Flexion, abduction, internal rotation	Tensor fascia lata, rectus femoris, gluteus medius—anterior, gluteus minimus
Knee	Extended—position unchanged	Quadriceps
Ankle/foot	Dorsiflexion, eversion	Peroneus tertius
Toes	Extension, lateral deviation	Extensor hallucis, extensor digitorum

FLEXION—ABDUCTION—INTERNAL ROTATION WITH KNEE FLEXION

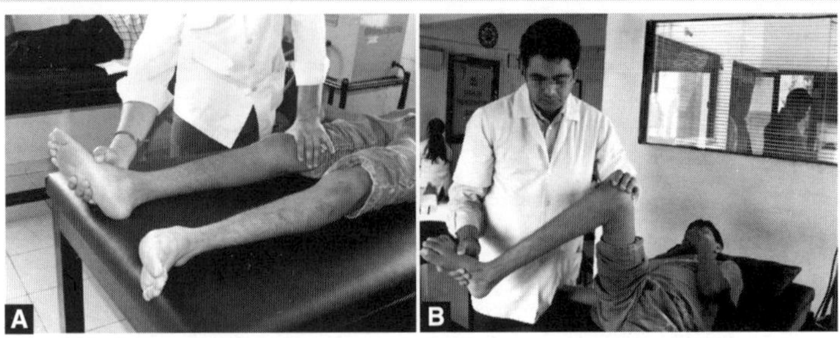

FIGURES 13.10A and B

Joint	Movement	Muscles : Principal components
Hip	Flexion, abduction, internal rotation	Tensor fascia lata, rectus femoris, gluteus medius—anterior, gluteus minimus
Knee	Flexion	Hamstrings, gracilis, gastrocnemius
Ankle/foot	Dorsiflexion, eversion	Peroneus tertius
Toes	Extension, lateral deviation	Extensor hallucis, extensor digitorum

FLEXION—ABDUCTION—INTERNAL ROTATION WITH KNEE EXTENSION

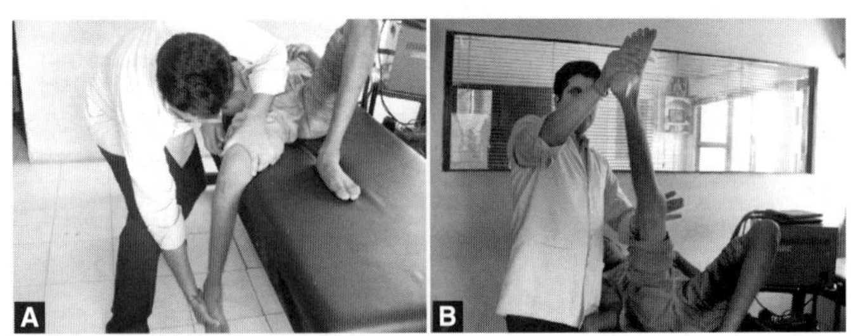

FIGURES 13.11A and B

Joint	Movement	Muscles : Principal components
Hip	Flexion, abduction, internal rotation	Tensor fascia lata, rectus femoris, gluteus medius—anterior gluteus minimus
Knee	Extension	Quadriceps

Ankle/foot	Dorsiflexion, eversion	Peroneus tertius
Toes	Extension, lateral deviation	Extensor hallucis, extensor digitorum

EXTENSION—ADDUCTION—EXTERNAL ROTATION

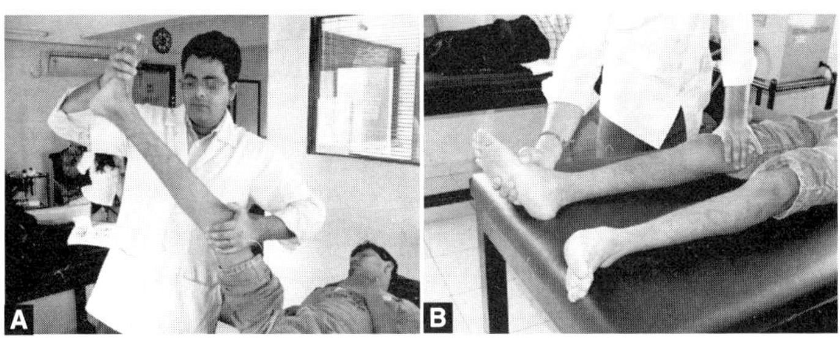

FIGURES 13.12A and B

Joint	Movement	Muscles : Principal components
Hip	Extension, adduction, external rotation	Adductor magnus, gluteus maximus, hamstrings, lataral rotators
Knee	Extension—position unchanged	Quadriceps
Ankle	Plantar flexion, inversion	Gastrocnemius, soleus, tibialis posterior
Toes	Flexion, medial deviation	Flexor hallucis, flexor digitorum

FLEXION—ADDUCTION—EXTERNAL ROTATION WITH KNEE FLEXION

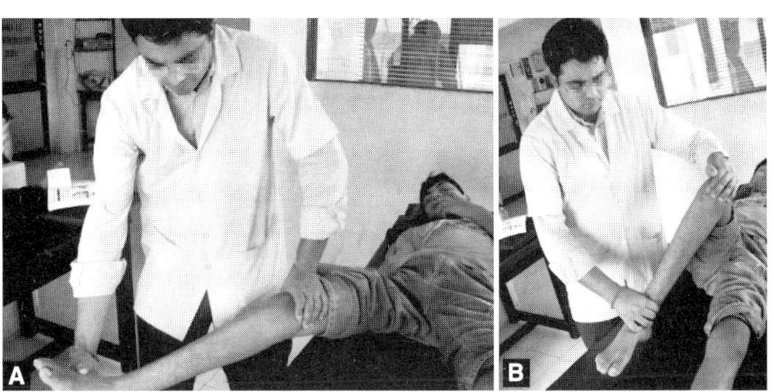

FIGURES 13.13A and B

Joint	Movement	Muscles : Principal components
Hip	Flexion, adduction, external rotation	Psoas major, iliacus, adductor muscles, sartorius, pectineus, rectus femoris
Knee	Flexion	Hamstrings, gracilis, gastrocnemius
Ankle/foot	Dorsiflexion, inversion	Tibialis anterior
Toes	Extension, medial deviation	Extensor hallucis, extensor digitorum

FLEXION—ADDUCTION—EXTERNAL ROTATION WITH KNEE EXTENSION

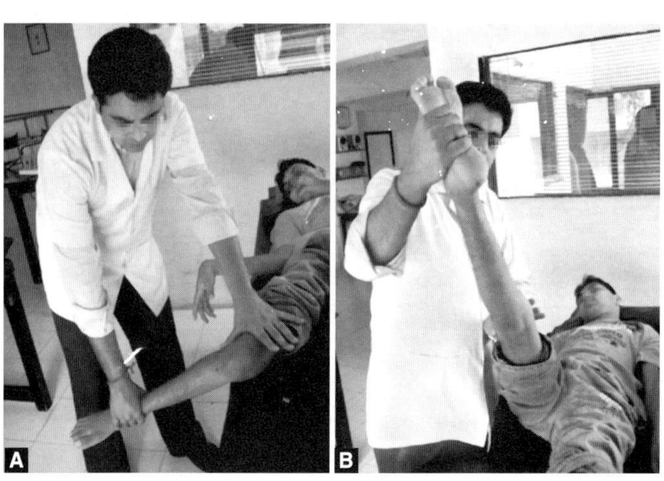

FIGURES 13.14A and B

Joint	Movement	Muscles : Principal components
Hip	Flexion, adduction, external rotation	Psoas major, iliacus, adductor muscles, sartorius, pectineus, rectus femoris
Knee	Extension	Quadriceps
Ankle/foot	Dorsiflexion, inversion	Tibialis anterior
Toes	Extension, medial deviation	Extensor hallucis, extensor digitorum

EXTENSION—ABDUCTION—INTERNAL ROTATION

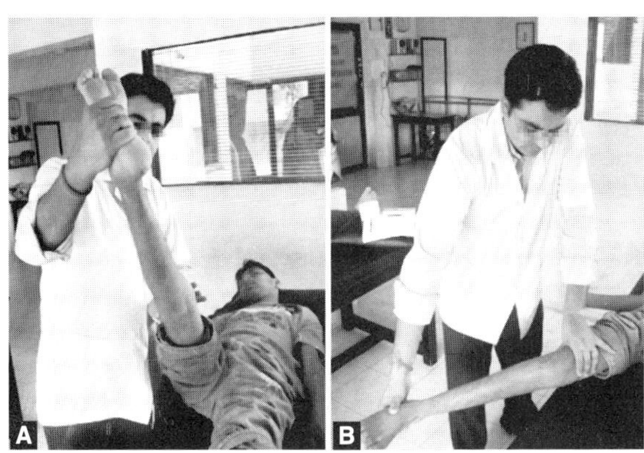

FIGURES 13.15A and B

Joint	Movement	Muscles : Principal components
Hip	Extension, abduction, internal rotation	Gluteus medius, gluteus maximus—upper hamstrings
Knee	Extended—position unchanged	Quadriceps
Ankle/foot	Plantar flexion, eversion	Gastrocnemius, soleus, peroneus longus and brevis
Toes	Flexion, lateral deviation	Flexor hallucis, flexor digitorum

EXTENSION—ABDUCTION—INTERNAL ROTATION WITH KNEE EXTENSION

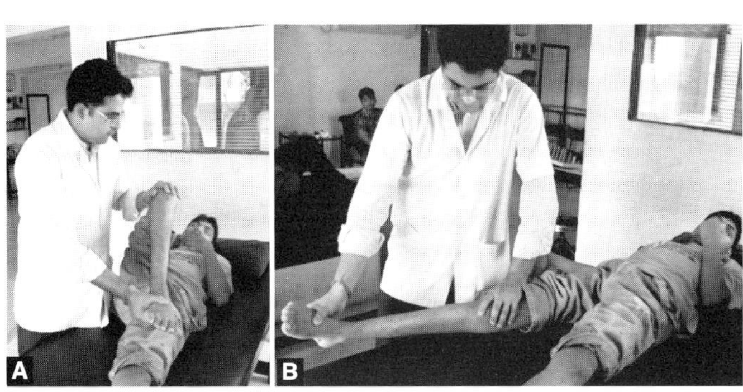

FIGURES 13.16A and B

Joint	Movement	Muscles : Principal components
Hip	Extension, abduction, internal rotation	Gluteus medius, gluteus maximus—upper hamstrings
Knee	Extended	Quadriceps
Ankle/foot	Plantar flexion, eversion	Gastrocnemius, soleus, peroneus longus and brevis
Toes	Flexion, lateral deviation	Flexor hallucis, flexor digitorum

EXTENSION—ABDUCTION—INTERNAL ROTATION WITH KNEE FLEXION

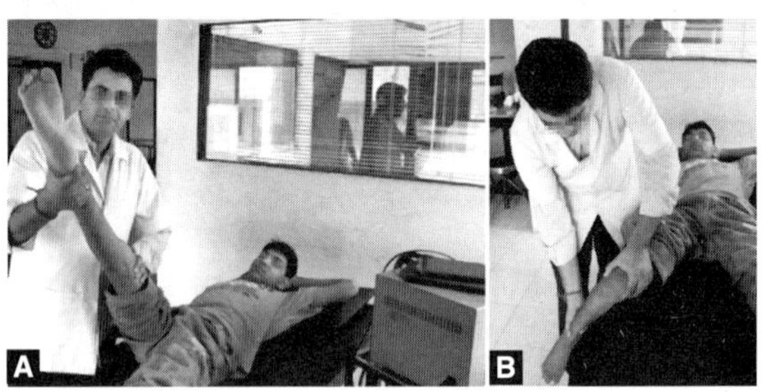

FIGURES 13.17A and B

Joint	Movement	Muscles : Principal components
Hip	Extension, abduction, internal rotation	Gluteus medius, gluteus maximus—upper
Knee	Flexion	Hamstrings, gracilis
Ankle	Plantar flexion, eversion	Soleus, peroneus longus and brevis
Toes	Flexion, lateral deviation	Flexor hallucis, flexor digitorum

BILATERAL SYMMETRICAL LEG PATTERNS: FLEXION—ABDUCTION WITH KNEE EXTENSION IN SITTING

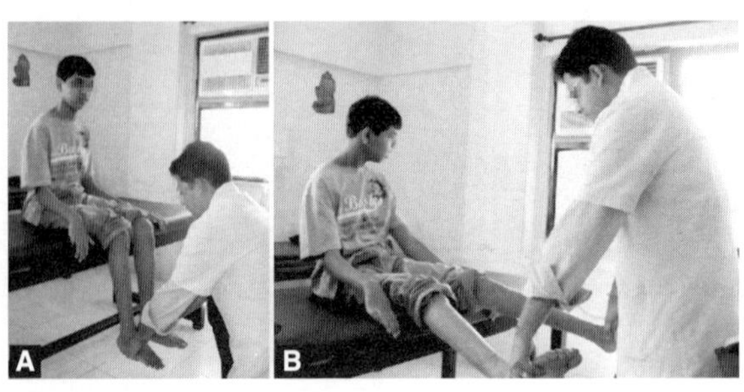

FIGURES 13.18A and B

These activities train lower limbs in a bilateral symmetrical pattern of activity. Mirroring of the movements on the affected side helps in irradiation.

BILATERAL ASYMMETRICAL PATTERNS: FLEXION—ABDUCTION WITH KNEE EXTENSION ON THE LEFT; EXTENSION—ABDUCTION WITH KNEE FLEXION ON THE RIGHT

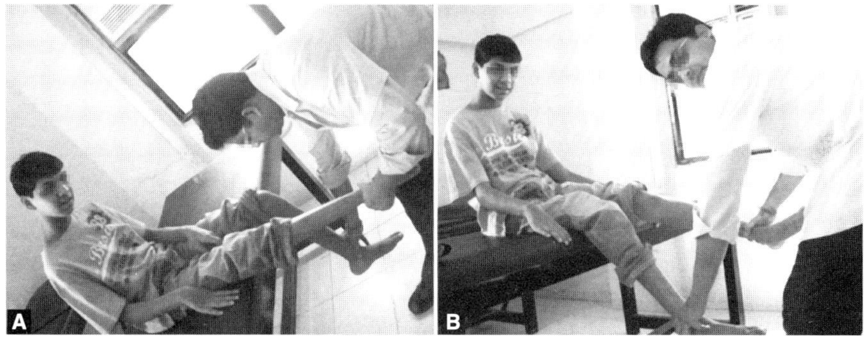

FIGURES 13.19A and B

These activities train lower limbs in bilateral asymmetrical pattern of activity and helps in dissociation of mass movement patterns. It is useful in gait training.

BILATERAL SYMMETRICAL PATTERN IN SUPINE—FLEXION—ABDUCTION

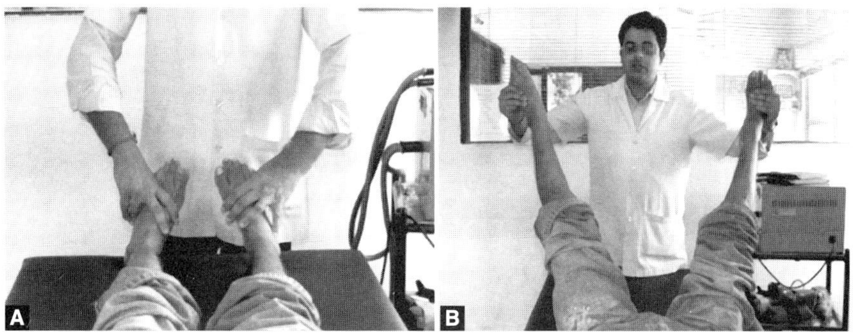

FIGURES 13.20A and B

LEG PATTERNS IN SITTING: EXTENSION—ADDUCTION WITH KNEE FLEXION

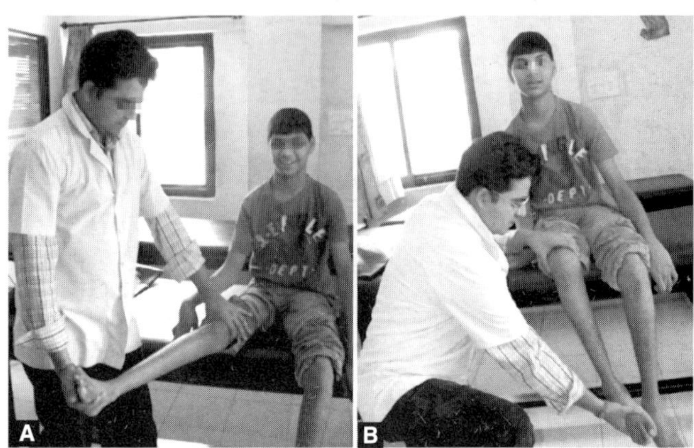

FIGURES 13.21A and B

This activity trains knee extension with dorsiflexion of ankle and knee flexion with planter flexion of ankle. It is useful in walking. Note the position of the hip too.

LEG PATTERNS IN SITTING: EXTENSION—ABDUCTION WITH KNEE FLEXION

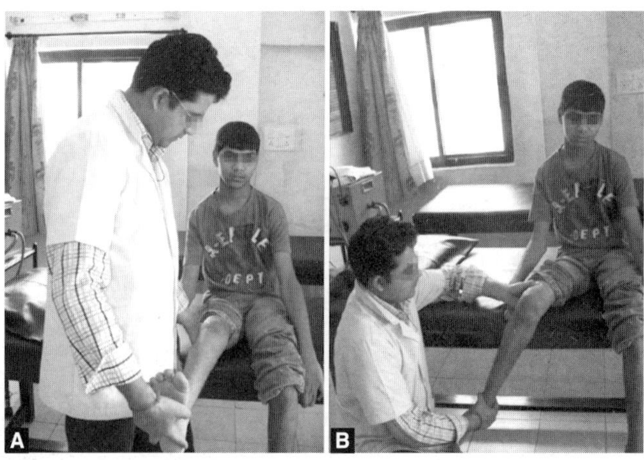

FIGURES 13.22A and B

FLEXION—ADDUCTION WITH KNEE EXTENSION

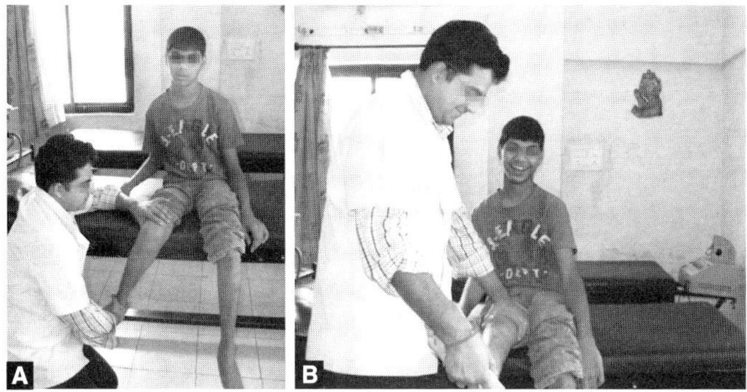

FIGURES 13.23A and B

PATTERNS OF TRUNK

Chopping in Lying

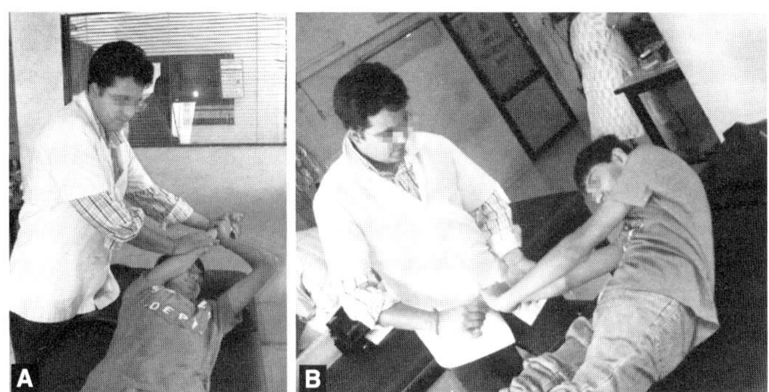

Figures 13.24A and B: Chopping from the left to the right with trunk flexion in lying

Chopping in Sitting

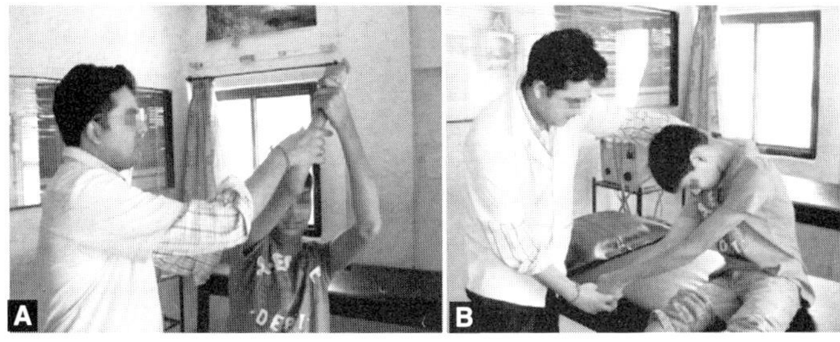

Figures 13.25A and B: Chopping from the left to the right with trunk flexion in sitting

BILATERAL LEG PATTERNS FOR TRUNK IN LYING

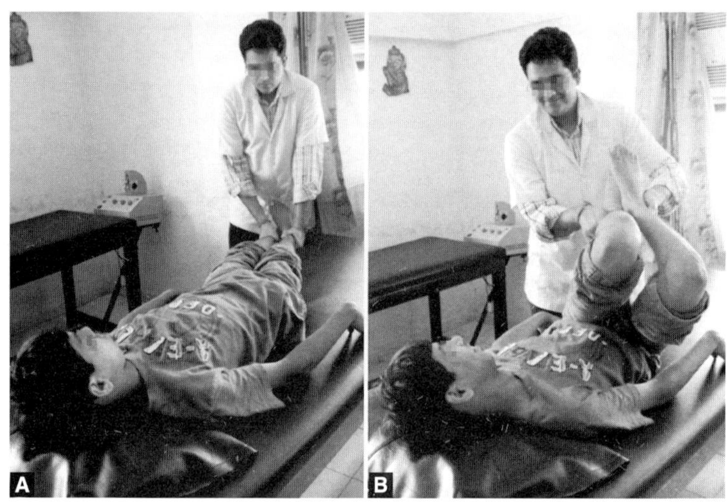

Figures 13.26A and B: Bilateral hip-knee flexion with flexion and rotation of trunk from left to the right side

BILATERAL LEG PATTERNS FOR TRUNK IN SITTING

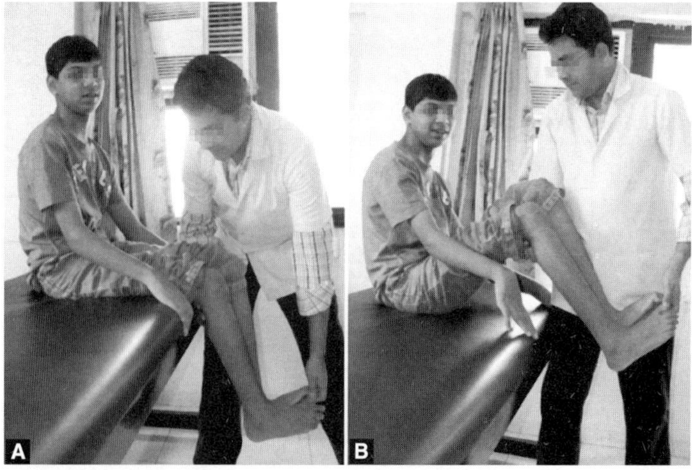

Figures 13.27A and B: Bilateral hip-knee flexion with flexion and rotation of trunk from left to right side in sitting

COMBINING PATTERNS FOR THE TRUNK

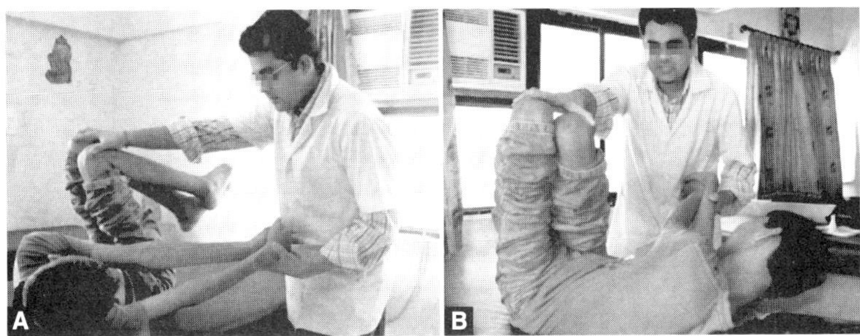

Figures 13.28A and B: Combination of hip-knee flexion with lower trunk flexion and rotation to the left with upper trunk rotation to the right side in lying

RESISTIVE PATTERNS ON MAT

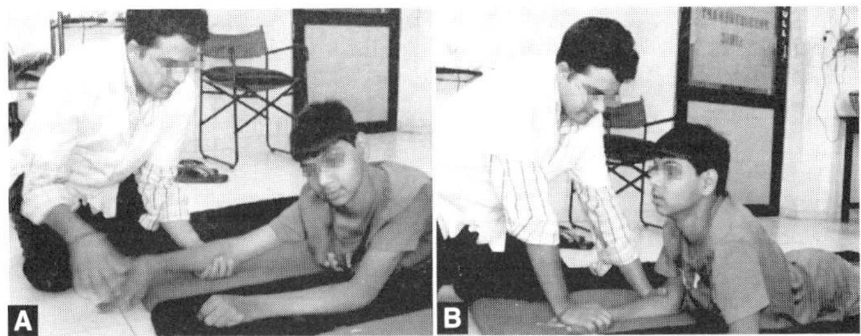

Figures 13.29A and B: Taking prone on elbows, right hemiplegia

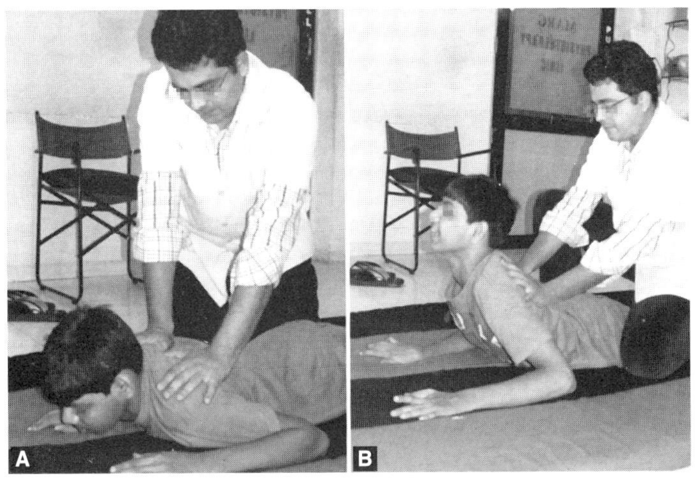

Figures 13.30A and B: Resisting upper trunk extension
Note; Similar resistance can also be applied to pelvis when the patient tries to come on all fours. The resistance provides facilitation to the contracting muscles and hence, quality of movement improves along with the strength

14

Orofacial Rehabilitation

RESPIRATORY AND OROMOTOR ACTIVITIES

Goals of early training include normalizing respiratory, facial, swallowing, and chewing functions. Patients on prolonged bed rest with marked deconditioning, marked paralysis, or dysarthria may experience impaired or shallow breathing patterns. Improved chest expansion can be achieved by effective use of manual contacts, resistance, and stretch to various chest wall segments. Diaphragmatic, basal and lateral costal expansion should be stressed. A pre-speech activity consists of having the patient maintain a vocal expression (e.g.; "ah") during the entire expiratory phase, since poor breath control often contributes to soft or vacillating production of sounds. Respiratory activities should be combined with other movement patterns whenever possible (e.g. inspirations with PNF reverse chop pattern and expiration with chop). During any sustained activity (isometric holding), breath control should be emphasized; the valsalva maneuver should always be avoided. This is especially important in stroke patients with documented concomitant cardiovascular problems.

Facial movements should be encouraged and facilitated whenever necessary. This may include the use of stretch, resistance, or quick ice to stimulate the desired function. Emphasis should be placed on the affected muscles in order to regain a balance of function. The use of a mirror may be helpful in treatment, providing the patient does not have visuospatial dysfunction.

The goals of oromotor retraining are: to improve strength, coordination, and range of oral musculature, to promote normal feeding through graduated resumption of activities, and to promote volitional control through effective verbal coaching. A key element is the attainment of an upright sitting posture with hips well back, symmetrical weight-bearing, and feet flat on the floor.

The head should be erect and in its normal position rather than extended or tipped back. This reduces the chances of aspiration or choking and promotes normal swallowing through appropriate alignment of the necessary structures. If the patient lacks adequate head control, the head should be supported either manually or with supports. Food should be positioned at an appropriate height and distance from the patient and in the patient's visual field. Adapted utensils, plate guards, and non-slip mats can be used to assist in the transfer of food to the mouth. Food should be at first semi-moist, progressing to foods rich in taste, smell and texture, qualities which assist in facilitating the swallowing reflex. Sensation, reflex activity (gag), and breath control are necessary. Facilitation techniques can be used to stimulate the muscles responsible for jaw opening and closing. Jaw movements can be stimulated by vibrating or pressing above the upper lip for closure and under the lower lip for opening. Jaw closure can also be assisted, when necessary, during feeding by holding the jaw firmly closed, using a jaw control technique. Tongue movements can be resisted manually or with a moist tongue depressor. Firm pressure to the anterior third of the tongue can be used to stimulate the posterior elevation of the tongue, necessary for swallowing. Sucking control and saliva production can be stimulated using small amounts of ice water or an ice cube. The therapist can also apply deep pressure on the neck above the thyroid notch to stimulate sucking. Resisted sucking can be promoted using a straw and very thick liquids, or by holding the open end of the straw against the finger. As sucking control proceeds, thinner liquids can be substituted. Patients with a hypoactive gag reflex may be stimulated briefly with a cotton swab to develop this response.

An additional consideration for successful feeding includes management of the environment. The patient's full attention should be directed to the task at hand by using appropriate and consistent verbal cues.

MUSCLES OF FACIAL EXPRESSIONS

While treating the facial muscles, use of the stretch reflex and resistance promotes muscle activity and increases strength. Proper grip and pressure will guide and facilitate the movements. Additional facilitation can be achieved by use of ice. Two to three quick short strokes with ice on the skin, overlying the muscles, on the tongue and inside the mouth facilitate movements. Use of bilateral movements is advocated when exercising the face. Contraction of muscles on the stronger or more mobile side will facilitate and reinforce the action of weaker side. Timing for emphasis, by preventing full motion on the stronger side, will further promote activity in the weaker muscles. The muscles of the face have many functions including facial expressions, jaw motion, protecting the eyes, aiding in speech and assisting in breathing.

The general principles in treatment of face include:

- Gross motions are mass opening and mass closing of mouth
- There are two general areas: The eyes and the forehead, the mouth and the jaw. The nose works with both
- Facial motions are exercised in diagonal patterns
- Bilateral treatment is advocated
- Strong motions in other parts of the body reinforce facial movements. For example, while doing heavy work with hands, facial expression changes
- A functional position is chosen for treating facial muscles
- A mirror can help in giving visual biofeedback.

Frontalis

Command: "Lift your eyebrows up, look surprised, and wrinkle your forehead."

Apply resistance to the forehead, pushing caudally and medially. This motion works with eye opening (Figure 14.1). It is reinforced with neck extension.

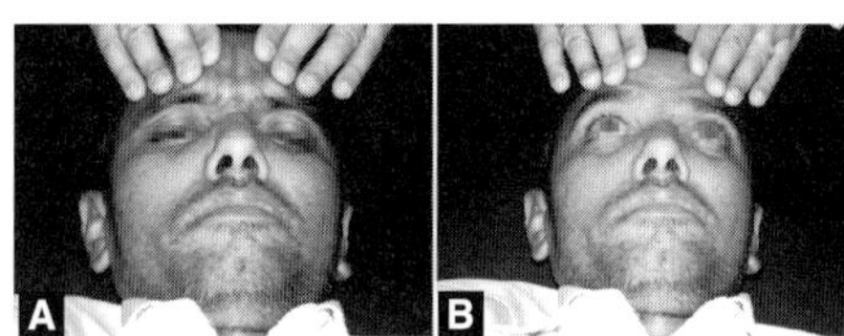

FIGURES 14.1A and B: (A) PNF for frontalis, starting position and (B) PNF for frontalis, end position

Corrugator

Command: "Frown, pull your eyebrows down."

Give resistance just above the eyebrows, diagonally in a cranial and lateral direction (Figure 14.2). This motion works with eye closing.

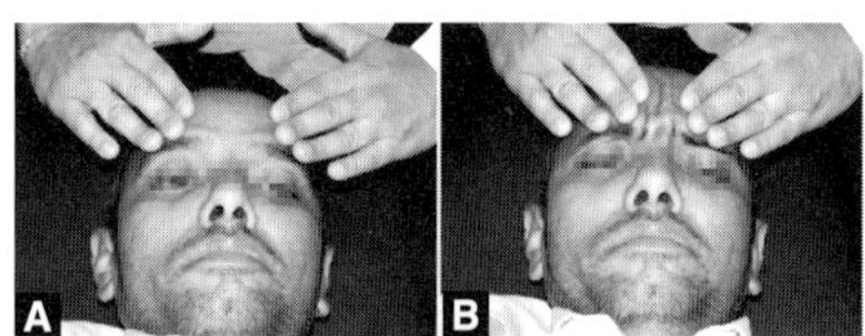

FIGURES 14.2A and B: (A) PNF for corrugator, starting position and (B) PNF for corrugator, end position

Orbicularis Occuli (Upper)

Command: "Close your eyes."

Give gentle diagonal resistance to the upper eyelids. Avoid putting pressure on the eyeballs (Figure 14.3).

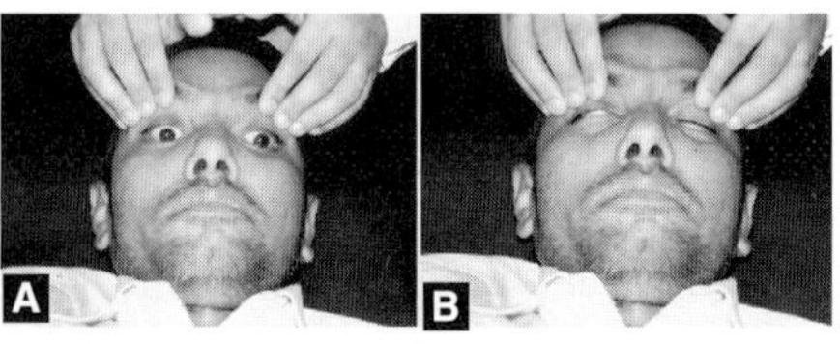

FIGURES 14.3A and B: (A) PNF for orbicularis occuli-upper, starting position and (B) PNF for orbicularis occuli–upper end position

Orbicularis Occuli (Lower)

Command: "Close your eyes."

Give gentle diagonal resistance to the lower eyelids (Figure 14.4). Again avoid putting pressure on the eyeballs.

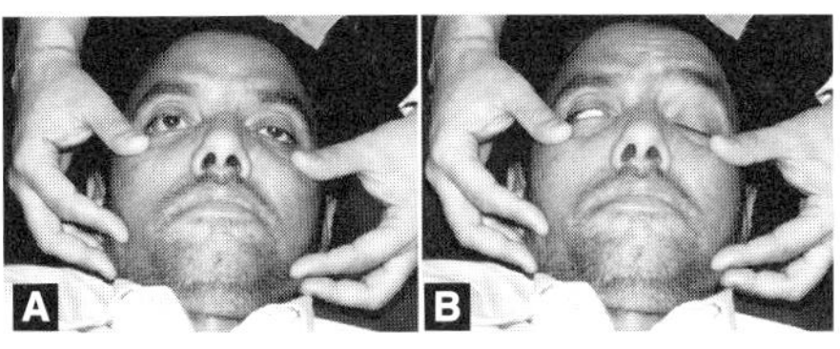

FIGURES 14.4A and B: (A) PNF for orbicularis occuli–lower, starting position and (B) PNF for orbicularis occuli–lower end position

Orbicularis Oris

Command: "Purse your lips, whistle, say 'prunes'."

Give resistance laterally and upwards to the upper lip, laterally and downward to the lower lip (Figure 14.5).

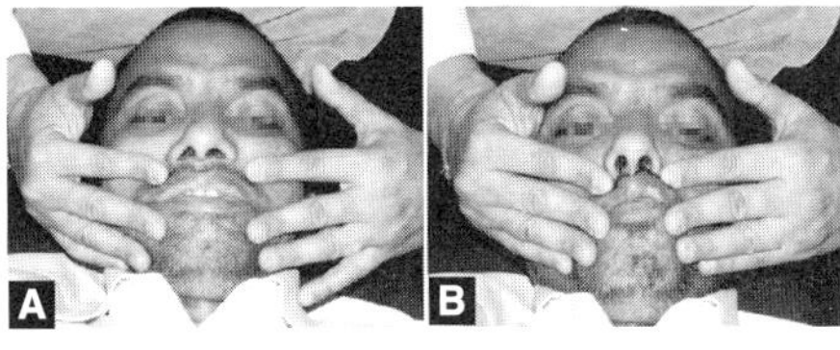

FIGURES 14.5A and B: (A) PNF for orbicularis oris, starting position and (B) PNF for orbicularis oris, end position

Mentalis

Command: "Wrinkle your chin."

Apply resistance down and out at the chin (Figure 14.6).

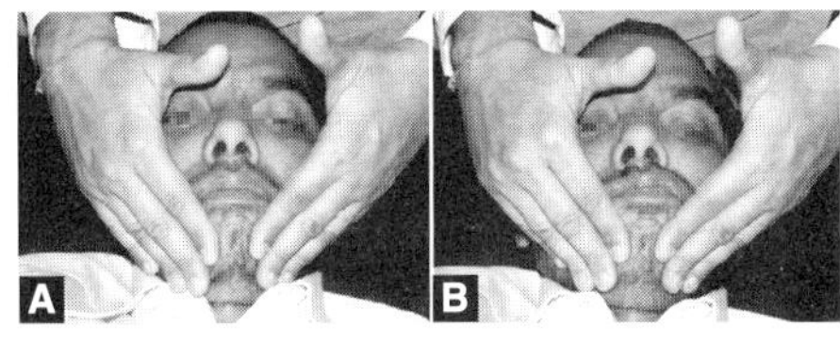

FIGURES 14.6A and B: (A) PNF for mentalis, starting position and (B) PNF for mentalis, end position

Levator Labii Superioris

Command: "Lift your upper lip, show your upper teeth."

Apply resistance to the upper lip, downward and medially (Figure 14.7).

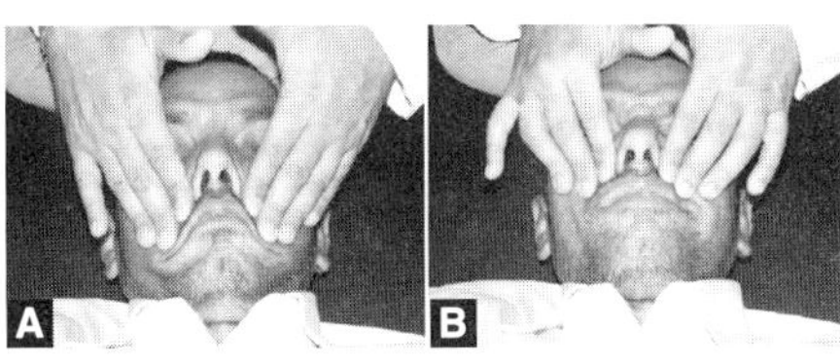

FIGURES 14.7A and B: (A) PNF for levator labii superioris, starting position, and (B) PNF for levator labii superioris, end position

Levator Anguli Oris

Command: "Pull the corner of your mouth up, a small smile."

Push down and in at the corner of the mouth (Figure 14.8).

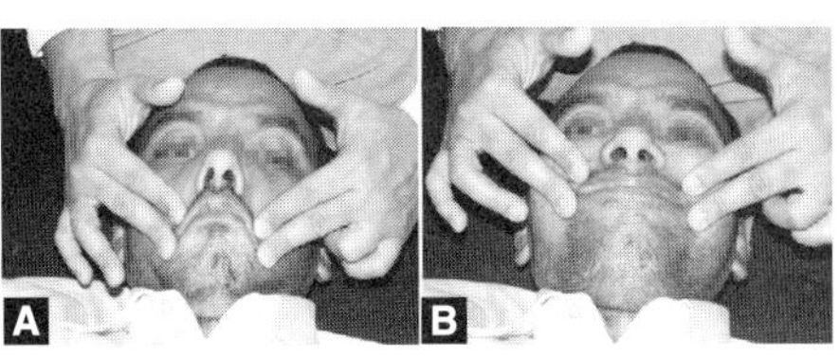

FIGURES 14.8A and B: (A) PNF for levator anguli oris, starting position and (B) PNF for levator anguli oris, end position

Depressor Anguli Oris

Command: "Push the corners of your mouth down, look sad."

Give resistance upwards and medially to the corners of the mouth (Figure 14.9).

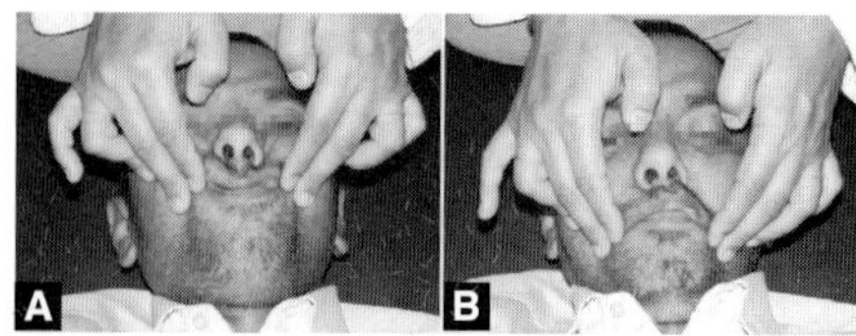

FIGURES 14.9A and B: (A) PNF for depressor anguli oris, starting position and (B) PNF for depressor anguli oris, end position

Buccinator

Command: "Suck your cheeks in, pull in against the tongue blade."

Apply resistance on the inner surface of cheeks with your gloved fingers or a dampened tongue blade. The resistance can be given diagonally upwards or diagonally downwards as well as straight out (Figure 14.10).

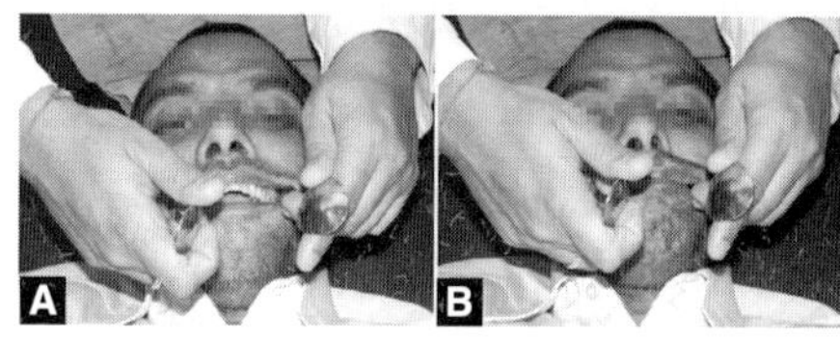

FIGURES 14.10A and B: (A) PNF for buccinator using a spoon, starting position and (B) PNF for buccinator using a spoon, end position

Procerus

Command: "Wrinkle your nose."

Apply resistance next to the nose diagonally down and out (Figure 14.11).
This muscle works with corrugators muscle and with eye closing.

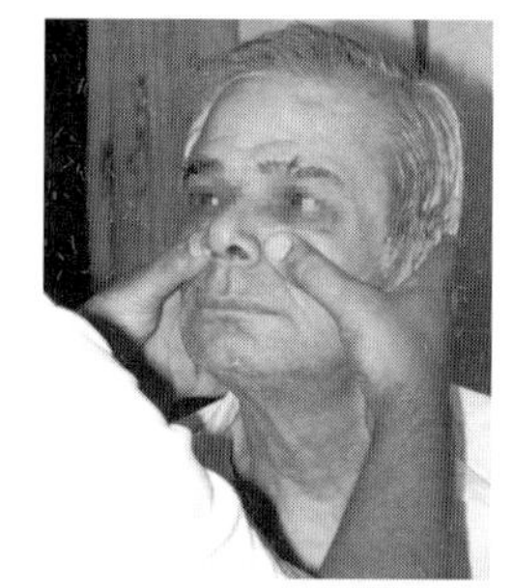

FIGURE 14.11: PNF for procerus

Zygomaticus Major

Command: "Smile."

Apply resistance to the corners of the mouth, medially and slightly downward (Figure 14.12).

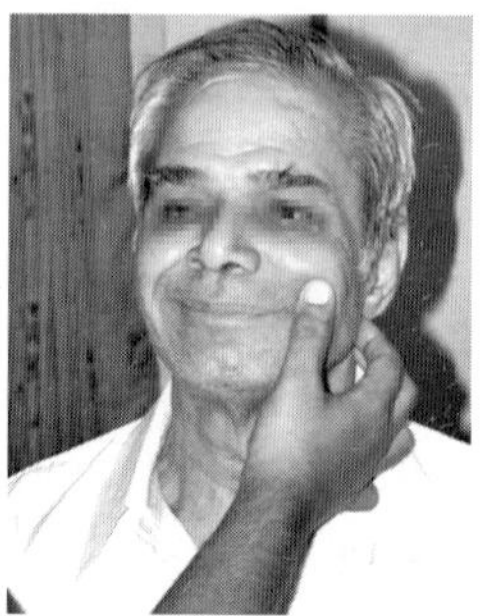

FIGURE 14.12: PNF for zygomaticus major

The functional activities as in mouth opening, combination of muscle contraction is required for achieving the desired motion. After carrying out the diagonal pattern of individual muscle activity, muscles can be trained in a group for some purposeful tasks. Smooth interplay of muscles is required for the coordinated task and unwanted activity in other part of the face should be inhibited by giving strong verbal commands and by visual biofeedback. Initially, the therapist actively assists these movements on both the sides for symmetry of motion. Gradually, only the affected side needs to be assisted till the patient is able to actively achieve the movement. In day to day life, individual contraction of facial muscle is rarely seen and almost always a combination of different muscles is responsible for carrying out various tasks. As the training progresses, unilateral activation of the facial movements on either side, i.e. affected and unaffected both is carried out and various complex expressions can be worked out upon with assistance from immediate family and friends, if need be, to ensure similar expressiveness to that of the premorbid state (Figure 14.13).

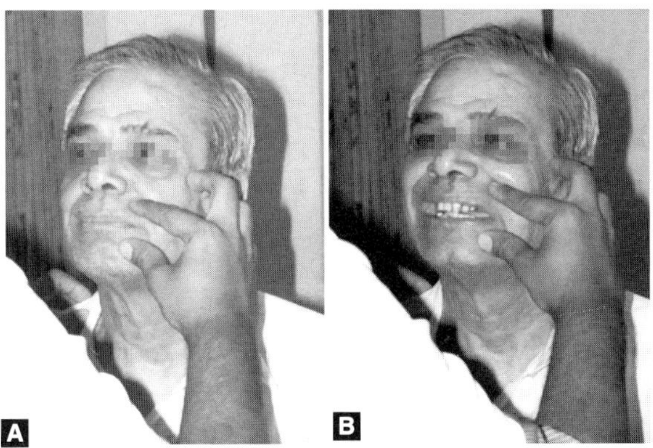

FIGURES 14.13A and B: Combined movement pattern as in showing the teeth

STIMULATION OF LIPS AND ORAL CAVITY (VIBRATION AND ICING)

Activities of chewing and swallowing need to be trained right from the initial stages. Even in patients with no apparent facial involvement, there may be overall decrease in tone of the muscles which may lead to difficulty in swallowing and controlling saliva in the oral cavity. Prolonged presence of a Ryle's tube

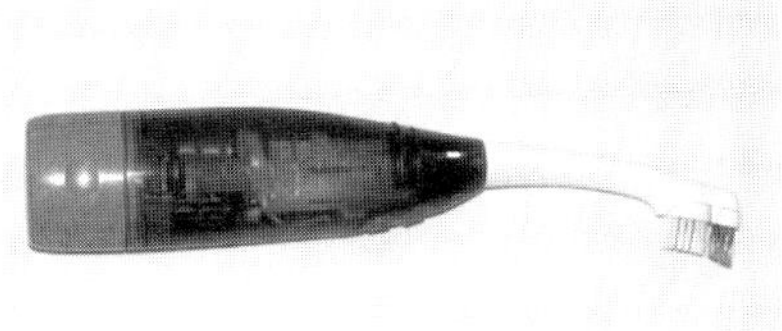

FIGURE 14.14: Tooth brush with vibrator

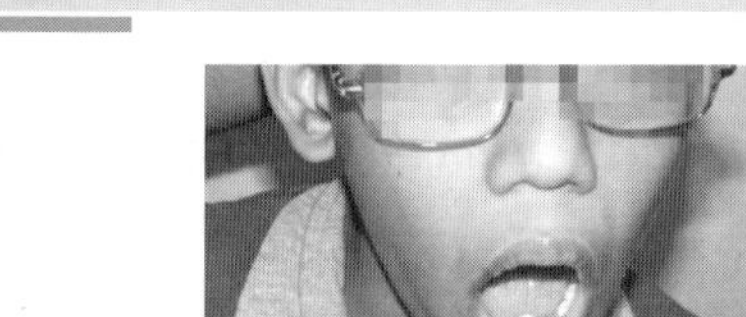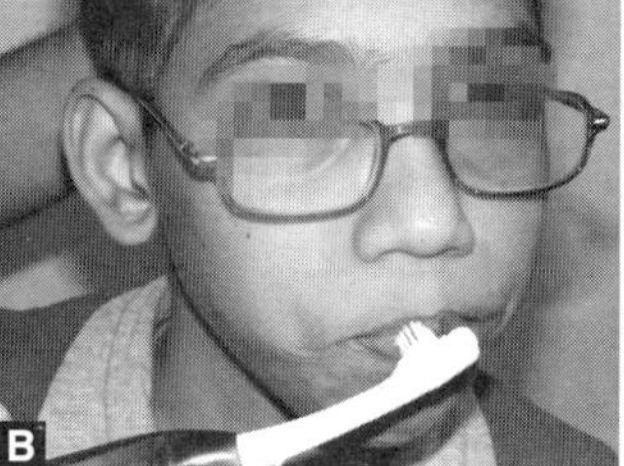

FIGURES 14.15A and B: (A) Vibrations on inside area of lips and (B) vibrations on outside area of lips

inhibits sucking and swallowing reflexes. The protocol of oral rehabilitation commences with sensory activation of the lips and oral cavity (Figures 14.14 and 14.15). Mechanoreceptors are activated with the use of vibratory sense. The vibrations can be provided by a hand held 'vibratory toothbrush' available easily in the market.

The vibrator is moved gently on the outer surface of the lips. Gradually, it is also moved on the inner surface of both the lips with mouth kept open. A 50 Hz frequency can be selected initially moving on to 100 Hz, if option is available. The second step of treatment is to apply vibrations in the entire oral cavity (Figure 14.16).

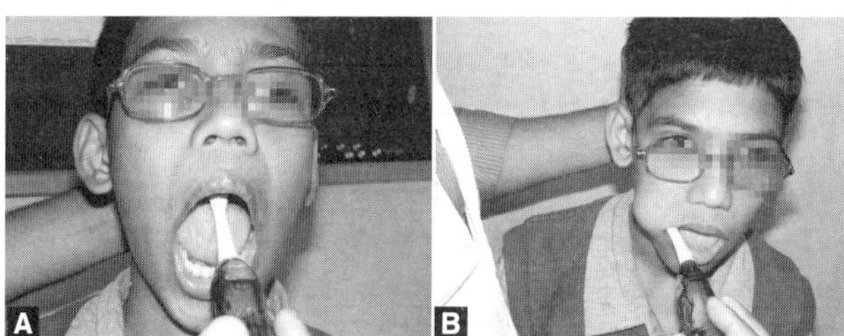

FIGURES 14.16A and B: Vibrations in the oral cavity

These techniques improve sensitivity of the oral cavity, reduce dribbling of saliva and improve the tone of lips and buccal cavity. Vibratory stimulation can also be used in improving sensitivity and tone and hence, the movements of the tongue. The vibrator can be moved on the entire tongue but care should be taken as stimulating the posterior area of the tongue may induce an exaggerated gag (Figure 14.17).

The vibrations applied over the tongue

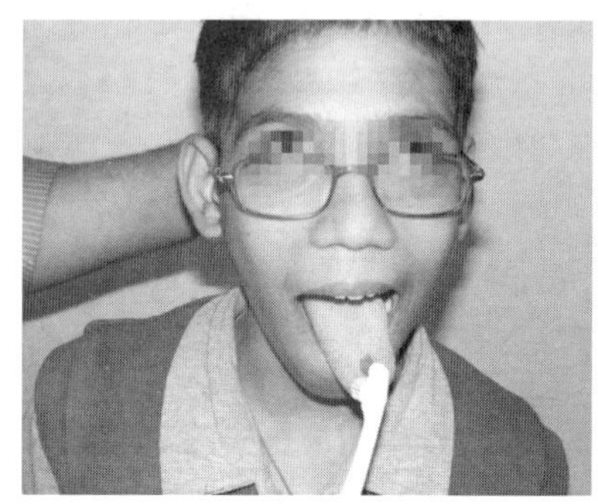

FIGURE 14.17: Vibrations on the tongue

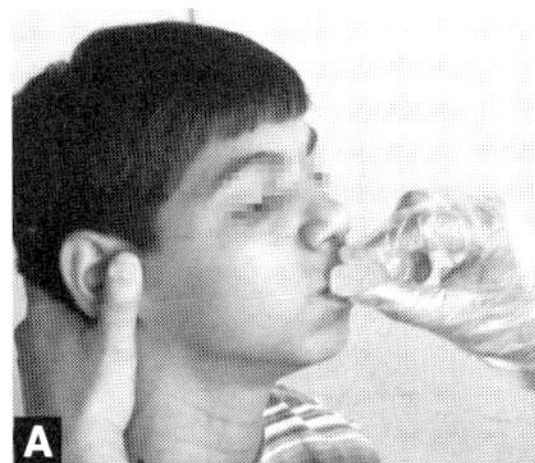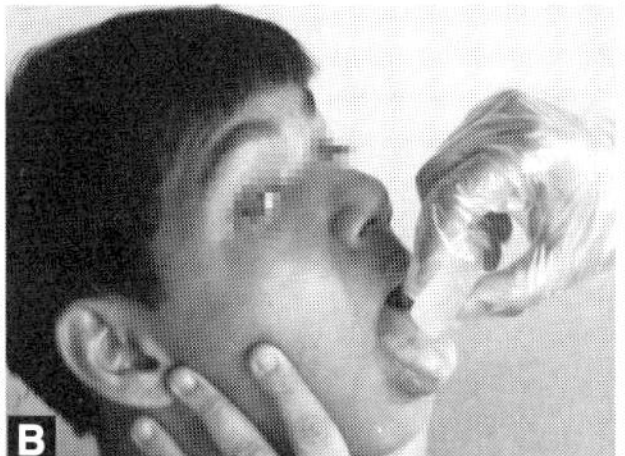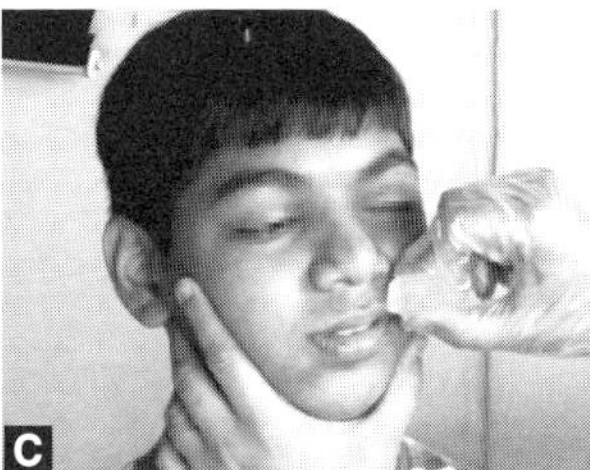

FIGURES 14.18A to C: (A) Icing over the lips, (B) icing on the tongue and (C) icing for facial muscles

are also effective in normalizing the tone of spastic tongue along with icing and passive stretching of the tongue.

Icing of the lips, oral cavity and the tongue has proved to be highly effective in improving the functions. Ice is applied over the lips, inside surface of the lips, inside the oral cavity and on the tongue (Figure 14.18). Quick ice facilitates the movements while, the prolonged ice is useful in reducing the tone of spastic tongue.

RESISTED TONGUE MOVEMENTS

Tongue is a muscle which has only one attachment, other side is free for movement and articulation with various parts of the oral cavity for production of different sounds. Twisting motion of the tongue prepares bolus of the food and its wave-like motion pushes the bolus near the esophagus. Weakness or spasticity in the tongue may produce difficulty in speech and difficulty in swallowing. Active exercises for the tongue help in normalizing the above mentioned functions.

Active exercises for the tongue are:
- Protrusion
- Taking tongue back
- Taking tip of the tongue to the right
- Taking tip of the tongue to the left
- Rotating the tongue in oral cavity
- Rolling the tongue up on the upper rows of teeth
- Rolling the tongue on the lower rows of teeth
- Making a 'U' shape with tongue as if a narrow tunnel
- Twisting the tongue

Majority of the tongue movements can be resisted to facilitate the functions. A use of a blunt spoon or a spatula is advised.

Upward motion is resisted by keeping the spoon on the distal part of tongue and pressing down, while the patient attempts to take the tongue up (Figure 14.19A). Side to side motions and protrusion can also be resisted by applying

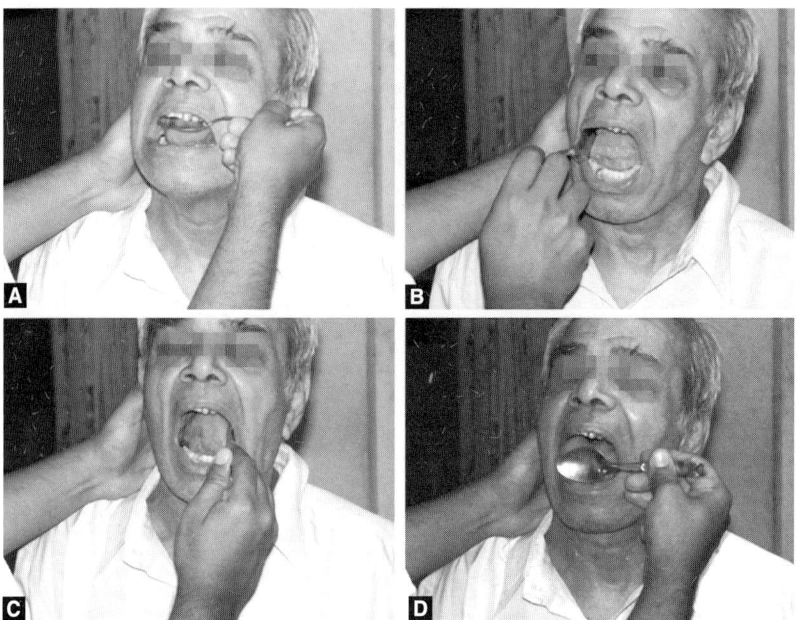

FIGURES 14.19A to D: (A) Resisted upward movements of tongue, (B) resisted left sided movements of tongue, (C) resisted right sided movements of tongue and (D) resisted protrusion of tongue

resistance in proper directions (Figures 14.19B to C). Backward movement of the tongue can be resisted by asking the patient to first protrude the tongue out of the mouth. Then, the tongue can be held by a sterile gauze with gloved fingers of the therapist. The patient then attempts to take the tongue back while the therapist applies resistance.

CHEWING AND DEGLUTITION

Chewing can be facilitated early by asking the patient to chew semi-hard substances like an apple or a carrot. Placing such food articles themselves facilitates the chewing action (Figure 14.20). Cutting and tearing can be practiced by the incisors (teeth in front) while grinding can be practiced by the premolars and the molars (teeth at the side and back).

All the activities of the tongue and chewing are carried out while the patient is in sitting position with the head kept erect. Facilitation of chewing can be carried out as described below.

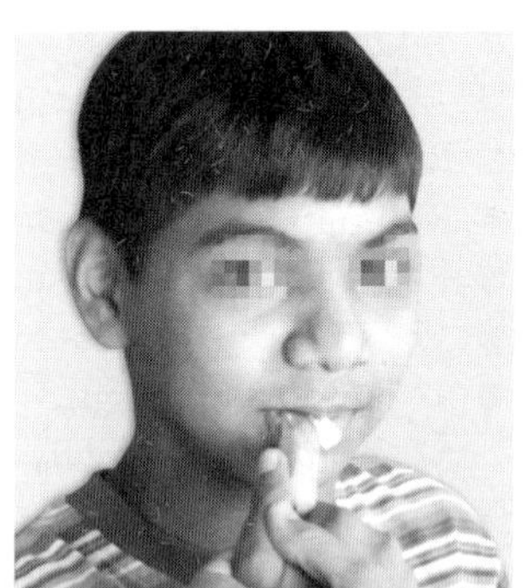

FIGURE 14.20: Chewing a juicy apple

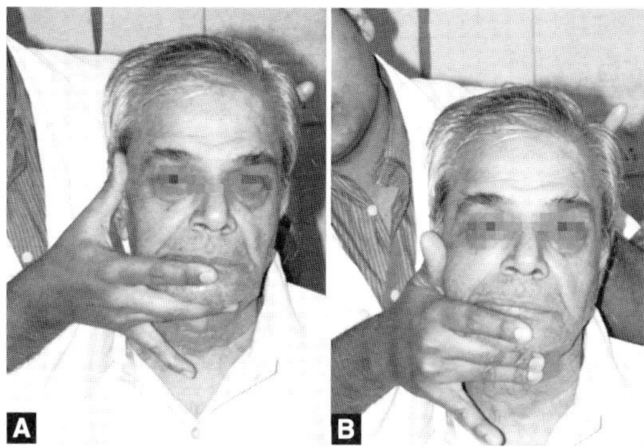

FIGURES 14.21A and B: Grip for facilitation of chewing and deglutition

The patient is sitting straight with adequate support. The head is supported by the therapist who is standing sideways and behind the patient. The therapist controls the movement of the head of the patient with left hand while the right hand is placed on the patient's jaws as shown in Figures 14.21A and B. The thumb is placed on the temporomandibular joint and index finger controls the opening and closing of the mouth and lower lip. Middle and ring fingers are kept on under surface of the chin on the mylohyoid muscle. Wave-like motion of the tongue in backward direction and contraction of the muscle of the floor of the mouth—mylohyoid whose action is to contract the floor of the mouth; is facilitated by applying a firm and gentle pressure in up and backward direction towards the esophagus while the mouth is closed. This movement is carried out initially with nothing in mouth except saliva and progression is made by introducing food articles of different sizes and textures.

ACTIVITIES FOR COORDINATION OF EYE MOVEMENTS

Activities which train eyeballs and which improve field of vision are started as and when required. Following an object only with the eyes without moving the head and neck, is started in the initial stages.

- The therapist holds a brightly colored object in front of the patient who is seated comfortably with the head and neck held straight. The therapist asks the patient to look to the object and keep the vision fixed. The therapist moves the object in various directions and asks the patient to look at it, without moving the head and the neck.
  - The therapist moves the object upward and hence, the patient has to move the eyeballs upwards to look at it (Figure 14.22).

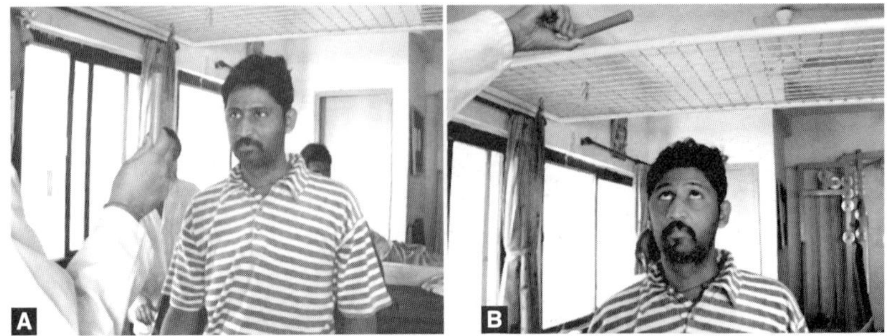

FIGURES 14.22A and B: Following an object with eyes upwards. neck is not moved

– The therapist moves the object downwards and hence, the patient has to move the eyeballs downwards to look at it (Figure 14.23).

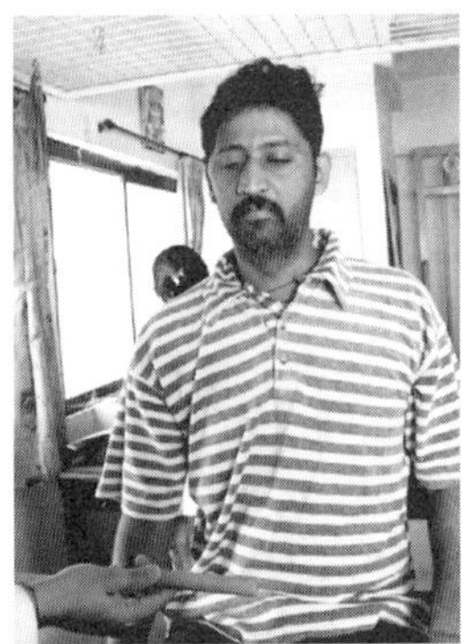

FIGURE 14.23: Following an object with eyes downwards

– The therapist moves the object to the right and to the left and hence, the patient has to move the eyeballs to the right and to the left, respectively (Figures 14.24A and B).

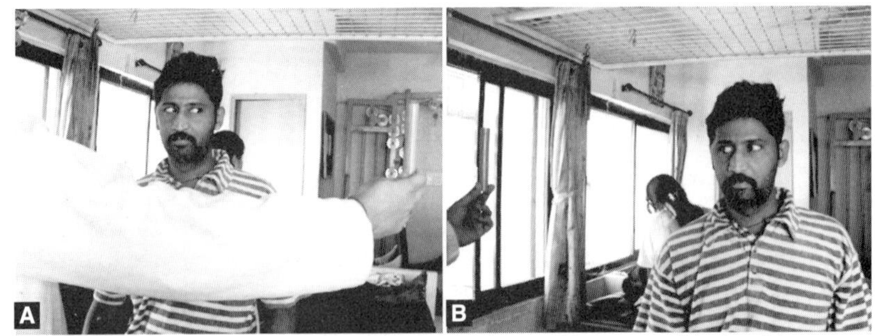

FIGURES 14.24A and B: Following an object with eyes side-to-side

– The therapist moves the object diagonally upwards and to the right and downwards to the left, and hence, the patient has to move the eyeballs accordingly upwards to the right and downwards to the left (Figures 14.25A and B).

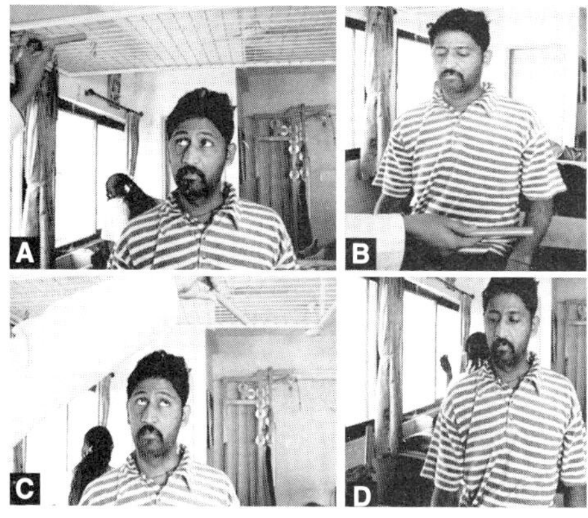

FIGURES 14.25A to D: Following an object with eyes-diagonally on either side: (A) up and to the right, (B) down and to the left, (C) up and to the left and (D) down and to the right

- The therapist then moves the object diagonally upwards to the left and downwards to the right and hence, the patient moves the eyeballs accordingly upwards to the left and downwards to the right (Figures 14.25C and D).

■ In another method, the therapist keeps the object immobile while the patient moves the head in various directions all the while looking at the stationary object. The neck is moved upwards, downwards, to the right and to the left, as shown in Figures 14.26A to D. Diagonal patterns can also be added later on as a progression to this activity.

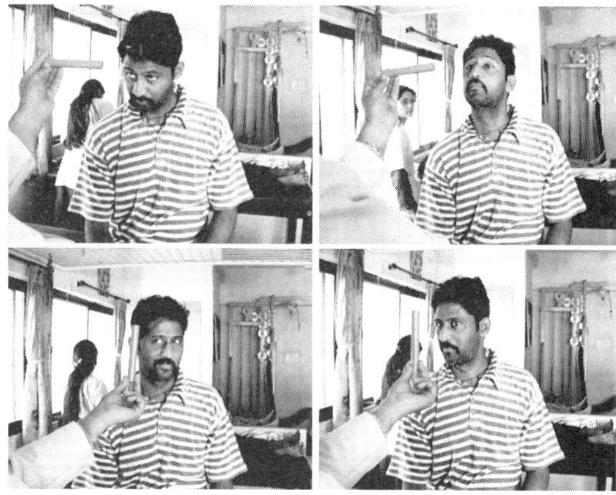

FIGURES 14.26A to D: Moving the head while constantly looking at an object (eyes fixed on the moving object): (A and B) up-down and (C and D) side-to-side

■ A beautiful smile is what the patients and their therapists work for isn't it? As shown in the Figure 14.27, proper smile will increase the confidence of the patient and one will feel confident to confront upcoming social interactions.

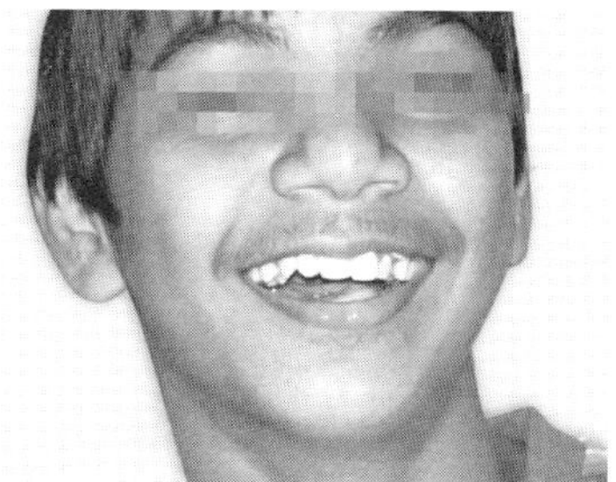

FIGURE 14.27: A beautiful smile at last

Perceptual Dysfunctions and Treatment

SOMATOSENSORY DYSFUNCTION

It includes disorder of sensation and perception.

Sensation: It refers to the activity from the peripheral sensory receptors, primary afferent sensory tracts and the appropriate 1° sensory cortex.

Perception: It refers to the integration of sensory impressions into psychologically meaningful information, i.e. it is a processing in the brain that transforms all the information from visual, auditory, tactile and kinesthetic channel into our immediate experiences of the world.

It is sometimes difficult to differentiate between the two:
- Sensation when impaired causes distortion of information from self and the environment.
- Perception when impaired causes dysfunction in understanding and interpreting information from self and from the environment.

Common Dysfunctions

- Impaired proprioception
- Impaired tactile sensation
- Astereognosis
- Asomatognosia.

Impaired Proprioception
- Difficulty in maintaining balance
- Appears to forget affected body parts
- Joint damage
- Asymmetrical posture.

Impaired tactile sensation:
- It affects motor activity, as sensory feedback is limited
- Functional perception is impaired
- Damage of affected part, particularly to skin breakdown resulting in bedsores
- Lack of awareness of body parts.

Astereognosis
- Astereognosis is defined as the inability to recognize the form and nature of common objects without looking at it. Integration of various sensory modalities is required.

Asomatognosia
- It is loss of knowledge and awareness of one's own body and position of the body and its parts in relation to themselves and objects in the environment.

Related deficits include:
- Right/left discrimination problem
- Impaired body part identification
- Finger agnosia
- Anosognosia (denial of one's illness)
- Unilateral neglect.

Unilateral neglect
- It is manifested by a failure to respond to or orient to stimuli presented contralateral to brain lesion
- It is commonly seen in (left) hemiplegics
- It is frequently seen in combination with visual field deficits
- Bizarre statements about limb found in unexpected places
- Naming the affected part
- 'Alien hand syndrome.'

Functional corelation
- Shaves only one side of his face
- Reading is also impaired
- Writing only on one side of paper.

PERCEPTUAL DISABILITIES: SITE AND SIDE OF LESION

See Table 15.1.

TABLE 15.1	Site and side of lesion and perception deficits	
Local vascular supply	**Left hemisphere deficits (dominant)**	**Right hemisphere deficits (non-domimant)**

Temporal lobe
  Internal carotid artery
  Posterior cerebral artery
  Middle cerebral artery
	Somatoagnosia
	Auditory agnosia
	Ideomotor apraxia
	Ideational apraxia
	Constructional apraxia
	Disorders of speech
	Acalculia
		Unilateral neglect
		Constructional apraxia
		Difficulty recognizing complex or incomplete visual stimuli

Occipital lobe Posterior cerebral artery	Visual object agnosia Simultagnosia Prosopagnosia Color agnosia Constructional apraxia Right homonymous hemianopsia Sensory aphasia Alexia Agraphia Acalculia	Visual object agnosia Color agnosia Topographical disorientation Depth and distance perception Prosopagnosia Dressing apraxia Left homonymous hemianopsia Symbol agnosia Complex visual hallucinations

Parietal lobe
  Internal carotid artery
  Anterior cerebral artery
  Posterior cerebral artery
  Middle cerebral artery
	Somatagnosia
	Right-left discrimination
	Finger agnosia
	Gerstmann's syndrome
	Visual object agnosia
	Visual spatial agnosia
	Astereognosis
	Ideomotor apraxia
	Ideational apraxia
	Constructional apraxia
	Aphasia
	Alexia
	Agraphia
	Acalculia
	Diminished logic
		Unilateral neglect
		Right-left discrimination
		Finger agnosia
		Anosognosia
		Spatial relations syndrome
		Figure-ground discrimination
		Form constancy
		Position in space
		Topographic disorientation
		Vertical disorientation
		Visual object agnosia
		Visual spatial agnosia
		Astereognosis
		Dressing apraxia
		Difficulty comprehending the emotional tone of language

Frontal lobe
  Internal carotid artery
  Middle cerebral artery
  Anterior cerebral artery
	Motor aphasia
	Agraphia
	Verbal apraxia
	Motor apraxia
		Motor amusia
		Motor apraxia

BODY SCHEME AND BODY IMAGE DISORDERS

Body image is defined as a visual and mental image of one's body that includes feelings about one's body, especially in relation to health and disease. The term body scheme refers to a postural model of the body, including the relationship of the body parts to each other and the relationship of the body to the environment. Body awareness is derived from the integration of tactile, proprioceptive and interoceptive sensations, in addition to the individual's subjective feelings about the body. An awareness of body scheme is considered one of the essential foundations for the performance of all purposeful motor behavior. The two terms, body image and body scheme, are often used interchangeably. Specific disturbances of body image and body scheme are somatagnosia, visual or unilateral spatial neglect, right-left discrimination, finger agnosia and anosognosia.

Somatagnosia

Somatagnosia, or impairment in body scheme, is a lack of awareness of the body structure and the relationship of body parts in oneself or in others. Patients with this deficit may display difficulty following instructions that require distinguishing body parts and may be unable to imitate movements of the therapist. Often patients report that the affected arm or leg feels unduly heavy. Lack of proprioception may underlie or compound this disorder. Body scheme impairment is also termed autopagnosia.

Clinically, the patient may have difficulty performing transfer activities because he or she does not perceive the meaning of terms related to body parts, for example, "pivot on your leg and reach for the armrest with your hand". Additionally, a patient with a body scheme disorder will have difficulty in dressing up. Patients may have a hard time participating in exercises that require some body parts to be moved in relation to other body parts; for example, "bring your arm across your chest and touch your shoulder.

The lesion site is the dominant parietal lobe, or posterior temporal lobe. Thus, this disorder is seen primarily with right hemiplegia. However, impairment in body scheme may also occur with left hemiplegia.

Assessment

■ The patient is requested to point to body parts named by the therapist, on himself or herself, on the therapist, and on a picture or puzzle of a human Figure. For example, "show me your feet. Show me your chin. Point your back." The words "right" and "left" should not be used because they may lead to an inaccurate diagnosis with right-left discrimination. Aphasia should be ruled out as a cause of poor performance.

■ The patient is asked to imitate movements of the therapist. For example, the therapist touches his or her cheek, arm, leg, and so forth. A mirror-image response is acceptable.

■ The patient is requested to answer questions about the relationship of body parts. For example, "are your knees below your head?" which is on top of your head, your hair or your feet?" for patients with aphasia, questions should be phrased to require a yes or no or true or false response. Patients with intact function in this area should respond correctly most of the time and within a reasonable period of time. Those patients with receptive aphasia are particularly likely to do poorly on tests for somatagnosia.

Treatment

■ The sensorimotor approach attempts to associate sensory input with an adaptive motor response. Facilitation of body awareness is accomplished through sensory stimulation to the body part affected. For example, the patient is asked to rub the appropriate body part with a rough cloth as the therapist names it or points to it.

■ With the transfer of training approach, the patient verbally identifies body parts, or points to pictures of them as the therapist touches them.

UNILATERAL VISUAL OR SPATIAL NEGLECT

Homonymous Hemianopia

It is defined as loss of vision in one-half of the visual field following lesions of the optic tract, the lateral geniculate nucleus or the visual cortex.

Functional Impairment

It decreases the patient's awareness of the environment and affects the performance of the motor task. Patient may demonstrate lack of appreciation or the need to scan or turn their head to affected side unless prompted or taught to do so. May bump into objects or be startled by their presence.

Visual Inattention

Lack of response to stimuli on the affected side when simultaneous stimuli are applied to both sides and there is no actual visual field defect. Patient will be able to see a visual stimulus placed on the side, contralateral to the lesion, but fails to perceive it, when there are simultaneous bilateral stimuli.

Unilateral spatial neglect, sometimes termed visual hemi-inattention when referring to the visual component, is the inability to register and to integrate stimuli and perceptions from one side of the body and the environment. This usually, although not always, affects the left side of the body, and for purposes of this discussion, we still assume that it is the left. The patient ignores the left side of the body and stimuli occurring in the left personal space. This may occur despite intact visual fields, or concomitantly with right or left homonymous hemianopsia; however, it is not caused by hemianopsia. Frequently, the patient has sensory loss on the affected side, which compounds the problem. Although, the patient with left-sided hemianopsia has actual loss of vision from the left visual field of both eyes, he or she may be aware of the problem and compensate by turning the head. The patient with visual neglect has intact vision but seems unaware of the problem and does not attempt to compensate spontaneously by turning the head. In extreme cases, the patient appears totally indifferent to the left side of the body and environment, and may deny that the left extremities belong to him or her. More time seems to be required in learning to compensate for this disability than with hemianopsia. There is great difficulty in integrating all stimuli from the left half of the body and personal space for use in ADLs. As with hemianopsia, the patient with visual spatial neglect often avoids crossing the midline visually or motorically. Current theories consider spatial neglect a disturbance of attention. It is important for the therapist to be familiar with this disorder as it is frequent clinical finding following a right hemisphere stroke.

Clinically, the patient ignores the left half of the body when dressing and forgets to put on the left sleeve or left pants leg. Often a male patient will forget to shave the left half of his face. The patient may neglect to eat from the left half of the plate and will start reading a newspaper from the middle of the line. Typically, the patient bumps in to objects on the left side or tends to veer towards the right when walking or propelling a wheelchair.

Assessment

- The patient is asked to copy simple drawings of a house, a tree, a person, and/or a clock. The drawings done by a patient with this deficit will have parts missing from the left half of the picture or be lacking in detail. Differentiate these drawings from those likely to be produced by a patient suffering from constructional apraxia, in which most parts would be present but not in correct relation to each other. In addition, many patients with constructional apraxia will improve when copying a model, but those with unilateral neglect will not.

- The patient is asked to read aloud. It should be noted if words are missed on the left half of the page or if there is hesitation at the beginning of a line.

Approach

- Use stimuli that are specialized for the right side of the brain, such as shapes and blocks, to enhance right brain activation.
- At the same time, minimize the presence of stimuli that are known to activate the left side of the brain, such as letters and numbers.
- Minimize the use of verbal instructions. Keep stimuli simple. Combine this with instructions to the patient to turn the head to the left, in order to anchor his or her attention to that side of space.
- Cognitive compensation (based on Weinberg and co-workers): The patient is taught to be aware of the deficit through the method of visual scanning. This technique is used to help the patient become aware of the imbalance in perception of the two sides of space. The patient practices turning toward the left and shifting the eyes to the left. With experience, the patient will begin to trust visual cues to guide action. For example, a patient does not shave properly on his left side. When asked to touch both sides of his face, or to look in the mirror, he will not notice that anything is amiss. However, after being trained to systemically scan the visual environment, starting with the left side of his face, the patient may notice the unshaven side in the mirror. At a later date, when asked to touch both sides of his face, he will confirm that one side is unshaven and take appropriate action.
- Using the functional approach, repeated practice is used in particular areas of difficulty in ADLS, such as transferring from a wheel chair or eating. Visuospatial deficits may interfere extensively with performance of ADLs.
- The following steps are recommended by Stanton and associates: Break down the activity in to small components. Have the patient practice each one in sequence until a criterion level has been reached; then taper the cues. Finally, arrange the activity in to larger components. Keeping ongoing records of progress will assist the therapist in guiding treatment appropriately. Encourage verbal self-cuing in verbally intact patients.

Adapting the Environment

- The patient is addressed and given demonstrations from the unaffected side. The nursing staff should place the patient's call button, telephone, and other essential paraphernalia on the unaffected side. A bold red line is drawn on the side of the page that is neglected. A mirror may be placed in front of the patient while he or she is dressing or ambulating to draw attention to the neglected side.

- Using the sensorimotor approach, the therapist stimulates the left side of the patient's body using a rough cloth, ice, or other material. The patient is reminded to watch what the therapist is doing. Next, the patient stimulates the affected side himself or herself while watching.
- In the transfer of training approach, the patient participates in tasks that make it necessary to look toward the affected side, such as watching television. For example, the television can be placed initially on the affected side. A brightly colored tape track may be placed along the floor and the patient may be instructed to walk or to guide the wheel chair along it.

RIGHT-LEFT DISCRIMINATION

A disorder in right left discrimination is the inability to identify the right and left sides of one's own body or that of the examiner. This includes inability to execute movements in response to verbal commands that include the terms "right" and "left". Patients are often unable to imitate movements.

Clinically, the patient cannot tell the therapist which is the right arm and which is the left. The right shoe cannot be discerned from the left shoe, and the patient is unable to follow instructions using the concept of right left, such as "turn right at the corner". The patient cannot discriminate the right from the left side of the therapist.

The lesion site is the parietal lobe of either hemisphere. A close relationship between aphasia and deficits in right-left discrimination has been reported. In non-aphasic patients, a relationship has been reported between general mental impairment and right left discrimination.

- The patient is asked to point to body parts upon *Command:* Right ear, left foot, right arm, and so forth. Six responses should be elicited on the patient's own body, on that of the therapist, and on a model or picture of the human body. To rule out somatagnosia, the patient should be tested first without the directional words.

Treatment

- In giving instructions to the patient, the words "right" and "left" should be avoided. Instead, pointing or providing cues using distinguishing features of the limb are more effective.
- Adapt the environment. The right side of all common objects such as shoes and clothing should be marked with red tape or any other color may be used.

FINGER AGNOSIA

Finger agnosia can be defined as the inability to identify the fingers of one's own hands or of the hands of the examiner. This includes difficulty in naming the finger upon command, identifying which finger was touched, and, by some definitions, mimicking finger movements. This deficit usually occurs bilaterally and is more common on the middle three fingers. Finger agnosia correlates highly with poor dexterity in tasks that require movements of individual fingers in relation to each other, such as buttoning, tying laces, and typing.

Finger agnosia may be the result of a lesion located in either parietal lobe, in the region of the angular gyrus, or in the supramarginal gyrus. It is often found in conjunction with an aphasic disorder, or with general mental impairment. Bilateral finger agnosia with right-left discrimination, agraphia, and acalculia is termed Gerstmann's syndrome. A portion of sauguet's test assessment is recommended.

- The patient is asked to name the fingers touched by the therapist, with the eyes open (five times) and if successful, with vision occluded (five times).
- The patient is asked to point to the fingers named by the therapist on the patient's own hands (10 times), on the therapist's hands (10 times), and on a schematic model (10 times).
- The patient is asked to point to the equivalent finger on a life-sized picture when each finger is touched by the therapist.
- The patient is asked to imitate finger movements for example, curl the index finger, and touch the thumbs to the middle finger.

Treatment

- To apply sensory integrative principles, the patient's discriminative tactile systems are stimulated. A rough cloth can be used to rub the dorsal surface of the affected arm, hand and fingers, and the ventral surface of the affected fingers. Pressure can be applied to the ventral surface of the hand.
- To use the transfer of training approach, the patient is quizzed on finger identification.

ANOSOGNOSIA

Anosognosia is a severe condition including denial, neglect, and lack of awareness of the presence of severity of one's paralysis. Presence of this disability may compromize rehabilitation potential greatly, because it limits the patient's ability to recognize the need for, and thus to use, compensation techniques.

Typically, the patient maintains that there is nothing wrong and may disown the paralyzed limbs and refuse to accept responsibility for them. The patient may claim that the limb has a mind of its own or that it was left at home, or in a cupboard. It has been observed that patients suffering from anosognosia have a tendency to cover the paretic arm.

The lesion is usually located in the non-dominant parietal lobe, in the region of the supramarginal gyrus.

- Anosognosia is assessed by talking to the patient. The patient is asked what happened to his arm or leg, whether he is paralyzed, how the limb feels, and why it cannot be moved.

- A patient with anosognosia may deny the paralysis, say that it is of no concern, and fabricate reasons why a limb does not move the way it should be.

- It is extremely difficult to compensate for this condition. Safety is of paramount importance in the treatment and discharge planning for patients suffering from anosognosia, because they typically do not acknowledge that they have a disability and will therefore, refuse to be careful.

SPATIAL RELATIONS DEFICITS

This group encompasses a constellation of deficits that have in common, a difficulty in perceiving the relationship between objects in space or the relationship between self and two or more objects. Research suggests that the right parietal lobe has the primary role in space perception. Thus, a spatial relations deficit most frequently occurs in patients with right-sided lesions and resulting left hemiparesis.

- Spatial relations syndrome includes disorders of figure-ground discrimination, form constancy, spatial relations, position in space, and topographical disorientation. Additional visuospatial deficits, such as depth and distance perception, will be discussed. Constructional apraxia and dressing apraxia are sometimes viewed as spatial relations problems.

Figure-ground Discrimination

A disorder in visual figure-ground discrimination is the inability to visually distinguish a figure from the background in which it is embedded. Functionally, it interferes with the patient's ability to locate important objects that are not prominent in a visual array. The patient has difficulty ignoring irrelevant visual stimuli and cannot select the appropriate cue to which to respond. This may lead to distractibility, resulting in a shortened attention span, frustration, and decreased independent and safe functioning.

Clinically, the patient cannot locate items in a pocket book or drawer, locate buttons on a shirt, or distinguish the armhole from the remainder of a solid colored shirt. The patient may not be able to tell when one step ends and another begins on a flight of stairs, especially when walking down. The predominant lesion is generally in the non-dominant parietal lobe but may be located in any part of the brain.

Assessment

- Ayres Figure ground test: The subject must distinguish the three objects in an embedded test picture, from a possible selection of six items. This test was standardized on children but may be useful as a clinical tool in identifying perceptual disorders in brain damaged adults. Normative data have been generated for normal adult males.
- Functional tests: A white shirt can be placed on a white sheet, and the patient is asked to point out the sleeve, buttons, and collar of a white shirt, or to pick out a spoon from an unsorted array of eating utensils. It is necessary to rule out poor eye sight, hemianopsia, visual agnosia, and poor comprehension, to improve the validity of these assessment techniques.

Treatment

- Compensation through cognitive awareness: The patient is taught to become aware of the existence and nature of the deficit. The patient should be cautioned to examine groups of objects slowly and systematically and should be instructed to use other, intact senses when searching for items such as clothing or utensils.
- Adaptation and simplification of the environment: Red tape may be placed over the Velcro strap of the shoe or orthosis to aid the patient in locating it. Few items should be placed in the patient's drawers or nightstand, and they should be replaced in the exact location each time. Brightly colored tape can be used to mark the edges on stairs.
- With the functional approach, repeated practice is used in each specific area of difficulty each practice session, incorporating verbal cues and touch as adjuncts to vision.
- Using the transfer of training approach, the therapist should arrange for practice in visually locating objects in a simple array, and progress to more difficult ones.

Form Consistency

Impairment in form consistency is the inability to perceive or to attend to subtle differences in form and shape. The patient is likely to confuse objects of similar shape or not to recognize an object placed in an unusual position. Clinically, the patient may confuse a pen with a toothbrush, a vase with a water pitcher, a cane with a crutch, and so forth. The lesion site is the parieto-temporo-occipital region of the non-dominant lobe.

Assessment

- A number of items similar in shape and different in size are gathered. The patient is asked to identify them. One set of items might be a pencil, pen, straw, toothbrush, watch, and the other might be a key, paper clip, coins, and a ring. Each object is presented several times in different positions. Visual object agnosia must be ruled out as a cause of poor performance by first presenting objects separately and asking the patient to identify them or to demonstrate how they are used.

Treatment

- With the transfer of training approach, the patient should practice describing, identifying, and demonstrating the usage of similarly shaped and sized objects. The patient should sort like objects and should be assisted to focus on differentiating cues.
- To achieve cognitive awareness and compensate for the disability, the patient must be made aware of the specific deficit. If the patient can read, frequently used letters and words are taught to the patient and the patient is encouraged to use vision, touch, and self-verbalization in combination when confused about objects.

Spatial Relations Deficit

A spatial relations deficit, or spatial disorientation, is the inability to perceive the relationship of one object in space to another object, or to oneself. This may lead to, or compound, problems in constructional tasks and dressing. Crossing the midline may be a problem for patients with spatial relations deficits.

Clinically, the patient might find it difficult to place the cutlery, plate, and spoon in the proper positions, when setting the table. The patient may be unable to tell the time from a clock because of difficulty in perceiving the relative positions of the hands. The patient may have difficulty learning to position his or her arms, legs, and trunk in relation to the wheelchair to prepare for transferring.

The lesion site is predominantly the non-dominant parietal lobe.

Assessment

■ The therapist draws a picture of a clock and then asks the patient to fill in the numbers and to draw in the hands to designate a particular time. Patients with poor eye-hand coordination can be requested to place markers in the appropriate positions instead of drawing numbers.

■ Two or three objects are placed on a piece of paper in a particular pattern. The patient is asked to duplicate the pattern.

■ To improve the validity of these assessments, unilateral neglect and hemianopsia should be ruled out as the causes of poor performance. If these are present, position the stimulus array appropriately.

Treatment

■ Using the transfer of training approach to improve the ability to orient oneself to other objects, the patient can be given instructions on positioning himself or herself in relation to the therapist or another object; for example, "sit next to me", "go behind the table", "step over the line". In addition, the therapist can set up a maze of furniture. Having the patient copy block or matchstick designs of increasing difficulty will increase awareness of the relationship between one object and the next.

■ With the sensorimotor approach, if the patient avoids crossing the midline, activities that require crossing the midline, both motorically and visually, can be incorporated into other therapeutic activities.

■ One specific activity is to have the patient hold a stick in both hands. The therapist guides it from the uninvolved side to the involved side. Later, the patient can progress to manipulating the stick with only verbal or visual cues, and finally to guiding it independently.

Position in Space

A deficit in the perception of position in space is the inability to perceive and to interpret spatial concepts such as up, down, under, over, in, out, in front of, and behind.

Clinically, if a patient is asked to raise the arm "above" the head during a ROM assessment or is asked to place the feet "on" the footrests, the patient may behave as if he or she does not know what to do.

The lesion is located in the non-dominant parietal lobe.

Assessment

- To assess function, two objects are used, such as shoe and a shoe box. The patient is asked to place the shoe in different positions in relation to the shoe box; for example, in the box, below the box, or next to the box.
- Alternatively, the patient is presented with two objects and asked to describe their relationship. For example, a toothbrush can be placed in a cup, under a cup, and so forth, and the patient is then asked to indicate the location of the toothbrush.
- Another mode of assessment is to have the patient copy the therapist's manipulations with an identical set of objects. For example, the therapist hands the patient a comb and a brush.
- The therapist then takes an identical set and places them in a particular relationship to each other, such as the comb on top of the brush. The patient is requested to arrange his or her comb and brush in the same way. Success in this task may represent sufficient ability to use position in space functionally.
- Figure-ground difficulty, apraxia, in coordination, and lack of comprehension should be ruled out when performing these assessments. Objects should be positioned to avoid compounding of results with hemianopsia unilateral spatial neglect.

Treatment

- To use the transfer of training approach, three or four identical objects are placed in the same orientation. An additional object is placed in a different orientation. The patient is asked to identify the odd one, and then to place it in the same orientation as the other objects.
- The sensorimotor approach used for treatment of spatial relations is similar to that used for treatment of disorders of position in space.

Topographic Disorientation

Topographic disorientation refers to difficulty in understanding and remembering the relationship of one location to another. As a result, the patient is unable to get from one place to another, with or without a map. This disorder is frequently seen in conjunction with other difficulties in spatial relations.

Clinically, the patient cannot find the way from his or her room to the physical therapy clinic, despite being shown repeatedly. The patient cannot describe the spatial characteristics of familiar surroundings, such as the layout of his or her bedroom at home.

The lesion site is the occipitoparietal lobe of the non-dominant hemisphere.

Assessment

- The patient is asked to describe or to draw a familiar route, such as the society in which he or she lives, the layout of his or her house, or a major nearby landmark. The impaired patient will be unable to succeed in this task.

Treatment

- Using the transfer of training approach, the patient practices going from one place to another, following verbal instructions. Initially, simple routes should be used, and then more complicated ones.
- Using the functional approach, important routes in the actual environment or in the patient's home are repeatedly practiced.
- Adapt the environment. Frequently travelled routes can be marked with colored dots. The spaces between the dots are gradually increased and eventually eliminated as improvement takes place.
- This is an example of taking a normally right-hemisphere task and converting it in to a left-hemisphere task. In this instance, we take the spatial task of remembering routes and substitute sequential landmarks to accomplish the goal of getting from place to place.
- To reinforce cognitive awareness, the patient should be instructed not to leave the clinic, room, or home unattended, because he or she may get lost.

Depth and Distance Perception

The patient with deficits in these areas experiences inaccurate judgment of direction, distance, and depth. Spatial disorientation may be a contributing factor in faculty-distance perception.

Clinically, the patient may have difficulty navigating stairs, may miss the chair when attempting to sit, or may continue pouring juice once a glass is filled.

This may occur with a lesion in the right, non-dominant hemisphere, particularly in the occipital lobe.

Assessment

- For a functional assessment of distance perception, the patient is asked to take or to grasp an object that has been placed on a table. The object may be held in front of the patient, in the air, and the patient is again asked to grasp it. The impaired patient will overshoot or undershoot.

- To assess depth perception functionally, the patient can be asked to fill a glass of water. A patient with depth perception deficit may continue pouring once the glass is filled.

Treatment

- Help the patient become aware of the deficit (cognitive awareness).
- Stress the importance of walking carefully on uneven surfaces, particularly the stairs.
- With the transfer-of-training approach, the patient is requested to place the feet on designated spots during gait training. Also, blocks can be arranged in piles 2 to 8 inches high. The patient is asked to touch the top of the piles with the foot. This is done to re-establish a sense of depth and distance.

Vertical Disorientation

Vertical disorientation refers to a distorted perception of what is vertical. Displacement of the vertical position can contribute to disturbance of motor performance, both in posture and in gait. Early on, in recovery, most post-CVA patients demonstrate some impairment in the sense of verticality. This is not influenced by the presence or absence of homonymous hemianopsia. Scores on one test for visual perception of the vertical position were found to correlate with differences in walking ability.

An example of the way in which a person with distorted vertically views the world and the way this may affect posture.

The lesion site is in the non-dominant parietal lobe.

Assessment

- The therapist holds a cane vertically and then turns it sideways to a horizontal plane. The patient is handed the cane and asked to turn it back to the original position. If the patient's perception of the vertical position is distorted, the cane will most likely be placed at an angle, representing the patient's conception of the world around him or herself.

Treatment

- The patient must be made aware of the disability. The patient should be instructed to compensate by using touch for proper self-orientation, especially when going through doorways, in elevators and on the stairs.

AGNOSIA

Agnosia is the inability to recognize familiar objects using one or more of the sensory modalities, while often retaining the ability to recognize the same object using other sensory modalities. All types of Agnosia represent impairment in the transmission of the sensory signal, to the conceptual level.

Visual Object Agnosia

Visual object agnosia is the most common forms of agnosia. It is defined as the inability to recognize familiar objects despite normal function of the eyes and optic tracts. One remarkable aspect of this disorder is the readiness with which the patient can identify an object once it is handled. Visual object agnosia may occur with or without hemianopsia. The patient may not recognize people, possessions, and common objects. Specific types of visual agnosia are described below.

Simultagnosia, also known as Balint's syndrome, is the inability to perceive a visual stimulus as a whole. The patient perceives an entire array on a part at a time. The lesion is in the dominant occipital lobe.

Prosopagnosia was traditionally considered to be the inability to recognize faces as being familiar. This phenomenon is now thought to be related to any visually ambiguous stimulus, the recognition of which depends on evoking a memory context, such as different species of birds or different makes of cars. Prosopagnosia is usually accompanied by visual field defects. Bilaterally symmetric occipital lesions are thought to be responsible for this deficit.

Color agnosia is the inability to recognize colors; it is not color blindness. The patient is unable to name colors or to identify them on command, although the ability to name objects is retained. Color agnosia is frequently associated with facial or other visual object agnosias. It is usually the result of a dominant hemisphere lesion. The simultaneous occurrence of left-sided hemianopsia, alexia, and color agnosia is a classic occipital lobe syndrome.

The lesions associated with visual object agnosias are thought to occur in the occipito-temporo-parietal association areas of either hemisphere; these areas are responsible for the integration of visual stimuli with respect to memory. The exact nature of the disability may be determined by the laterality of the lesion. Color agnosia frequently accompanies diffuse dementia.

Assessment

■ To asses this disorder, several common objects are placed in front of the patient. The patient is asked to name the objects, to point to an object named by the therapist, or to demonstrate its usage. It is important to rule out aphasia and apraxia.

Treatment

■ Using the transfer of training approach, drills can be used to practice discrimination between faces that are important to the patient, in discrimination between colors and common objects.
■ The therapist should assist the patient in picking out salient visual cues for relating names to faces.
■ With compensation techniques, the patient is instructed to use intact sensory modalities such as touch or audition to distinguish people and objects.

Auditory Agnosia

Auditory agnosia refers to the inability to recognize non-speech sounds or to discriminate between them. This rarely occurs in the absence of other communication disorders.

The patient with auditory agnosia cannot tell, for example, the difference between the ring of a doorbell and that of a telephone, or between a dog barking and thunder.

The lesion is located in the dominant temporal lobe.

Assessment

■ Assessment is usually carried out by a speech therapist.
■ The patient is asked to close the eyes and to identify the source of various sounds. The therapist rings a bell, honks a horn, rings a telephone, and so forth, and asks the patient to identify the sound (verbally or by pointing to a picture).

Treatment

■ Treatment generally consists of drilling the patient on sounds, but this has not been found to be particularly effective.

Tactile Agnosia or Astereognosis

Tactile agnosia, or astereognosis, is the inability to recognize forms by handling them, although tactile, proprioceptive, and thermal sensations may be intact.

This condition commonly causes difficulties in ADLs, in as much as many self-care activities that are normally done in the absence of constant visual monitoring require the manipulation of objects. If tactile agnosia is present in combination with unilateral neglect or sensory loss, performance in ADLs may be severely hampered.

If a patient is handed an object (key, comb, safety pin) with vision occluded, the patient will fail to recognize it.

The lesion is in the parieto-temporo-occipital lobe (posterior association areas) of either hemisphere.

Assessment

- The patient is asked to identify objects placed in the hand by examining them manually without visual cues.

Treatment

- With the transfer of training approach, the patient practices feeling various common objects, shapes, and textures with vision occluded. The patient is instructed to immediately look at the object for visual feedback and note special characteristics of the object.
- To achieve cognitive awareness, the patient is made aware of the deficit and is instructed in visual compensation.

Olfactory Agnosia

It is the inability to recognize familiar smells.

The smell of gas, of smoke and of burnt food is ignored and this has implications for safety.

APRAXIA

Apraxia is a disorder of voluntary learned movement. It is characterized by an inability to perform purposeful movements, which cannot be accounted for by inadequate strength, loss of coordination, impaired sensation, attention difficulties, abnormal tone, movement disorders, intellectual deterioration, poor comprehension, or uncooperativeness. The patient is unable to accomplish the task even though the instructions are understood. Many patients with apraxia also present with aphasia, and the two disorders are sometimes difficult to distinguish.

Ideomotor and ideational apraxias are generally thought to be the result of dominant hemispheres lesions and may be particularly difficult to assess in the patient with aphasia. Although aphasia and apraxia often occur together, there is not a strong correlation between the severity of the aphasia and the severity of the apraxia. Apraxia is a disorder of skilled movement and not a language disorder. Dressing apraxia and constructional apraxia occur with lesions in either hemisphere.

Ideomotor Apraxia

Ideomotor apraxia refers to a breakdown between concept and performance. There is a disconnection between the idea of a movement and its motor execution. It appears that information cannot be transferred from the areas of the brain that conceptualize to the centers for motor execution. Thus, the patient with ideomotor apraxia is able to carry out habitual tasks automatically and describe how they are done but is unable to perform a task upon command and is unable to imitate gestures. Patients with this form of apraxia often perseverate, that is, they repeat an activity or a segment of a task over and over, even if it is no longer necessary or appropriate. This makes it difficult for them to finish one task and then to go on to the next. Patients with ideomotor apraxia appear most handicapped when requested to perform tasks that require use of many implements and that have many steps. This form of apraxia can be demonstrated separately in the facial areas, upper extremity, lower extremity, and for total body movements. Patients with apraxia are often observed to be clumsy in their actual handling of objects. Impairment is often suspected when observing the patient in ADLs or during a routine motor assessment.

■ Several examples of ideomotor apraxia follow: the patient is unable to "blow" on command. However, if presented with a bubble wand, the patient will spontaneously blow bubbles.

■ The patient may fail to walk if requested to in the traditional manner. However, if a cup of coffee is placed on a table at the other end of the room and the patient is told, "Please have some coffee", the patient is likely to transverse the room to get it.

■ A male patient is asked to comb his hair. He may be able to identify the comb and even tell you what it is used for; however, he will not actually use the comb appropriately when it is handled to him. Despite this observation in the clinic, his wife reports that he combs his hair spontaneously, every morning.

■ A female patient is asked to squeeze a dynamometer. She appears not to know what to do with it, although her comprehension is adequate, the task has just been demonstrated, and it is clear that she has adequate strength. The lesion is generally found in the dominant supramarginal gyrus.

Assessment

- The Goodglass and Kaplan test for apraxia is comprised of universally known movements, such as blowing, brushing teeth, hammering, shaving, and so forth. It is based on what the authors consider a hierarchy of difficulty for patients with apraxia. First the patient is told, "Show me how you would bang a nail with a hammer." If the patient fails to do this or uses his or her fist as if it were a hammer, the patient is asked, "Pretend to hold the hammer". If the patient fails following this instruction, the therapist demonstrates the act and asks the patient to imitate it. The patient with apraxia typically will not improve after demonstration but will improve with use of the actual implements. Ability to correct oneself on following verbal suggestions is considered to counter indicative of apraxia.
- The therapist sits opposite the patient. The patient is asked to imitate different postures or limb movements. The patient with apraxia is unable to imitate postures.

Treatment

- Anderson and Choy suggest the modification of instructional sets as follows: Speak slowly and use the shortest possible sentences. One command should be given at a time, and the second command should not be given until the first task is completed. When teaching a new task, physically guiding the patient through the task is necessary. It should be completed in precisely the same manner each time. When all the individual units are mastered, an attempt to combine them should be made.
- A great deal of repetition may be necessary.
- Family members must be advised to use the exact approach found to be successful in the clinic.
- Performing activities in as normal an environment as possible is also helpful.
- Using the sensorimotor approach, multiple sensory inputs are used on the affected body parts in order to enhance the production of appropriate motor responses.

Ideational Apraxia

Ideational apraxia is a failure in the conceptualization of the task. It is an inability to perform a purposeful motor act, either automatically or on command, because the patient no longer understands the overall concept of the act, cannot retain the idea of the task, and cannot formulate the motor patterns required. Often the patient can perform isolated components of a task but cannot combine them into a complete act. Furthermore, the patient cannot verbally describe the process of performing an activity, describe the function of objects, or use them appropriately.

■ Sharpless claims that ideational apraxia is unusual complication of stroke and is often present concomitantly with agnosias.

Ideational apraxia is typified by the following behavior: When presented in the clinic with a toothbrush and toothpaste and told to brush the teeth, the patient may put the tube of toothpaste in the mouth, or try to put toothpaste on the toothbrush without removing the cap. Furthermore, the patient may be unable to describe verbally how tooth brushing is done. Similar phenomenon may be evident in all aspects of ADL and so may limit the safety and potential independence of patient. It has been shown that patients with ideational apraxia test poorly in the clinical situation and appear more able to perform ADLs at the appropriate time and in a familiar setting.

The lesion causing ideational apraxia is thought to be in the dominant parietal lobe. This deficit also may be seen in conjunction with diffuse brain damage such as cerebral arteriosclerosis.

Assessment

■ The tests for ideational apraxia are essentially the same as those for ideomotor apraxia. The major difference to be expected in response is that the patient with ideomotor act spontaneously and automatically at the appropriate time, but the patient with ideational apraxia is unable to do so.

Treatment

■ The treatment techniques used are the same as those for ideomotor apraxia.

Constructional Apraxia

■ Constructional apraxia is characterized by faulty spatial analysis and conceptualization of the task. Normal constructional skills encompass the capacity to understand the relationship of parts to a whole. This ability is critical in activities such as drawing, dressing, building from a model, copying block design and the like. Performance of these complex tasks requires a combination of visual perception, motor planning, and motor performance.

- Thus, constructional apraxia is most evident in the inability to produce two-or three-dimensional forms by drawing, constructing, or arranging blocks or objects spontaneously or upon command. It hampers the patient's ability to manipulate the environment effectively because of an inability to construct things from components parts. Although able to understand and to identify the individual components, the patient cannot place them in to a correct, meaningful relationship.

- This deficit is found in patients with lesions to either hemisphere, but upon testing, there is a difference in the quality of their responses. Patients with right-sided lesions appear to be more severely affected that those with left brain involvement. They clearly lack the visuospatial ability to succeed in a task. Additionally, they lack perspective, are unable to place a figure in the appropriate position in space, and seem unable to analyze parts in relationship to each other.

- Patients with left-hemisphere damage seem to lack the analytic or planning ability necessary to initiate and perform movements in sequence to complete a constructional task. In a study by Mcfie and Zangwill, the left-lesioned group (in contrast to the right-lesioned group) rarely presented with unilateral neglect or topographic disorientation but often demonstrated impairment in constructional tasks in conjunction with general intellectual impairment.

- The presence of constructional apraxia is thought to be related to body scheme disorders, and often results in difficulty in dressing and diminished performance in other ADL skills.

- Constructional apraxia is demonstrated, for example, by a patient who understands all about sandwiches and what they are for but is unable to assemble one, even with all ingredients laid out in front of them.

Lesions are located in the posterior parietal lobe of either hemisphere. Constructional apraxia is more common and more severe in patients with right-hemisphere lesions. Right-sided lesions that results in constructional apraxia tend to be less diffuse than left-sided lesions.

Assessment

- The patient is asked to copy a drawing of a house, a flower, or a clock face.
- The patient is requested to copy geometric designs (e.g., circle, square, or t-shape).
- The patient is instructed to copy block bridges, matchstick designs, or pegboard configurations. Initially, only three pieces are used in a jigsaw and a progression is made to use more.

- Visuoconstructive difficulties found with right and left-sided lesions demonstrate qualitative differences, as described above. In response to the assessment materials, patients with right-sided damage tend to draw on the diagonal and neglect the left side of the page. They draw pieces of the picture without any coherent relationship to each other. Thus, their drawings tend to be complex, yet unrecognizable. They have immense difficulty with copying or constructing anything in three dimensions, are not helped by the presence of a model or by landmarks in a picture, and do not generally improve with practice.

- In contrast, the drawings of patients with left-hemisphere damage are usually more recognizable. They are characterized by great simplicity. Patients with left-sided lesions draw slowly and hesitatingly, are often unable to draw angles, and have general difficulty in execution. In contrast to that of right-hemisphere stroke victims, their performance often improves with the aid of a model, the use of landmarks in drawings, and with repeated trials. Short-term visual memory impairment is thought to be associated with constructional apraxia in patients with right-sided lesions.

- Verbal and comprehension difficulties, poor manual dexterity, and the presence of homonymous hemianopsia must be ruled out during assessment for this disorder.

Treatment

- With the transfer of training approach, the patient is asked to practice copying geometric designs, both by drawing and by building. Initially, simple patterns are used, progressing to the more complex. Patients with left-hemisphere lesions may benefit from the use of landmarks, and then their gradual withdrawal as skill improves.

Dressing Apraxia

Dressing apraxia is inability to dress oneself properly owing to a disorder in body skin or spatial relations rather than difficulty in motor function.
  For example, patients put on clothes upside down inside out, etc.
  The lesion site is non-dominant occipital or parietal lobe.

Assessment

- An assessment technique includes clinical observation; constructional apraxia and dressing apraxia has a high degree of correlation.

Treatment

- To develop a sequence and pattern for dressing which patient practices daily. A key to successful performance is proper positioning of garments, color codes for right and left, start buttoning from bottom and to color code inside and outside of garments.

COGNITIVE DYSFUNCTION

Cognition

It is an ability of the brain to process, store, retrieve and manipulate information. Attention, orientation, memories are the basic process upon which are built the higher cognitive functions. Higher cognitive functions include:
- Fund of knowledge
- Ability to manipulate old knowledge (e.g. calculation)
- Problem-solving
- Social awareness
- Abstract-thinking.

Attention

It is an ability to focus on specific stimulus without being distracted. Evaluation: Digit repetition, random letter test, etc.

Orientation

Orientation to time, place and person is evaluated.

Memory

The ability to process, store and retrieve information depends on intact memory system. Weschler memory scale is commonly used by neuropsychologist. We, as therapists, need to evaluate the status of immediate memory, STM and LTM to plan any relearning program for the patients. Memory dysfunctions are commonly seen after frontal lobe lesions.

Assessment

- Immediate memory: Digit repetition
- Ask the patient to remember four words (e.g. brown, honesty, tulip, eye) and then test this immediate recurs after 5 minutes, 10 minutes and 30 minutes. This examines verbal memory.

Visual Memory

It is assessed by pointing to four objects in the room and having the patient recall them immediately, after 5 minutes and at the end of the session.

Problem-solving

It requires both an intact fund of knowledge and the ability to manipulate and apply this information to new or unfamiliar situations. A deficit in problem solving will affect all phases of the patient's daily life.

Functional Problems

- Unable to figure out which bus to take
- How to plan a meal
- Experiences difficulty in social situations.

Assessment

- Proverb interpretation, e.g. Rome was not built in a day
- Social awareness
- Mathematical problems
- Conceptual series completion
- Verbal similarities.

Emotional Dysfunction

- Depression denial, anxiety and fear may occur as a result of the CVA
- Lesions of left or right hemisphere may produce differences in effective behavior
- Lesions to right are thought to 'release' talking whilst lesions to left are thought to reduce talking (Kolb and Whisaw, 1980)
- Always differentiate between depressive catastrophic reaction occurring with left hemisphere lesion versus indifference reaction with right hemisphere lesion.

Clinical Co-relation

- Attention seeking and dependent on external support
- Try to isolate themselves
- Afraid of physical exertion
- Irritable
- Easily distractable.

STRATEGIES TO IMPROVE COMMUNICATION IN A PATIENT HAVING SPEECH DISORDER

- Cut down on outside distractions
- Speak slowly and look at the person you are talking to
- Use simple and concrete language
- Do not change topics quickly
- Use short and clear sentences
- Try to convey only one idea at a time
- Pause between phrases
- Use less ambiguous phrases
- Do not shout. (If you suspect hearing loss, arrange for a hearing test)
- Check whether the patient understands you
- Check whether you understand the patient
- Encourage the patient
- Do not pretend that you understand
- Do not expect too much of yourself. The important thing is to keep trying. So that the patient does not experience social isolation and lack of human contact.

THERAPEUTIC GUIDING TECHNIQUES

In the cases of brain damage in children and adults, guiding the patient's hands and body during performance of actual tasks and learning of the movement have proved amazingly successful by this unique technique, perceived and developed by a Swiss neuropsychologist Dr Félicie Affolter over many years. This technique has proved appropriate at any stage of treatment. The technique enables the patient to improve both his physical and cognitive abilities (Affolter 1981 and 1991). To facilitate the learning process the task must be goal, oriented and clearly identified by the patient. The most elementary motor processes can be influenced by specific cognitive states such as expectations, goal and knowledge of the result. Goal-oriented tasks help to inhibit spasticity and task must be selected in real life situation and involve problem-solving activities. The activity should be planned at the patient's level of performance, this is judged by observing the patient's performance. The patient's attention span and understanding of the activity are prerequisite for effective learning. Considering the complex processes involved in learning, therapies based on reflex responses do not help the patient to relearn to function adequately and independently. In the normal development of an infant, various reflexes become modified and are organized into goal-directed activities (Piaget 1969).

Criteria for Optimal Learning

- Interaction with the environment through tactile kinesthetic channel
- To work with tacto-kinesthetic inputs in real life situation
- Successful performance of the problem-solving tasks
- Repetition with variation
- Meaningful goal-oriented activities.

In the treatment of cognitive and perceptual deficits, apraxias and agnosias, the treatment aims at the root of the problem to achieve maximum lasting recovery.

The patient who is unable to learn through his environment because he cannot feel or move normally, the therapist aims to achieve the necessary interaction by guiding the patient's hands and body to ensure the maximum tactokinesthetic input in inhibited postural patterns.

Considerations for guiding technique:
- Position of the patient and the therapist
- Stability
- Quiet environment
- Activities are guided in non-verbal realm or in a soothing voice. Avoid loud strong commands that distract the patient
- Alternating activities with both hands

Guiding is not only invaluable as treatment intervention but provides important information for the continuous assessment of patient's level of performance at his optimal level.
- The patient is quiet
- His eyes are directed towards the task
- His muscles relax and unwanted motor activity is reduced to minimum
- Spasticity reduces and if hypotonus present alert tension is felt
- The therapist may feel forward movement in appropriate direction and active participation or notice a slight movement of his head towards the object require for the next step in the task. Close observations during the activity will reveal improvement or the difficulties encountered by the patient.
- The ability to feel through an intermediary tool or an object and its use permits skillful activities like surgery, painting, etc.

The concept of therapeutic guiding makes a big difference to the patient during his full course of rehabilitation. These techniques enable him to achieve more positive outcome and better adjustment in the society. There should be no limits placed on what the patient can achieve.

Complications and their Management

Hemiplegia is a condition which is manifested due to variety of causes which are enumerated before. After the onset of these symptoms, complications may occur which are as follows. The management of the complication becomes a daunting task because of the fact that the one half of the body is paretic and the patients usually are apprehensive about their recovery.

SHOULDER PAIN

The painful shoulder is one of the most distressing of the problems faced by the hemiplegic patient. The pain has been described as affecting 70% of hemiplegic patient. (Caldwell et al, 1969).

To carry out the treatment successfully, it is important to review "the three areas" in the shoulder joint complex which is inherently a very mobile joint and the stability is partly compensated by the surrounding musculature (Zinn 1973).

■ The mobility of scapula on thorax

■ The normal scapula-humeral rhythm and the factors influencing the shoulder joint mobility and stability

■ Muscular attachments—the various muscles acting in harmony as the stabilizers and prime movers. These muscles have their attachments to cervical, thoracic and lumbar spine and the rib cage. The upper extremity can function effectively only on a stable trunk. The abdominals stabilize the trunk on thorax, and during the movement of the arm, there is a constant subtle activity in the trunk flexors and extensors. The shoulder problems are divided in to 3 main groups:

1. The subluxated shoulder

2. The painful shoulder
3. The shoulder hand syndrome.

Associated shoulder pain is the most common of the complications post hemiplegia. The causes are: The decreased tone around the hemiplegic shoulder. The shoulder joint has only muscular attachment with the scapula. The stability of the shoulder is compromised for the mobility. Usual subluxation is inferior subluxation. The other cause is malhandling of the patient in the initial stage. Turning on the hemiplegic side with the shoulder trapped in the internal rotation under the body can cause severe shoulder pain. When the patient is assisted for sitting up in the bed or during turning, if the affected upper limb is pulled abruptly, it can harm the shoulder. The loosely hanging hemiplegic upper limb during sitting and standing will have effect of gravity and, in turn can damage the shoulder due to lack of tone in muscles around shoulder and scapula.

The best approach to this problem is the prevention. Education regarding the handling of the patient to the nursing staff and the relatives of the patient can prevent the problems to a great extent. If the problem has already occurred, then early electrical stimulation to the shoulder and scapular muscles with the shoulder subluxation strap will ease out the problem. The pain can be taken care of by the transcutaneous nerve stimulation (TNS) (Figure 16.1) and interferential therapy (IFT). If not treated

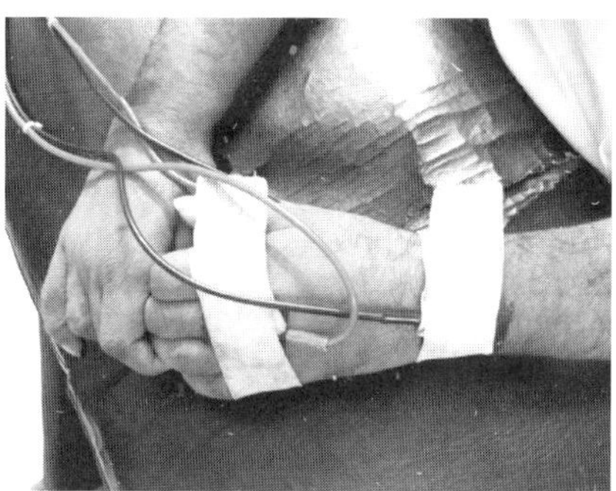

FIGURE 16.1: TNS for reflex sympathetic dystrophy (RSD) left upper limb, left hemiplegia

early, it can cause traction on the brachial plexus and can result into shoulder hand syndrome and sudek's osteodystrophy. Early weight-bearing with proper handling of the part and joint approximation will improve the tone around the shoulder joint and will stabilize the shoulder. Ice application is a vital therapy for pain relief. Quick ice will facilitate the muscles.

THE SUBLUXATED SHOULDER

The subluxated shoulder occurs in early stages of stroke when:
- The stabilizing biomechanical factors are disturbed; the position of scapula on thorax is in relation to the glenohumeral joint
- Loss of head, neck and truncal activity.

Inferior subluxation is a very common feature, subluxation itself is not painful, but it may progress to a painful shoulder. Maintenance of scapula rotation on thorax and full pain free mobility of the glenohumeral joint will avoid the pain in the joint.

Treatment Aim is Threefold

- Proper positioning and handling techniques in bed and in sitting position
- Passively orient the position of scapula in relation to glenohumeral joint
- Restore normal locking mechanism and stimulate muscle activity in hypotonic trapezius, deltoid, supraspinatous, sternomastoid and truncal muscles.

Slings

Do not place the subluxated arm in sling for the immobilized arm interferes with the body image; reinforces flexor tone impairing postural support and impending gait pattern (Voss 69). Neurologist Oliver Sacs (1995) mentions after undergoing surgery for his right shoulder, "I am adapting, learning all the while with my toes to learn a new balance pattern'.

Causative Factors

As described above, improper handling of the shoulder girdle in the acute stage of stroke is the main cause of pain when the arm is elevated without proper protraction of scapula and external rotation of the humerus, this results in delayed rotation of the scapula and the greater tuberosity of the internally rotated arm impinges on the acromian causing pain and joint limitation beyond 90°–100°. Improper positioning in bed when the patient directly lies on his shoulder joint or is pulled from the shoulder during transfers are also common factors. If the causative factors are not eliminated, constant trauma increases pain beyond patient's tolerance.

Treatment

The therapeutic approach is to gently mobilize the scapula and glenohumeral joint (Maitland techniques), gentle mobilization of adverse neuromuscular tension (Butler techniques). As the pain reduces, gently perform passive movements in small ranges, mobilize the shoulder through the pelvis girdle rotations to normal side in supine-lying. If the sensations are intact, warm sponges, TENS and ultrasound can be used, taping and ice help in reducing pain considerably. Approach is to work on head-neck orientation, encourage truncal activity, gentle mobilization of the scapula to achieve normal scapulo-humeral rhythm by inhibiting spasticity and facilitate muscle activity.

Pulleys

It has been assumed that pulleys and shoulder wheel aid to maintain and increase joint mobility, but on the contrary, the patient traumatizes his own shoulder in attempt to force the internally rotated and inactive arm in to elevation and abduction without adequate scapular rotation. (Najenson et al, 1971), (Devise, 86). There are three disadvantages of pulleys and shoulders wheel.

- Loss of scapular stabilization
- Loss of external rotation
- Compensatory extension and lateral rotation of the spine decreasing glenohumeral mobility.

SHOULDER HAND SYNDROME (REFLEX SYMPATHETIC DYSTROPHY)

- Occurs most commonly in first 3 months, about 12.5% of hemiplegic patients are affected (Davies), swollen hand is associated with pain in the shoulder, its dull aching pain, causative factors are the imbalance of muscle tone and loss of selective muscle activity constantly places the wrist in flexion and ulnar deviation. The swelling on the dorsum of the hand is caused by the obstruction of venous drainage. The inflamed hand is swollen with skin discoloration, a marked hard, tender ganglion-like prominence appears in the center of the dorsum of the wrist. There is marked tenderness of wrist and fingers with limitation of joint ranges, the MP and IP joints are in extended position with loss of index finger-thumb space. There is associated loss of supination and shoulder girdle mobility. This can also lead to carpal tunnel syndrome in few cases.
- Over stretching of tight painful flexors tendons while-weight-bearing exercises or forceful passive movements of the wrist and fingers predisposes the hand in inflammatory reaction of shoulder hand syndrome.
- **Treatment approach** is to prevent all the causative factors, should the patient complain of pain or discomfort, the therapist should immediately change his treatment techniques.
- Main aim is to reduce edema, pain and joint stiffness. Rest the wrist in neutral cock-up splint. Position the forearm well in chair and elevate the arm about heart position in bed. The arm should never be left to hang down. The therapy session should be totally pain-free. Icing and compressive crepe bandage aid in reducing swelling.

■ Contraindications

Therapists dread soft tissue contractures and tend to be too vigorous while treating swollen hand, this feature inflames the joints. The rule here is too little rather than too much (Davies, 1977). Self-ranging flexion, elevation and abduction exercises are contraindicated.

■ Conclusion

Importance of understanding the exact nature of shoulder problem, early detection, careful supervision of handling and treatment, techniques, systematic evaluation and with symptom specific treatment this painful complication can be avoided. In spite of prophylactic measures should this problem arise, they can be overcome if detected early, and never ever working in to pain for mobilization or weight-bearing. The treatment strategies are based on interrelationship between orthopedic and neurological factors. Once the pain is under control, there is good steady progress and the patient is motivated partner.

FRACTURES

Hemiplegic patients can fall due to lack of balance and can fracture their limbs. If the bone is broken on the hemiplegic side, then the immobilization can deprive the patient of the physiotherapy and the recovery is delayed. It can cause additional stiffness, and pain can increase spasticity and thus, further complicating the matter. If the fracture is on the uninvolved side, it may render the normal side useless of any functional activity and dependence of the patient increases. With lower limb fractures, it may take around 4 to 6 months for the patient to get back to normal functional activities. Commonest sites of fractures are: neck humerus, radial head, Colles', intertrochanteric and neck femur.

Patient and careful approach of the physiotherapist will improve the condition. For the prevention, the patient should be not left alone, while he does not get enough balance to handle himself.

THALAMIC PAIN SYNDROME

This condition is of severe burning pain which the patient is unable to bear due to thalamic lesions. There are severe unpleasant sensations on one half of the body. This condition is unfortunate and difficult to handle. Apart from the drugs, TNS and IFT, desensitization and application of pressure over body parts can be used effectively. Weight-bearing on the affected site can ease out the symptoms. A very patient approach on the part of the physiotherapist with enough care is required for effectiveness.

OUTBURST OF LAUGHING AND CRYING

As such, the thalamic pain syndrome and the outbursts of laughing and crying are both thalamic lesion problems. In certain thalamic lesions, the patient cannot have control on the emotions. The emotional discharges are uncontrolled and hence, the patient becomes emotionally viable even with a slight stimulus or many a time, with no stimulus at all. This condition is very disturbing for the patient and is embarrassing too. The people around might feel that the patient has lost the mental balance but it is not the case. The patient's intelligence has no effect due to this problem. Autosuggestions and understanding can control these symptoms at a long run. The patient needs to count, the number of times a day, this outburst occurs and cautiously try to minimize the outbursts. Meditation and chanting of mantras will help to cope up with the situation.

TIGHTNESS-CONTRACTURES-DEFORMITY

Moderate-to-severe spasticity on the affected site coupled with the lack of proper stretching exercises right from the acute stage may produce tightness of the muscles in which the resting length of the muscle is decreased. If a faulty exercise like resisted exercises of the spastic muscles is done without complete stretching of the muscles, the tightness of the muscles will increase fast. The tight muscles will have a newer length and hence, the length tension relationship of the muscular action on the joint is altered and the efficiency of the muscular contraction is further lessened. This is a vicious cycle. The tight muscles can be relaxed and newer better length is achieved by adequate stretching of those muscles. These exercises are continued for maintenance of normal length of the tissues. Splints help to keep the part in a position where tightness can be prevented.

If muscular tightness is not tackled with, it may permanently have decreased length which does not increase even with passive stretching. This is known as contracture. There is no therapy for contracture and hence, they should be prevented at all cost. If the contractures have already occurred, surgical intervention of muscle tissue lengthening can be done but, with little effect due to the spasticity. Night splints can be used for maintenance of the muscular and soft tissue length. If contractures are neglected, the other structures like the ligaments, joint capsule, cartilage of the joint, will lose their physiology and the deformities of the joints and the entire affected limb will set in. This is not uncommon in rural India, where physiotherapy services are unavailable. Deformities alter the normalcy of the body parts totally and the patient's chances to recover as before diminish. Counseling, training to adjust to newer body challenges will help to cope up with this difficult situation to some extent.

The treatments includes ice application for pain relief and decrease in spasticity pre and post physiotherapy sessions, splintage for positioning of the body parts in a stretched condition, stretching exercises to maintain muscle length, passive exercises to maintain and increase range of motion of joints and surrounding structures and active motor control activities to prevent spastic muscles to over contract. All the spasticity relieving methods should be incorporated, as early as possible, to prevent this dangerous complication, which impairs the patient's normal recovery phase.

PUSHER'S SYNDROME

Pusher's syndrome is a very severe condition which is characterized by the fact that the patient will take the weight on the hemiplegic side by 'push' from the sound side. The push from the sound side is so strong that the patient totally leans on the hemiplegic side and falls over in sitting position. Even in lying, the patient pushes on to the bed with the sound side and hence, the midline orientation which is of paramount importance, is lost. As the therapy becomes difficult right from the initial stages, the prognosis is poor. The patient takes a long time to register the normal postural reflex mechanism, which is a base for all the motor activity. As in lying and sitting, when the patient is brought to standing, the push from the sound side will not allow the patient to stand erect without support. Many a times, the push is so strong that even with support, it is difficult for the therapist to make the patient do any activities in sitting or standing position.

Treatment for the pusher's syndrome is extremely difficult for the reasons discussed above. Moreover, the patient usually exhibits other perceptual problems which complicate the matter further. The line of treatment would be to make the patient be in midline in all the activities and postures right from the initial stages. Strategies which incorporate manual shifting of the weight on to the sound side and dynamic trunk control with the vestibular ball are employed. Visual feedback for the midline orientation with strong verbal commands is often necessary.

Associated Problems

Associated conditions like the speech involvement make it difficult for the patient to communicate effectively and hence, the frustration which may generate from it may cause increased spasticity in affected limbs, depression and hence, delayed recovery.

■ Prolonged bedrest in severe cases of disability causes pressure sores. If they are not treated timely, they may lead to infection and septicemia and may even lead to death. Pressure sores or the bed sores can be prevented by skin breathing, i.e. turning the patient frequently, once in 45 minutes to 1 hour. This will ease out the pressure on the dependent site and skin circulation will improve. Devices such as air bed, water bed, and ripple bed can minimize the chances of pressure sores but, nevertheless, turning the patient frequently and keeping good hygiene of the part has no alternative.

   Other complications of prolonged lying are pneumonitis and deep venous thrombosis. The pneumonitis can be prevented by early chest and pulmonary physiotherapy in form of deep breathing, coughing and huffing, segmental breathing exercises, incentive spirometry and percussions and vibrations. After the complication has already occurred, postural drainage along with suction and above mentioned physiotherapy will dilute the secretions and help in clearing the lungs of the secretions.

   Deep venous thrombosis or the DVT can be prevented by regular rhythmic contractions of the muscles of the lower limbs, especially calf muscles. It will maintain the venous return and will not allow the blood to become stagnant. On an hourly basis, passive physiotherapy of the lower limbs can be given in all patients to minimize the risk. The ripple stocking will prevent this complication. Post DVT, a very careful approach is employed and the experienced physiotherapist will do movements so as not to create further complication.

■ Complications of the general systems are dealt with by the experts of that system effectively. Timely referral will take care of the same.

17

Adjunct Therapies

BIOFEEDBACK

Electromyographic biofeedback (EMG-BFB) may be used to improve motor functions in patients with hemiplegia. This technique allows patients to alter motor unit activity based upon audio and visual feedback information. Thus, firing frequency can be decreased in spastic muscles, or increased, along with recruitment of additional motor units, in weak, hypoactive muscles. Patients in the chronic stage or patients in late recovery for whom spontaneous recovery is more or less complete have consistently demonstrated positive results that may be attributed to biofeedback therapy. Benefits include improvements in ROM, motor control, function, and relaxation. Most studies indicate that its greatest effectiveness is achieved when it is used as an adjunct to regular therapy in a combined approach. Following an initial training period, EMG-BFG can also be self-administered, allowing patients to practice on their own.

Successful biofeedback applications in the trunk and lower extremity have focused on improving posture and balanced control of ankle and knee muscles. Programs typically begin training in the more dependent postures (e.g. sitting) and gradually progress to more upright postures. Dynamic control using feedback during gait has also been utilized. Electromyography or electrogoniometric information can improve control of the limb and eliminate problematic gait deviations such as genu recurvatum or limited dorsiflexion in swing. Limb load devices that give feedback about the amount of loading or weight-bearing on the hemiplegic limb have also been effective in improving gait. Patients receiving this training demonstrate more normal weight-bearing and stance times on their affected limb and increased swing times on their unaffected limb. Upper extremities applications in stroke rehabilitation have largely focused on relaxing the spasticity of muscles such as pectoralis major, biceps, or wrist and finger flexors. Significant improvements in initiating voluntary finger extension have also been reported following upper extremity biofeedback training.

ELECTRICAL STIMULATION

Neuromuscular electrical stimulation (NMES) may be used with patients recovering from stroke to facilitate voluntary motor control, to temporarily reduce spasticity, and/or to substitute for an orthosis. Neuromuscular electrical stimulation has been shown to increase the ability of muscle to exert force, by preferentially activating the fast-contracting motor units. Effective treatment results in stroke rehabilitation have been reported using NMES to improve dorsiflexor function, wrist extension function, and spasticity reduction associated with antagonist muscle activation. The term functional electrical stimulation (FES) refers to the regular use of ES in functional tasks. Functional electrical stimulation to the posterior deltoid and supraspinatus muscle has been used in patients with stroke to re-establish glenohumeral alignment and reduce subluxation. It has also been used to assist dorsiflexor function in place of an AFO or as an adjunct. Patterned FES, in which a multichannel program was developed from individual profiles of EMG and anthropometric measurements yielded significant improvement in active ROM of paralyzed limbs. Since this group of patients had limbs that have been paralyzed for more than six months, the results suggest a significant CNS learning effect from FES.

Electrical stimulation has a very distinct role in the field of physiotherapy. Its importance has been stated in many research works and it enjoys a respectable position in our field. Its effect on maintenance of the physiology of tissues after a lower motor neuron lesion is very well accepted. Its effect in gaining

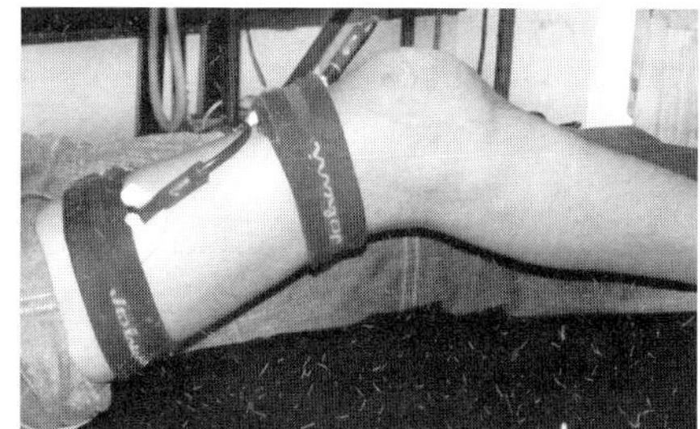

FIGURE 17.1: Electrical stimulation to knee extensors, right hemiplegia

the near normal tetanic contractions using the faradic type of current is well-known (Figure 17.1). TNS or the transcutaneous electrical nerve stimulator is highly effective in relieving the pain in any part of the body. It also can activate the sensory system of the body and help in restoring the lost sensations post hemiplegia.

However, its role in gaining back the lost motor functions post hemiplegia has always been very controversial. Many physiotherapy clinics across the globe freely use the faradic or the galvanic type of electrical stimulation regularly on their patients. Sometimes, due to lack of time on the part of the physiotherapist compeled to use the electrical stimulation more than the specialized techniques of neurophysiotherapy.

While electrical stimulation may be effective in gaining the motor control back as many studies suggest, its judicious use is strongly advocated. If electrical stimulation is given wrongly, it may prove to be harmful rather than beneficial e.g. faradic stimulation given to the flexor of the wrist and fingers and elbow flexors may increase spasticity and complicate the case further and delaying the recovery of the wrist and fingers extensors and elbow extensors, respectively.

Thus, electrical stimulation should be used cautiously and is to be used as an adjunct to the neurophysiotherapeutic techniques and not as a replacement.

TENS and interferential current therapy are highly effective in reducing the pain which is present in large numbers of the patients in shoulder region. They are also effective in reducing the pain and improving the circulation in the cases of shoulder hand syndrome. Interferential current therapy also helps in influencing the sympathetic nervous system and hence, decreasing the symptoms of the shoulder hand syndrome like burning, hypersensitivity, pain, etc. TENS and Interferential current therapy help in reducing the dreadful symptoms of the condition called Thalamic Pain Syndrome. They are effective in reducing the discomfort resulting from the subluxated shoulder.

The sensory activation post stroke can be influenced positively by the use of sensory amplitude electrical stimulation and neuromuscular electrical stimulation in the early stages.

Thus, electrical stimulation is a good tool for gaining the motor control and sensory activation in the patients suffering from hemiplegia if used along with the neurophysiotherapeutic techniques, even in as chronic cases as five years post stroke.

New researches are going on in the world in this field using different methods. One of the methods is intracranial electrical stimulation, where, tiny electrodes are placed on the brain and the part to be stimulated is triggered with external unit. It is explained elsewhere in this thesis.

Another method is EMG triggered electrical stimulation in which, the sensory electrodes are kept at the surface of the muscle to be stimulated, and, the patient is asked to perform the task of that muscle. The signals of the muscular contraction initiation are taken up by the machine via sensory surface electrode and when the desired threshold is reached, the machine gives electrical stimulation to that muscle to complete the movement. This method is unlike the conventional electrical stimulation, which is passive in nature. Here, in this method, the electrical stimulation of the muscle is only done when the patient tried to perform the task of that muscle. Thus, it is an augmenter of the patient's own efforts and not a mere passive stimulation. The effectiveness of this method is under scanner and hence, its results would be out soon.

At some places in the world, neuroprosthesis have been used, to a lesser effect. They are devices to be fixed inside the nerves and they stimulate the nerve when need be. The research on this topic is far too less to comment upon.

One more method of stimulation is the functional electrical stimulation, (FES), which is an effective way of gaining desired motor activity at a desired time. The patient is fitted with the stimulator while engaging in the task simultaneously. For example, the long extensors of the wrist and fingers are stimulated for opening of the fingers while doing hand functions. The stimulation is done when the patient attempts to open the fingers when need be to either release the object or to grasp it. It can be effectively used while walking when the muscles which are responsible for say dorsiflexion are stimulated at the time of initial swing. The timing of the start of the impulse is highly important in this technique.

ISOKINETICS

Isokinetic training may be used to improve the timing of reciprocal movements of the lower extremities required for gait. The therapist should initially preset movements to utilize slower speeds as control improves. If consistency in maintaining a steady rhythm is problematic, a metronome can be used to pace the activity. With some types of equipment, the patient's position can be modified to approach a more upright standing position. A rate of movement approaching 1 cycle per second, which is within normal parameters for heel-strike to heel strike, should be the desired end point of treatment.

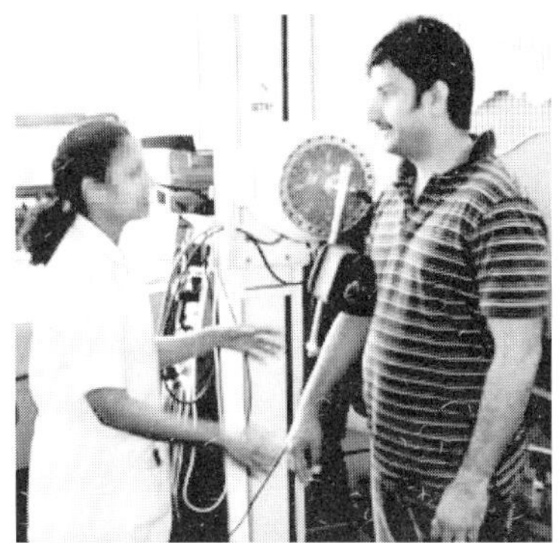

FIGURE 17.2: Isokinetic machines 'primus', right scapula dysfunction (orthopedic case)

Isokinetic training may also be valuable in stabilizer muscles of upper limb (Figure 17.2). These muscles are difficult to rehabilitate but with the help of isokinetic workout, this task can be simplified.

MUSIC AS THERAPY

Music can be of great assistance in gaining the rhythm of the movement. Soothing music can decrease the spasticity in the muscles and improve functions in the agonists. It provides a sense of general relaxation and global reduction in the muscular tone. The pulse rate stabilizes and hence, the patient is able to concentrate more effectively on the task at hand. Some ragas of Indian classical music and rhythmic chanting of vedic mantras can influence the mind and body complex of the individual and take them to a newer height. They can increase the inner strength of the individual and help cope up with the situation. These methods also relax the therapist and the work efficiency increases with the decrease in stress levels. Music also provides with the entertainment which is of vital importance for both the therapist and the patient.

EXERCISE CONDITIONING

Patients with stroke demonstrate decreased levels of physical conditioning following periods of prolonged immobility and reduced activity. The energy costs to complete many of the functional tasks in their daily lives are higher than normal owing to the abnormal ways in which they perform these activities. Many patients also demonstrate concomitant cardiovascular disease and may be recovering from acute cardiac events at the same time. These patients can benefit from an organized exercise program to improve cardiovascular fitness as part of their rehabilitation. The geriatric survivor with compromised cardiovascular function can benefit from an ambulation program regulated by signs and symptoms of activity intolerance. Other stroke survivors should be able to engage in a more traditional exercise conditioning program (Figure 17.3).

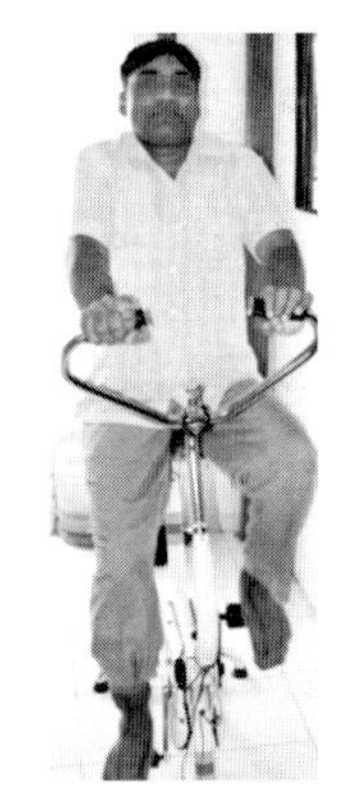

FIGURE 17.3: Bicycle ergometry for exercise conditioning, left hemiplegia

To ensure patient safety, patient should receive a thorough evaluation before starting a program. Adequate supervision, monitoring, and safety education about warning signs for impending strokes and heart attack are also important considerations. Considerations for prescription should be based upon individual abilities and the interest of the patient. The components of an exercise program should include type of exercise, frequency, intensity, and duration. Warm up and cool down sessions should include stretching and strengthening elements as well as aerobic elements of increasing or decreasing intensity, typical aerobic elements include cycle ergometry of arm and leg, walking, and stair climbing. A frequency of 3 to 5 days a week with an intensity of 60 to 85% of the age predicted maximal heart rate, 50 to 80% of maximal oxygen consumption or REPE (ratings of perceived exertion) value of 12 to 13 should provide an adequate training stimulus. The duration will vary depending upon the frequency and intensity of the activity. The use of training diary is an excellent way to keep track of prescriptive elements, objective measurements (heart rate, RPE, blood pressure), and subjective reactions (perceived enjoyment).

Conditioning programs for stroke patients can yield significant improvements in physical fitness, functional status, psychological outlook, and self-esteem. Regular exercise may also have the additional benefit of reducing risk from recurrent stroke. Finally, patients who participate in a regular conditioning program may more successful in adopting continuing, lifelong exercise habit and in moving beyond the disabilities of the stroke.

ROBOTICS AND COMPUTER-AIDED THERAPY

The role of robotics and computer-aided therapy is a very novel concept in the field of medicine and in the field of neurorehabilitation. As the studies suggest, there is marked improvement in the arm functions after the use of robot in the motor relearning post hemiplegia. It may take a while this technique arrives in India but the advancement always brings about a radical change in the way we look at the problem. The use of computers and its feedback is also effective in gaining the motor functions post hemiplegia. There are programs which help the patient use their paretic limbs more effectively. The use of surface electrodes which are attached to the computer show the contraction as the graphical representation on the screen. The patient can thus follow the graph and the desired repetitive contractions can be achieved. Virtual reality method which employs computer generated life-like images in the controlled environment can be used as a precursor to the functions in the actual environment. The patient first practices the functions on the virtual images in the virtual world and then, the real world functions can be safely started.

Other newer technique is stem cell therapy which is in its nascent stage. The results of the same are eagerly awaited by medical persons as well as general population equally.

CONSTRAINT-INDUCED THERAPY

Constraint therapy is a newer invention in the field of the rehabilitation of hemiplegic hand. After gaining a reasonable motor recovery in the post hemiplegic hand, most patients find it difficult to use their upper extremity in activities of daily living. This is known as 'learned disuse' of the body part. This occurs due to the inhibition of that specific part, here, the upper extremity. To tackle this problem of learned disuse, the patients are well, almost, forcibly made to carry out the active hand usage in a controlled environment.

The patients are kept in a room with minimum or no external disturbances like sound or visual stimuli so that mental distraction is minimum and there is full concentration in the task which is given. The normal hand is kept in a splint so that they cannot use that limb and hence, cannot substitute for the hemiplegic hand. The patient is given a series of tasks which are ranging from simple prototype active movements of the hand to a more complex set of activities of daily living. They are encouraged to carry out the same with full zeal and force. The sessions are carried out for 5 to 6 hours a day, 3 to 4 times a week, and the progress is monitored every fortnight. Recent studies have shown remarkable improvement in the functional ability in the individuals with the problem of learned disuse in 3 to 4 weeks of time.

Limitations

This therapy can only be used in the individuals with some amount of active motor control in hand. The patients many a times become irritable at the limitations of their performance and get frustrated. In patients with gross spasticity, the hypertonia increases in the entire body, rendering the therapy useless.

MOTOR RELEARNING

Motor relearning is a technique developed in Australia and in the recent times, a lot of studies are going on to find out the efficacy of the same in the treatment of hemiplegia.

This technique concentrates on the fact that the repetition of the movements produces the required memory anagrams in the brain and hence, the motor function of the part improves. The patients with hemiplegia are made to do the exercises a number of times a day till they become proficient in doing the same. The numbers of repetitions are designed according to the tolerance of the patient. Maximum numbers of repetitions are selected for each activity and patient is asked to do the same several times a day. This treatment is continued till the patient can easily perform the task assigned.

These exercises can be simple active movements of the joints in the acute stage to progressing towards more complex functional activities including various muscles and joints interplay.

HYDROTHERAPY

Hydrotherapy is a specialized approach of treatment for the patients suffering from hemiplegia. As the name suggests, water is used for the therapy.

Hydrotherapy or exercises underwater use the principle of buoyancy of water. The force of the buoyancy of water is the force which is opposite to that of the force of gravity. If any object is placed in the water, the water will exert the force of buoyancy on that object, in opposite direction to that of the force of gravity. Thus, the effective weight of the body will decrease when in water, as compared to its effective weight on land. Physiotherapy also uses the force of buoyancy in the favor of the patient. If the hemiplegic patient is placed underwater, the effective weight of the patient will decrease. Thus, the patient will have to carry that much less load of the moving limbs. When the limbs become light in weight, it is easier to move them. This will ensure decreased effort on the part of the patient with increased efficiency. The spasticity decreases with the decrease in the effort, which will in turn improve the motor function.

Water is also a good tactile stimulator and hence, the sensory integration can be carried out underwater effectively. Underwater exercises can be relaxing and entertaining for most of the patients.

In the initial stages when the patient is unable to move by himself, the patient is lowered in the water with the use of a waterproof plinth which is lowered in the water by the use of chains attached to a pulley device. For the safety, the patient is tied onto the plinth with the straps. The patient is then asked to perform the movements underwater on the plinth itself keeping the head and neck outside the line of water. The buoyancy of water will provide assistance to the moving limbs if the movement is done against gravity. This will register the movements in the brain in the antigravity direction which is not possible for the patient in the initial stages. The endurance will improve as the patient can perform the activities underwater for a longer duration than on land due to weightlessness of the body.

In the later stages, more active protocol can be employed and the recovering limbs can be subjected to resistance by the water itself if the movement is made in the direction of gravity. Gait training can be done in the gravity eliminated plane underwater, effectively.

Apart from the various advantages of the exercises underwater, there are many disadvantages of the same. The temperature of the water should be neither high nor low to accommodate the patient. The water should be very clean so that the chances of cross infection can be avoided. The maintenance for keeping the water warm and clean is too high for the most of the rehabilitation clinics across India. The patient safety is also of a paramount importance as one little negligence may prove extremely dangerous. A tie up with the swimming pool can be done, but the unavailability of the trained staff and the sadistic approach of the swimming pool attendants does not go in patient's favor and hence, the patient cannot be sent to the pool which is not run by rehabilitation personnel.

A small effort on the part of the physiotherapy community with the help from the local government and non-government organizations can solve the problem of non-commissioning of the hydrotherapy units in India and the patients can reap the benefits of exercising underwater even in our country.

ORTHOSIS IN HEMIPLEGIA

An orthosis is an external appliance worn to restrict or assist motion or to transfer load from one area to another. Term orthosis appears to be since after World War II. In case of hemiplegic patient orthosis are basically required when persistent problems prevent normal and safe walking.

Factors Responsible for Using Orthosis

- Instability
- Weakness of ankle, foot, knee
- Extent of spasticity
- Sensory deficit of limb.

Types of Orthosis

- Temporary
- Permanent
- Static
- Dynamic.

Orthosis Used in Hemiplegic Patients (Figure 17.4)

- AFO
- KAFO
- Wrist cock-up splint
- Pressure splints
- Air stirrup ankle brace

Functions of Static Splints

- It provides immobilization to the joint
- It maintains joint in correct alignment preventing tightness, contracture and deformity
- It provides support and stability to the lax joints
- It maintains the corrected or improved ROM gained by therapeutic measures
- It provides stability to proximal joint to facilitate action of distal joint, e.g. cock-up splint to stabilize weak wrist extension and to facilitate finger flexion.

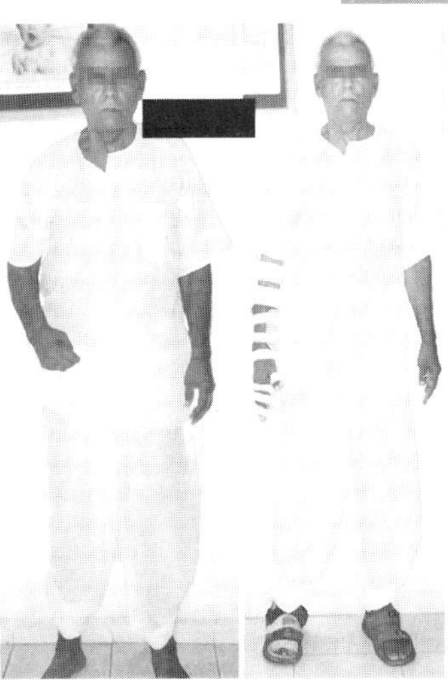

FIGURE 17.4: Note the use of elbow extension splint, cock up splint, AFO, right hemiplegia

Functions of Dynamic Splint

- It provides resistance to tendons providing easy gliding, preventing adhesion and stimulating circulation thereby, assist in reducing edema.
- It provides mobility to stiff joints by controlled sustained low load stretching. Constant stretch lengthens shortened musculotendinous units and tight articular structures as well.
- It provides re-education to weak or paralyzed muscles with synchronization of active efforts
- It protects overstretching of weak muscles by strong pull of normal opposing muscle group.

Static splints commonly used in hemiplegic are:
- Upper limb splints
  - Cock-up splint
  - Opponens splint

 – Functional position splint
 – Safe position splint
- Lower limb splint
 – Posterior knee splint or cast
 – AFO.

Dynamic splints commonly used in hemiplegic are
- Upperlimb splints
 – Dynamic wrist flexion-extension splint
 – Dynamic thumb splint
- Lowerlimb splints
 – Dynamic AFO
 – Dynamic KAFO.

Upperlimb Splints

Cock-up Splint

It maintains the wrist in 25–30 degrees of extension. In case of lack of extension, control at MP joints, outriggers may be applied to make it dynamic, e.g. radial nerve.

Opponens Splint

It maintains the web space of the thumb, thus holding the thumb in maximum opposition.

Functional Position Splint

It is mainly a positioning splint,, maintaining flexion at MP and PIP joints fixed at 40–50 degrees and the thumb in abduction and opposition.

Safe Position Splint

It is resting or positioning splint. The wrist is fixed in slight dorsiflexion, MP joints in 90 degrees of flexion, PIP and DIP joints in neutral extension and thumb is placed in abduction and opposition to allow ROM at the CMC joint. The hand is safe from developing flexion contracture and to promote functional use at larger stage. This is useful to prevent contractures following burns.

Dynamic Wrist Flexion-extension Splint

It allows both the movements of flexion and extension at the wrist with a provision to maintain any of these movements fixed at desired range.

Dynamic Thumb Splint

A dynamic thumb splint can be fabricated as a low profile splint which keeps the thumb in opposition, maintaining the web space.

Lowerlimb Splints

Posterior Knee Splints or Cast

It offers stability to unstable joints due to derangement; it facilitates the function of weight-bearing and ambulation, the lower extremity splinting is in the form of orthosis. It provides the needed functional stability to the unstable joint.

AFO

It consists of foundation, ankle control and super structure.

Foundation
Consists of shoe, plastic or metal component.
- Insert
    - An insert or footplate foundation is used to provide best control of the foot.
    - Insert is usually used in shoes, close high on the dorsum of the foot to retain the orthosis.
    - Orthosis with an insert is relatively light-weight as it is made up of thermoplastic material.
    - It is appropriate if the shoe to be worn on orthosis is not of proper heel. If the heel is low, upright will incline posteriorly , increasing tendency to wearer's knee to extend. If the heel is high, patient might experience knee instability.
- Metal stirrup
    - It is steel stirrup, U-shaped fixture riveted to the shoe through shank.
    - A solid stirrup—maximum stability of orthosis on the shoe.
    - A split stirrup—it is heavier than solid stirrup or the foot plate.

Ankle Control
To control ankle motion by limiting plantar flexion or dorsiflexion or by assisting motion.
- Posterior leaf spring:
    - It is used as dorsiflexion assistance arising from plastic insert.
    - Upright is bend backwards slightly during early stance.
    - During swing phase, plastic recoils to lift the foot.
    - Narrow plastic permits greater motion.

- Klenzak joint—steel dorsiflexion spring assistance:
  - The coil spring compresses during stance and rebounce during swing.
  - Tightness of the coil can be adjusted but orthosis is noticeably bulkier than post leaf spring.
  - Both assistance will yield slightly into plantar flexion at heel contact, affording the wearer protection against excessive knee flexion.
- Posterior stop—plantar flexion resistance:
  - To prevent toe drag through plantar flexion resistance, preventing the foot from plantar flexion so that during swing phase foot drag will not occur to catch the toe and stumble.
  - It imposes flexion over the knee during early stance and prevents lax knee from hyperextending.
- Anterior stop:
  - It limits dorsiflexion which helps during later stance.
  - Plastic anterior spring extending from mid-dorsum of foot to proximal margin of the orthosis.
- Plastic solid ankle foot orthosis:
  - It limits foot and ankle motion
  - It compensates for lack of plantar flexion in early stance.
  - It may be divided into 2 section at ankle through hinged known as hinged solid ankle-foot orthosis providing sagittal motion, achieving foot flat position in early stance.

Super Structure

Uprights

- Solid ankle and hinged ankle AFO have posterior shell, extending from medial to lateral midline of the leg, thus providing excellent medial lateral control and broad surface to minimize pressure.
- Uprights have calf bands which must not impinge on peroneal nerve.
- Anterior band part of solid AFO imposes posteriorly directed force near the knee, enabling AFO to resist knee flexion.
- Tone reducing orthosis in hemiplegics consist of foot plate and broad uprights designed to modify reflex hypertonicity by applying constant pressure to the plantar flexors and invertors.

Merits of AFO

- AFO is usually prescribed to control deficient knee and ankle foot function.
- Posterior leaf spring helps to control foot drop.
- Modified AFO has wider lateral brim and provide additional control of calcaneal and forefoot inversion and eversion.
- Solid ankle-molded AFO helps in maximum stabilization through its wider lateral trim lines.

- Posterior stop can be added to limit plantar flexion, with spring assist, can be added to assist dorsiflexion.
- An ankle set in 5 degrees dorsiflexion limits knee hyperextension, while an ankle set at 5 degrees plantar flexion, stabilizes the knee during mid stance and prevents knee buckling.

Air Splints/Inflatable Pressure Splints

- It stabilizes and helps in maintaining the extremity in elongated position.
- Inhibition of tone, for example, spastic elbow flexors, is provided.
- Splints also helps in control unwanted associated reactions, and assist in early weight-bearing.
- Patients with a flaccid, hypotonic limb benefit from the use of pressure splints to provide increased sensory input. When used along with weight-bearing, tone is facilitated.
- Long or full limb pressure splints also assist in controlling edema, a common problem of paralyzed limb. Positioning with elevation is an important consideration.

Demerits

Disadvantage of metal devices include heavier weight, less cosmetic appearance, and increased difficulty in putting it on.

The type of orthosis may change with continuing recovery.

With limited reimbursement, ordering a new orthosis may create problems and speak to the need to anticipate changes when ordering the device, its change in prescription and discontinuing the use of the device.

Orthotic training includes donning and doffing instructions, skin inspections, and education in safe use of the device during gait.

BOTULINUM INJECTIONS FOR SPASTICITY

Physical and occupational therapists play important roles in the evaluation and management of patients receiving botulinum toxin type A (BTX) injections for spasticity. Having a thorough working knowledge of this intervention will allow therapists to refer appropriate patients for such injections. The sudden decrease in muscle tone brought on by BTX enables the therapist to focus on functional treatment goals and implement interventions quickly and effectively.

Before BTX injection, patients need to be extensively evaluated by the therapists to quantify baseline function for effective outcomes determination.

Since a decrease in spasticity in one area can precipitate functional changes in other associated or unanticipated areas, the evaluation must include areas beyond those being injected. After injection, and once the patient's response is ascertained, the evaluation may be modified for future injections to the same region.

With patients affected by chronic spasticity, it is helpful to evaluate and treat the patient as a "new" patient after injection. Injections will interrupt synergistic patterns and affect neighboring or more distant muscle groups. With local spasticity suddenly reduced, the patient may present with a different clinical and functional picture and may be a candidate for therapeutic interventions not previously possible. Motivated by the sudden decrease in spasticity, patients frequently stop taking oral and antispasmodics despite previous instruction to the contrary. Therapists need to reinforce that patients must continue taking their medication until after post-injection assessment as directed by their physician.

Evaluation

A patient receiving BTX should be evaluated thoroughly before the first injection. The scales and techniques chosen can be adapted to either the occupational or physical therapies, as well as to the type of clinical setting. Pre and post-injection measurement consistency is essential for effective comparisons. Because the measures themselves may influence tone during the clinical visit, it may be important to run the testing series in the same order and position each time. Below is a list of evaluation tools and techniques that are available for the adult patient about to receive BTX treatment.

■ **Modified Ashworth Scale (MAS)**

Performed for all muscle groups in the extremity with increased muscle tone, whether these muscles will be injected or not. Spasticity reduction in one area may affect muscle tone in neighboring areas, particularly where synergies are involved.

■ **Pain Score**

Executed for the entire extremity to be injected, as well as for the specific region being injected. In left gastrocnemius injections for example, the lower extremity is rated for pain, as in the left ankle region. The patient is asked to rate the amount of pain in the affected region on scale from 1 to 13.

■ **Spasm Frequency (SF) Score**

All muscle groups with spasm within the extremity to be injected are graded. Spasticity and spasm reduction in one muscle group may result in a decreased SF in neighboring muscles.

■ Bilateral Adductor Tone

This measure is performed on all patients receiving lower extremity injections who exhibit increased tone in the adductors of the leg. The assessment is performed with the patient supine. The examiner abducts the legs simultaneously and grades the amount of effort needed.

■ Range of Motion (ROM)

ROM is assessed following the MAS assessment and measure of bilateral adductor tone so as not to influence existing muscle tone. Active and passive ROM is assessed goniometrically in the injected extremity. Consistency should be maintained in order and position of assessment pre- and post-treatment so as not to influence muscle tone or bias outcome assessment. Positions can be modified, however, so as to evaluate the upper extremity in sitting and the lower extremity in supine. This minimizes positional changes that may influence muscle tone.

■ Joint Resting Angles

Goniometric measurements can be taken of joint resting angles altered by spasticity. Joint position may be noted in various functional positions, e.g. sitting, standing, or immediately following ambulation. Documentation may be supplemented with photographs or videotape. It should be kept in mind that injections may interrupt synergistic patterns and reduce resting angles at neighboring joints.

■ Strength

Strength may be assessed in related areas where normal muscle tone is present. The accepted method of assessment is conventional manual muscle testing. The numerical scale used is a 6 point ordinal scale assessment strength from 0 (no contractile abilities) to 5 (strength through the full ROM with maximal resistance). Dynamometer testing can objectively determine grip strength where normal muscle tone is present.

■ Motor Control

Motor control is assessed where muscle tone is altered. Unfortunately, standardized assessments for motor control that can be tested for validity and reliability have yet to be devised for use in the neurologic patient. Most available measures, including Brunnstrom and Fugl-Meyer, focus on assessment in the post-stroke patient. These methods, which are not widely used, are based on the premise that stroke recovery follows a predictable pattern from reflex movement, to volitional movement within synergistic patterns, and then to volitional movement out of synergy. Bobath's method grades the ability to move out of synergistic patterns as it relates to functional importance.

When measured goniometrically, the previously described active movement (active ROM) indicates available volitional movement. EMG evaluation can document available active muscle contraction and may help indicate the functional potential of opposing antagonists or neighboring muscle groups.

■ **Fine Motor Coordination and Dexterity**

The score for the finer functions and dexterity of the hand should be taken prior to the injections and timely evaluation of the same post injections should be taken to find out the effect of the same.

Order for Evaluation of Muscles in the Patient with Spasticity

Assessment in the patient with spasticity is complicated by the effect of the evaluation procedures on muscle tone; the examination influences what it is measuring. The proper order of evaluation can minimize this influence, and performing the evaluation in the same order each time ensures consistency of effect between successive examinations. Muscle tone is assessed before any functional or other clinical assessments requiring movement or handling of the patient. The upper extremity precedes the lower, right precedes left. The upper extremity is evaluated in the sitting position. As indicated below, the shoulder rotators, pronators, supinators, wrist flexors/extensors, and finger flexors are assessed with the elbow in 90 degrees of flexion. Other muscle groups are assessed with the elbow extended.

The following order of muscles may be considered:

With elbow extended, evaluate:
■ Shoulder flexors
■ Shoulder extensors
■ Shoulder adductors
■ Shoulder abductors

With elbow flexed, evaluate:
■ Shoulder internal rotators
■ Shoulder external rotators
■ Elbow flexors (shoulder at 0 degree flexion)
■ Elbow extensors
■ Pronators (elbow flexed 90 degrees)
■ Supinators
■ Wrist flexors
■ Wrist extensors
■ Finger flexors

The patient is positioned in supine for assessment of all muscle groups of the lower extremity except the knees flexors. The right side is assessed first, followed by the left. The patient is then positioned prone for assessment of the right, then the left knee flexors.

The following order of muscle may be considered:

Supine
- Hip flexors
- Hip extensors
- Hip adductors
- Hip abductors
- Knee extensors
- Ankle plantar flexors
- Ankle dorsiflexors
- Ankle invertors
- Ankle evertors.

Prone
- **Knee flexors**

The modified Ashworth scale assessment is executed first, followed by the bilateral adductor tone measure, if required. Goniometric measurements for active and passive ROM follow muscle tone assessment. All other aspects of evaluation may then be executed. This specific order of assessment may not fit all patients, therapists, or clinical settings. Of primary importance, however, is that movement of the trunk and limbs be minimized when assessing tone and that consistency be maintained between assessments.

- **Balance Skills**

Balance skills are assessed for patients receiving either upper or lower extremity injections. One useful test, which has shown good inter-rater reliability and validity, is the timed-up and go test, based on the initial get up and go test developed by Mathias. The patient is asked to rise from an arm chair, walk a line 3 meters across the floor, turn around, and return to the chair. The score is given as the number of seconds it takes to complete the task. The patient is allowed to wear his usual footwear and use his usual assistive device. This test is easily performed in any clinical setting and has direct functional importance.

- **Activities of Daily Living (ADL)**

All ADL skills are to be assessed before either upper or lower extremity injections. When appropriate, the caregiver may be questioned regarding type and amount of assistance required by the patient. Aspects of the functional independence measure (FIM) and the Barthel index may be used for grading ADL function. The Barthel Index is a questionnaire aimed at the three functional areas of self-caring (drinking, eating, grooming, dressing), bowel and bladder continence, and mobility including transfers (chair, tub and toilet), ambulation and stairs. Scoring is from 0, indicating total dependency, to 100, indicating total independence. Snow and Tsui developed a "Hygiene Score" which may be used for patients requiring caregiver assistance for perineal hygiene tasks. This measure allows documentation of changes in the amount of assistance required for complete care for patients receiving BTX injections in the lower extremity. The Berg balance scale assesses balance in a variety of functional skills and may be used to provide standardized functional data related to a patient's ADL abilities. This test scores 14 skills of a total of 56 points and includes such tasks as transfers, getting in and out of a chair, aspects of standing (stance and balance), forward reaching, and retrieving objects from the floor.

▉ Transfers

Transfers can be influenced by a reduction in spasticity and, therefore, are assessed.

Effects and Benefits

The Botulinum toxin is injected in the spastic muscle for the reversible paralysis of the spastic muscles. This will ensure the relaxation of the spastic muscles. Due to spasticity, even the resting posture of the limbs is not correct and if it is allowed to stay put same way, can lead to contractures and deformities. The relaxation of the muscles will ease out the process of stretching of the muscles and hence, prevent deformities. Hygiene of the part improves with the improvement in the posture of the limb, e.g. hygiene of the palm in spastic long flexors of forearm. The reduction of the spasticity of the agonists will facilitate the recovery of the agonists and help in speedy recovery of the patient.

Therapeutic Exercise

Das and Park, Dengler et al, Hesse et al., Dunne et al., Pierson et al., and Yablon et al., all have conducted studies demonstrating improved active or passive ROM following BTX treatment. Simpson et al. showed improved grip strength following injections in the upper extremity hemiplegic stroke patient. All investigators demonstrated decreased muscle tone in the injected muscles, which has important implications for therapeutic exercise intervention. After injection, a priority for therapeutic intervention is strengthening and facilitation of the opposing and neighboring muscle groups. Treatment goals include maximizing the patient's abilities in the antagonists, to further reduce spasticity are reciprocal inhibition and reinforce more normal mobility and position. These muscles can be chronically over-stretched and atrophied from disuse, and may be initially at a mechanical disadvantage after injection, requiring a longer response time.

Once spasticity is decreased, stretching and flexibility exercises for the spastic agonists may begin where indicated. New increases in passive or active range of motion may be possible. This may enhance therapy participation, function, or the execution of home programs by the patient or caregiver. In spasticity patients, decreased mobility and abnormal movement patterns may lead to under-stimulated proprioceptors and mechanoreceptors. Following spasticity reduction, stimulation can be provided via weight-bearing activities, vibration, proprioceptive neuromuscular facilitation, and a variety of other techniques. Many patients may now tolerate developmental or Bobath type activities that had not been possible before, such as quadruped and kneel-standing. Benefit may also be gained from re-educating balance and stability in such positions, as well as in standing and sitting.

The role of the injections is only to reduce the tone of the muscle and this means that more work needs to be done before its beneficial effects reach the patient. The assessment provides the background of the matter. After mapping the muscle of the muscles to be injected, the patient is prepared. The patient is informed regarding the merits and the demerits of the treatment and consent for injecting is taken. The muscles are then marked and exact site of injections is finalized. The toxin is diluted according to the dose suggestions and the type of the muscle. The injection is then given intramuscular. It is advisable that complicated and small muscles should be injected under the guidance of Electromyography or EMG.

One week post-injections, the patient is kept in an immobilizer for a period of 2 to 3 weeks. If the patient is uncomfortable with the immobilizer or if it is contraindicated, the patient is advised to stretch the injected muscle frequently throughout the day so that spasticity can reduce faster and relaxation and newer resting length of the muscle is obtained.

Vigorous physiotherapy in form of stretching, facilitatory exercises, weight-bearing and adjunct therapy are started immediately for many times in a day and patient is taught the same. The peak effect of the injections is approximately gained at one month and the effect lasts for about 4 to 6 months. There are subjective variations due to the dose of the drug, its antibody formation in the body, amount of stretching and physiotherapy. During this time, the patient is instructed and motivated for complete cooperation in physiotherapy. The injections can be repeated after the antibody response decreases in the blood which is after a six months of time.

The effect of botulinum toxin is best got in the patients who have got at least some amount of recovery in the agonist muscles. Otherwise, the spasticity may decrease in the injected muscle, but patient may not get the desired motor recovery and hence, may feel dejected and unsatisfied with the treatment.

OTHER ALLIED THERAPIES

In India, there are many systems of medicine which the patient undergoes when ill. These are the allopathy, homeopathy, ayurveda and unani to name a few. In today's world, any system of medicine which is not Allopathy is known as alternative medicine. But, this author differs from this general view. The systems which are listed above are existing since many years and the encouraging results and the scientific approach which they possess qualify them to be known as 'Allied Therapies' and not 'Alternative Therapies'. The discussion of the importance of these therapies is way beyond the scope of this study and hence, they will be enumerated below. It is the observation of this author as well as many other clinicians practising for neurological rehabilitation that the physiotherapy and rehabilitation has no alternative and hence, all the patients should undergo rehabilitation programs regardless the system of medicine they pursue. This will secure the patient of the basic motor and sensory awareness and rehabilitation would be complete in nature.

List of Therapies

- Ayurveda
- Allopathy
- Homeopathy
- Unani medicine
- Aroma therapy
- Reiki
- Pranic healing
- Accupressure
- Accupuncture
- Color therapy
- Gem therapy
- Crystal therapy

- Water therapy
- Mud therapy
- Naturopathy
- Magnet therapy
- Psychic healing
- Doraa-dhaagaa
- Meditation
- Sujok therapy
- Medicinal oil massage and tissue manipulation
- Traditional system of medicines of adivasis
- Chakra balancing therapy
- Stone therapy
- Pendulum therapy.

The list is endless due to the extent in which the hemiplegic patient tries to get the recovery from this dreadful condition. We respect all the methods of the patient care but firmly advocate the judicious use of all these therapies. The patient should be the central theme of the treatment and not the system of medicine which the patient uses.

Hemiplegia Care at Home

INTRODUCTION

When the patient gets discharge from the hospital, the patient may not be able to even turn to sides actively. In such a case in India where rehab hospitals are few in number, the patients are treated at home (Figure 18.1). All the arrangements for the patient care are done at the patient's residence. Physiotherapy services are arranged at the earliest on the reference of the consultant. The patient, if affording, will have the services of the nursing support staff. Sometimes, if the patient is in a vegetative state, a separate room, especially for the patient with the adjustable bed and ripple or the air or water mattress is arranged for. Physiotherapy is started at the home with the available resources. Usually, it is the physiotherapist who arranges for the required things. The therapist is the one who spends most of the time with the patient and hence, in the initial stages, the therapist becomes a clinical psychologist for the patient as well as the patient's relatives. Physiotherapist will educate the patient and the relatives regarding the importance of rehabilitation.

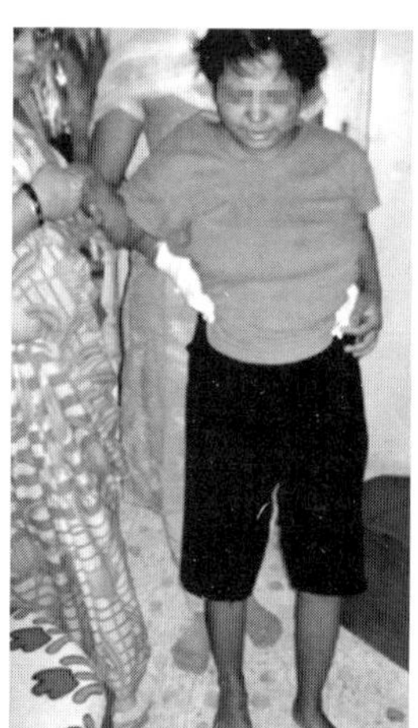

FIGURE 18.1: Assisted gait training at patient's home, helped by relatives

MERITS OF HOME TREATMENT

There are some advantages of the patient being treated at home.

- The patient initially is very nervous and anxious and has just returned from the hospital, which is a traumatic experience. After coming back to home which is a familiar environment, the patient's mood improves and it manifests on his recovery.

■ The patient may be disabled physically and hence, may not have enough strength for attending the physiotherapy and rehabilitation department. Physiotherapy at home will provide the best solution for this problem.

■ The physiotherapist would be treating only one patient at a time while at patient's home. This gives the therapist enough attention and focus on a single patient only, which is mandatory for the patient in the acute stage.

■ Home physiotherapy program is safer than the rehab department for the patient in the early stages.

DEMERITS OF HOME TREATMENT

Where there are merits, there are bound to be demerits. The demerits of the home treatment are as follows:

■ If the patient is treated at home, lot of arrangements for the patient are needed like the bed, mattress, physiotherapy and other rehabilitation services, etc.

■ For the physiotherapist, there are no equipments which may be useful.

■ The patient does not go for the rehabilitation or for recreational outing and will get confined to the home.

■ The patient will not have contact with other patient of similar condition and this will decrease the patient's communication.

■ Arranging everything for the patient is costly monetarily, for the relatives of the patient.

■ The patient may sometimes get used to confinement in the home and may not like to go out and mix with people even if they are physically fit to do so.

Brocklehurst suggested that social factors are the most significant elements which influence the doctor in his decision to treat the stroke patient at home. It has been claimed, however, that many doctors lose interest in the stroke patient, once the acute phase of the illness has passed and that most patients in the community receive very little, if any, long-term rehabilitation (Mulley and Arie, 1978).

There are a number of approaches to the treatment of the stroke patient, each with their enthusiastic advocates; here, we shall discuss different techniques which are usually selected empirically and tailored to fit the needs of the individual patient and his family. The methods used are similar to those employed in hospital. Within the home, there are not the comprehensive facilities available in hospital; this factor along with problems of space, equipment, old and infirm relatives and unsuitable beds all create special challenges for the domiciliary physiotherapist when treating the stroke patient at home.

TREATMENT PLAN

Before treatment commences, it is essential that a plan is prepared with a detailed assessment of the patient including physical dependency, communication problems, mental state, social background and medical diagnosis.

This initial record can be based on a number of different functional tests. No particular system of recording is wholly satisfactory and there is no general acceptance among physiotherapists as to which is most suitable. The ideal system needs to be easy to complete, simple, and reproducible by different physiotherapists on the same patient. The importance of accurate recording cannot be overstated.

As well as this initial assessment, there should be a continuous monitoring of progress, by a physiotherapist in order to have an unbiased assessment of the patient's achievement.

PROBLEMS ASSOCIATED WITH HOME-BASED TREATMENT

These can be considered under a number of headings which are not listed in any order of importance as the circumstance may alter from patient-to-patient—psychological, social environment, equipment, communication, diagnosis, supporting, services.

Psychological Problems

Following hemiplegia, a major problem can be depression which may be severe, and long-standing. Lipsey et al. (1984) estimated that depression can affect between 30% and 60% of post-stroke patients. It is, therefore, essential that the domiciliary physiotherapist is aware of the signs and symptoms of depression so that the concerned doctor is alerted.

It will be appreciated that an affective disorder such as depression involves an increase in intensity of normal emotions and that the boundary between normal and abnormal is imprecise. There are certain behaviors that are characteristic of the depressed state:

1. **Depressed mood:** The major complain in most cases. This state is reflected in the posture, facial expression, speech and general appearance of the patient.
2. **Difficulty in sleeping:** Either difficult to get to sleep or early morning awakening, there may be a loss of the sleep architecture in many of the patients. The ratio of the REM and NREM sleep patterns change.

3. **Loss of energy:** Patient feels tired and drained, may even imagine he has some serious disease.
4. **Loss of interest:** Patient loses interest in work, home, social activities, sex.
5. **Loss of concentration:** Patient is unable to concentrate, memory is unreliable. Pre-occupation with morbid self-doubt or guilt feelings.
6. **Loss of appetite:** Most patients lose their appetite, although younger people may over eat as a compensation for feelings of inadequacy.

Transference is a term used to describe the development of an emotional attitude in a patient towards a therapist. It is not unusual for a patient to experience powerful feelings of love, hate and so on with regard to the physiotherapist. The patient may also have certain fantasies about the physiotherapist and it is important that the therapist is able to appreciate that such events are a normal consequence of many therapeutic relationship.

Apart from the psychological problems experienced by some hemiplegic patients, there are also psychological problems for the physiotherapist when faced with a large contingent of such patients in the community. The work is usually heavy and demanding both in terms of time and effort, with the likelihood of emotional demands on the physiotherapist which are, on occasions, more exhausting than their physical counterparts.

The fact that the majority of the stroke patients are aged 65 and over adds additional stress, as many patients of this age are suffering from more than one pathological condition or present with a serious social problem, unconnected with the stroke.

As the domiciliary physiotherapist is working in comparative isolation, it is probable that the therapist is faced by more difficulties and the need to accept more responsibility for the patient than other medical staffs.

Social Problems

In the hospital, the patient is a part of a process which ensures that patients are fairly strongly regimented with regard to their treatment. If a physiotherapist shows the ward staff how to position the patient in a certain way, this will usually be implemented whether the patient is able to agree or not. In the home, the roles are reversed—the physiotherapist is a guest and if the patient does not wish to comply with the treatment procedures, he may refuse. It is vital that the domiciliary physiotherapist should gain the confidence and cooperation of the patient and his family, as early as possible, in the treatment course.

The physiotherapist will be teaching the family certain exercises and routines. In such a situation, it is not unusual for the physiotherapist to be seen as part of the family and professional standing of the physiotherapist should be retained in order that role boundaries do not become unclear.

In dealing with any patient, a friendly reserve should be adopted and it should be remembered that the dividing line between normal professional concern and friendship is easily misread. Making friends with a patient can lead to worry or even guilt; it is important to remember that some patients will misinterpret sympathy or similar attitudes which can lead them to develop unrealistic expectation about the clinical interaction. In this context, 'friend' is taken to mean a person with whom a mutual need of satisfaction can be realized. It is reasonable for the physiotherapists to express hopes, values and so on and to give support to the patient but the clinical interaction should not be used to support or satisfy own needs or anxieties.

Problems with the Environment

The treatment of the hemiplegia patient will normally require very little equipment. The main item of equipment missing in the home is a set of parallel bars, a vestibular ball and a high mat. It is often difficult, if not impossible, to get elderly person with hemiplegia down on to the floor and the appropriate treatment will therefore, be given while the patient is on his bed. Tables or chairs can sometimes be substituted for the parallel bars. Full length mirrors are not always available in the home but lengths of mirror which can be screwed to the wall can be obtained quite cheaply and are well worth the investment.

With an efficient community store, there should be few problems with aids such as chairs, commode, bath seats and transfer boards and so on.

Communication Problems

As physiotherapist is working single-handed within the community, it is probable that the therapist will experience problems arising from extended or non-existent lines of communication. To establish lines of communication is hardwork and, initially, can be very time-consuming. These lines of communication are well-established within the hospital but, in many areas, may be virtually unknown within the community. The general practitioner (GP), nurse may have established communication procedure but often the physiotherapist can find the self-having to contact these individuals separately which can prove both difficult and frustrating. Message left with a third party are rarely delivered correctly and the domiciliary physiotherapist may have no option other than to spend months establishing effective lines of communication with the colleagues in the community.

Diagnosis

Quite often the diagnosis which the domiciliary physiotherapist receives may be no more than telephone message saying 'Mr X, CVA, please treat'. There are always exceptions, but sometimes, it is difficult to contact the doctor on the day when he is needed. The establishment of group practices adds to this problem as some doctors may work only on certain days in the practice and cannot be contacted.

An additional task which, increasingly, is allotted the domiciliary physiotherapist is the request from a consultant for the opinion as to whether the patient requires hospital admission for rehabilitation. This type of work is an example of the role extension possible within the community and adds greatly to the challenge presented by this type of work.

Supporting Services

Often the physiotherapist is the first person to recognize a particular need in a family and then the therapist is faced with how to arrange for certain supporting services for the patient and his family. In areas, where there is no community, occupational therapist, the physiotherapist may have to request for alterations to be made within the home. This is an area of responsibility which ought to be extended to domiciliary physiotherapist who is trained to recognize such a need and, more importantly, probably one of the first experts to visit the patient.

SUGGESTED SOLUTIONS

All the above problems can be alleviated, if not prevented, provided a number of basic steps are taken at the commencement of treatment. If the preparation of the treatment plan, following the initial visit, is based on the problem-oriented assessment approach, this will allow the various problems to be listed in order of importance and enable the physiotherapist to define the role with regard to each separate problem. In this way, the total problem presented by any patient can be broken down into separate tasks, some which are the province of other specialties, and this will prevent the physiotherapist from attempting to do too much for any patient. The domiciliary physiotherapist will often be faced with a 'problem patient' who is excessively demanding of difficult. It is probable that the same patient is just as much a problem for the doctor or the nurse as is for physiotherapist. The sense of isolation, which is sometimes experienced by the domiciliary physiotherapist, can be helped by regular attendance at the weekly meetings and by regular visits to the consultants. Many consultants meet at intervals to hold clinical discussions. Such meetings are worth attending. The social atmosphere encourages a good working relationship between the disciplines. Many consultants welcome the physiotherapist's call at their clinic when they are more than willing to discuss the patient and compare notes.

PHYSIOTHERAPIST

The routine which is adopted for the patient nursed at home is broadly similar to that used in hospital. The extension of physiotherapy into the community has enabled many stroke patients to remain at home and there is evidence to suggest that patients receiving their rehabilitation at home, recover equally well as those treated in the hospital. In hospitals which do not have a stroke unit, there can be difference of expertize within the different wards and it is sometimes difficult to engage the cooperation equally of all ward staff. In this respect, the domiciliary stroke patient is at an advantage as provision of care is directed and monitored by the domiciliary physiotherapist.

Early Stages

Treatment will begin as soon as possible, following the hemiplegia and will include positioning, passive movements and care of the chest. The domiciliary physiotherapist will have access to intermittent positive pressure breathing (IPPB) machines, ultrasonic nebulizers and chest suction equipment; if required can also arrange the supply of a tipping frame. If there is a chest infection present, it is possible for the therapist to visit the patient frequently during the early stage of recovery.

A full range of passive movement should be given each day and the relatives will be shown these routines. Positioning of limbs should be taught and it is helpful to fix diagram or pictures of the correct positioning above the patient's bed. Relatives are usually most anxious to be of assistance at this stage of rehabilitation and time spent in careful teaching is well-rewarded.

It is important to remember that edema of the hand is found in 16% of all hemiplegia patients; it is due to insufficient drainage from the lymphatic and the tendency for patients to forget the arm, allowing it to hang over the side of a chair. Passive movement and ultrasound can be used to eliminate this edema which, if left, can rapidly become organized due to its high protein content (Howell, 1984).

Positioning

Co-operation between the physiotherapist and the nurse is essential to ensure that the patient is placed in the correct position following routine nursing procedures. It is also important that the relatives receive consistent advice from both professions as there is nothing as detrimental as conflicting instructions.

It is essential that the nurse and the relatives are shown how to lift the patient up and down, and in and out of the bed. It must be repeatedly stressed that they should not support him underneath his affected arm as this can lead to the painful shoulder syndrome commonly found in the stroke patient. Provided the nurse, physiotherapist and family work closely together, it is possible to give a consistent service to the patient in the home.

Bridging

This simple procedure, which is taught to the patient and to his relatives from the earliest possible time following his stroke, makes it much easier to manage the patient in bed and facilitates such nursing procedures as sheet changing, care of pressure areas and use of the bedpan.

Rolling

The ability to turnover in bed indecently provides considerable stimulus to the patient and will contribute to an improvement in his morale. When it is appreciated, many stroke victims suffering from depression which is often linked with the inability to move without help, it can be seen that any independent movement will be important to the patient.

Bridging and rolling can be taught easily to the relatives and their use will make nursing considerably easier in the early stage of recovery.

Exercise Routine

The program of exercise will closely follow that outlined previously, although there may be occasional modifications depending upon the time available to the physiotherapist. Many of the procedures can be broken down into sections and then taught to the relative, for example re-education of balance can be taught in sequence starting with head control and progressing to the other elements descried. It is possible for most relatives to cope with this 'sectionalized' approach and it ensures that the patient will be given a continuous and consistent treatment, even if it should be spread over a longer period with less direct professional input. The programmer of exercise assumes a bilateral approach to the restoration of function which constantly reinforces the awareness of the affected side. In the community where the patient is either too old or too frail, his relative(s) is/are incapable of cooperating in the rehabilitation, the method adopted may have to concentrate on making the patient mobile by using the support of a walking aid, perhaps utilizing some form of knee brace, such as the Swedish knee cage, or an ankle support.

The resulting pattern of walking is cumbersome and effectively prevents a retune to independence as the patient can never carry anything or, while standing, manipulate any utensil. There may be occasion when the use of a below knee leg iron is justified, especially in cases where the patient is unaware that the ankle is inverted and suffering repeated minor trauma.

Walking

When the patient achieves reasonable standing balance, walking can be attempted even before he has mastered the ability to swing his affected leg. The timing of this event will depend upon a number of factors including the morale of the patient and his family, his walking pattern and the space available within the home.

Advice

It is recognized that the patient and his relatives will seek advice from the physiotherapist at all stage of his recovery. It is probable that the domiciliary physiotherapist is the person with whom the patient most readily relates and from whom advice most often will be sought. The advice which the physiotherapist is expected to provide is wide-ranging and the therapist should beware of offering advice which is contradictory to that of the other professionals calling on the patient.

As far as advice on physical exercise is concerned it is probable that the physiotherapist is the person most suitable to provide it. In cases where advice on medication, social or psychological matters is required, the doctor or the social worker can be approached by the physiotherapist and asked for their opinions. It has been found that the patient is more likely to talk with the physiotherapist than most other professionals, possibly because of the special bond which develops during the course of treatment.

A delicate area is that of sexual activity. There have been a number of instances where a stroke patient has suffered a second one following such activity. Physiotherapists are often asked for their advice on whether such normal pursuits should be attempted. The fact that the patient should ask for advice of this nature suggests he should be encouraged to follow his desires, as the object of treatment is the restoration of function where possible. It is helpful to be reminded that doctors, when faced with similar questions, are no more experienced than most physiotherapists.

Factors which Influence Recovery

Patients who recover their muscle function within the first 2–3 weeks can be considered to have good prognosis for rehabilitation. Neurological recovery is thought to begin at some point between the first and seventh week following the onset of the hemiplegia, with little neurological improvement following the 14th week. Functional recovery is closely linked with neurological recovery; it has been suggested that much of the early recovery including that of the upper limb, may be due to the restoration of circulation to ischemic areas of the brain with late recovery attributable to the transfer of function to undamaged neurons (Tallis, 1984; Thomas, 1984). One finding suggests that improvement can occur in performance 2 years after the stroke (Langton-Hewer, 1979). Factor which militate against recovery include severe spasticity, loss of sensation and mental confusion with inability to cooperate with the rehabilitation exercises. This author has managed to see the recovery of post stroke hemiplegia after 10 years with proper physiotherapy in three to four cases.

The attitude of the relatives within the home is most important. Patient with many of the problem listed above can be maintained at home provided there is good family support. Such families will require long-term support from the domiciliary physiotherapist and it is common practice to keep such patients on the list of regular visits for periods of three more years. There may not be any physical improvement in such cases but the weekly or fortnightly visit by the physiotherapist has been shown to be a significant factor in keeping the seriously impaired stroke patient at home. Any claim that the recovery of the stroke patient can be attributed mainly to circulatory and neurological factors can be questioned by examining a stroke patient who has been neglected for some reason. His limbs will be fixed in abnormal positions; contractures, pressure sores and incontinence will complete the picture and will all contribute to a severe nursing problem. The psychological state of the patient is an important factor in recovery and the sudden change in physical circumstance will, depending on his personality type, lead to depression or anxiety. The patient will worry about his future, especially with regard to his work and finances, and married patients may be concerned about a possible loss of attractiveness where their partner is concerned. All of these worries will depend upon the ability of the patient to be aware of his condition and are absent in a patient suffering from anosognosia. When these worries are superimposed upon either a speech defect or a perceptual difficult, the physiotherapist needs constant patience and the ability to give continual reassurance.

Most physiotherapists will have had experience of a hemiplegia patient who has been excessively agitated or who has struck out at them. These patients are depressed and it should be remembered that this depression is natural and, when the patient adjusts to his changed condition, should improve within a few months. However, in one study, two-thirds of patients who were depressed at the initial evaluation remained so seven to eight months later (Lipsey et al, 1984). The best therapy is improvement and any change for the better, no matter how minimal, must be highlighted by profuse praise and encouragement. There can also be a loss of self-esteem with a refusal to accept a changed body image, is anything to the extent that the patient will deny that there is anything wrong with him. This state of mind is a serious impediment to progress and the use of portable video equipment may help the patient to adjust his self-concept.

The domiciliary physiotherapist must be able to advice on dressing, and in so doing must remember that attempts at dressing with a paralyzed side will involve twisting movement which can, in turn, cause muscle strain with subsequent pain. Cooperation with the occupational therapist over such matters as how best to put on socks, stockings, trousers, as well as what dressing aids are available, is to be recommended most strongly.

Toilet problems are common; one useful hint is to place a small table by the lavatory pedestal to hold sheets of loose toilet paper. Although washing is often difficult, self-help must be encouraged. A bath seat is essential, and support rails and uprights can be obtained by the relatives. Patients can be taught to dry themselves by using several small hand towels rather than a large bath towel which would be difficult to handle.

The economic, social and emotional effects experienced by the family as a result of stroke may be expressed in feelings of helplessness and frustration, often projected on to the physiotherapist in the form of criticism or by excessive demands for additional treatment. To counter this, family should be involved in all stages of the rehabilitation and should be encouraged to express their fears and anxieties. The family should also be prepared for the eventual termination of physiotherapy treatment and this process should commence from the first visit. The house-bound stroke patient is not able to mix with other stroke patients as is possible in hospital; such mixing in the ward encourages social skills and will facilitate interaction among the patients. In the case of the stroke patient at home, the physiotherapist will have to ensure that this element to rehabilitation is not overlooked and the therapist may have to advise the family how best to achieve it. The tendency for the family to be protective and over-indulgent to the patient needs to be guarded against.

Although recovery is ultimately dependent upon the underlying pathology, it is evident that the sooner the treatment begins, the better the outcome. The age of the patient is not significant although it has been claimed that the younger patient will have a stronger motivation to get better. Elderly patients are as likely to respond as well to treatment as younger ones.

Severe spasticity if present, may be helped by drugs or by various surgical procedures, while muscle weakness in sometimes treated by electrical stimulators, such as the peroneal stimulator used in cases of foot drop. The painful shoulder, common to many stroke patients, is a constant problem for the domiciliary physiotherapists. It can be treated with positioning, ice, heat, interferential therapy or ultrasound. Connective tissue massage is useful in domiciliary treatment, while support from slings or the use of figure-of-eight bandages may provide some relief. Maitland mobilization can be effective. In some units, biofeedback has been used with varying degrees of success (Williams, 1982).

Discharge

There are certain guidelines governing the discharge from treatment of the stroke patient, and these include:
1. Pressure of new referrals
2. The wishes of the patient and his family
3. Level of progress
4. Availability of follow-up services
5. Lack of further improvement.

For physiotherapists, the lack of progress is likely to be the point at which discharge from treatment is considered. It should be remembered that the idea of 'discharge' is stressful for the patient and his family may respond by demanding further treatment, convinced that improvement will occur. Emotional language if often employed: 'left to rot', 'thrown out' commonly being used to express the fear felt at such a time. Because the domiciliary physiotherapists are often required to face this situation alone, the therapist can experience acute discomfort and personal feelings of guilt. In order to avoid such problems, it is essential that the family is prepared for eventual discharge from the very first visit. This will require continual reinforcement on each subsequent visit and a possible routine is suggested:

1. Explain the nature of the illness and the possible plan of treatment.
2. Reassurance regarding the provision of other supporting services.
3. Praise and encouragement for the relatives.
4. Provide some indication regarding the probable number of weeks' duration of treatment.
5. This routine should be repeated on each visit so that the family is conditioned to expect the eventual termination of treatment. There may be cases where treatment will continue indefinitely on a restricted basis as described earlier.

As soon as the patient is able to walk upto the door, the encouragement is made to take the patient out of the home as soon as possible. The patient can practice the walking in the surroundings with the home-visiting physiotherapist initially and then by themselves with the help of the relatives or professional help. The patient can go out for the recreational activities and the problems encountered are listed. These problems are discussed with the physiotherapist and solution for the same is found out. The patient may start going for physiotherapy in the clinic as soon as possible. This will decrease the cost of the rehabilitation in a longer run. If the patient is affording, twice a day exercise protocol is used where, once the patient goes to the clinic and second time in the day, the physiotherapist would go for their home visits. As patient become more and more independent, the home visits should be stopped and the patient is advised to use the time for their professional activities.

The patient is taught to become independent of the physiotherapist so that the treatment protocol is followed even in their absence. Many a times, young physiotherapists migrate to foreign countries for better future and in turn, jeopardizing the future of the patient. The patients usually get attached to a physiotherapist who has treated him in the acute stages and with the therapist leaving the patient; the patient will feel lonely, left out and insecure. So, it is a duty of the therapist to see that the proper rehabilitation is carried out in their absence; whether the patient is shifted to clinic for better functioning, or the therapist migrating to some newer venues.

In social country like India, the strong social backdrop is a double-edged sword. The relatives of the patient can become extremely cooperative at some stage with the therapist and the patient and they can also become hostile with the therapist and the patient at other stage. The therapist, therefore, should gauge the social vibes of the patient's environment and find out a suitable way of treating, dealing and communicating.

Orthopedic Management of Stroke

INTRODUCTION

The orthopedic management of stroke can be divided into three distinct time periods:

1. Period of acute injury
2. Period of physiologic recovery
3. Period of functional adaptation to residual deficits.

The Period of Acute Injury

Initial efforts should be directed toward the medical stabilization of the patient. The orthopedic surgeon is rarely involved in the acute care of the stroke patient. In some situations, the orthopedic surgeon may be asked to assist with splinting extremities to prevent limb deformities.

The Period of Physiologic Recovery

Spontaneous neurologic recovery occurs primarily during the first 6 months following a stroke. This is particularly true for recovery of muscle function. During this subacute phase, limb flaccidity changes to spasticity. When spasticity becomes pronounced, temporary measures are used to prevent contracture taking place. These measures are used till spontaneous neurologic recovery is taking place.

The Period of Functional Adaptation to Residual Deficits

Generally, the patient is neurologically stable after 6 months. Decisions can then be made regarding surgery to correct limb deformities and rebalance the muscle forces. This is the time of greatest contribution by the orthopedic surgeon.

EVALUATION

Improving extremity function requires detailed evaluation of all factors causing the impairments.

Assessment of Cognition and Communication

An evaluation of cognition and communication skills is done during the physical examination. The patient must be capable of following simple commands and should also be able to cooperate with a postoperative therapy program. In addition, the patient should have sufficient cognition to incorporate the improved motor function into their use of the extremity. Adequate memory is needed to retain what is taught during postoperative therapy.

Sensory Evaluation

Intact sensation is essential to functional use of the hand. The basic modalities of pain, light touch, and temperature must be present. Two-point discrimination is a valuable predictive test. A patient rarely uses the hand for functional activities, if the discrimination is greater than 10 mm. Proprioception and kinesthetic awareness of the limb in space are also important. Kinesthetic awareness is tested in a hemiplegic individual by placing the spastic limb in a position and asking the patient to duplicate this position with the sound limb while keeping the eyes closed. Stereognosis is not a practical test in spastic patients. They lack the fine motor control necessary to manipulate an object in the hand. It is helpful to observe the patient's spontaneous use of the hand. Visual perceptual deficits add increased problems involving motion of the limb and even awareness of the limb itself.

The ability to maintain balance and ambulate depends on adequate sensation in the foot and ankle. The basic modalities of light touch and pain sensation are essential. Proprioception must be present at the level of the ankle joint for good balance reactions.

Evaluation of Motor Control, Spasticity and Contracture

In a neurologically impaired patient, it is frequently difficult to distinguish between the many potential causes of limited joint motion. The possibilities include increased muscle tone, a myostatic contracture, lack of motor control, or the lack of patient cooperation secondary to diminished cognition.

Evaluation focuses on the following characteristics of the involved muscles: voluntary or selective control, spasticity and contracture.

Ask five specific questions:
1. Does the patient have voluntary control over a given muscle?
2. Is the muscle spastic to passive stretch?
3. Is the muscle, as an antagonist, activated during active movement generated by an agonist?
4. Does the muscle have increased stiffness when stretched?
5. Does the muscle have fixed shortening (contracture)?

When many muscles cross a joint, the characteristics of each muscle may vary. Because each muscle may contribute to motion and movement of the joint, information about each muscle's contribution is useful to the assessment as a whole. Treatment depends on such information

Spasticity often masks underlying motor control. First, establish passive range of motion of each joint. Test by slow extension of the joint to avoid the velocity-sensitive response of the muscle spindle. When spasticity is significant and passive joint motion is incomplete, it is necessary and advisable to perform an anesthetic nerve block to assess whether a myostatic contracture is present. Alternatively, examine the patient under general anesthesia.

The degree of spasticity within selected muscles can be graded clinically in response to a quick stretch as mild, moderate, or severe.

Motor control can be graded in the extremity using a clinical scale. The extremity may be hypotonic or flaccid and without any volitional movement (grade 1). A spastic extremity may be held rigidly without any volitional or reflexive movement (grade 2). Patterned or synergistic motor control is defined as a mass flexion or extension response involving the entire extremity. This mass patterned movement may be reflexive in response to a stimulus but without volitional control (grade 3). It is also possible for a patient to initiate mass patterned movement volitionally (grade 4). Although patterned movement can often be volitionally initiated, it is a neurologically primitive form of motor control and of no functional use. Selective motor control with pattern overlay is defined as the ability to move a single joint with minimal movement in the adjacent joints when performing an activity slowly (grade 5). Rapid movements or physiologic stress make the mass pattern more pronounced. Selective motor control is defined as the ability to move a single joint or digit volitionally independently of the adjacent joints (grade 6).

Grade	Motor Control	Features
1	Flaccid	Hypotonic, no active movement
2	Rigid	Hypertonic, no active movement
3	Reflexive mass pattern	Mass flexion or extension response to stimulation

4	Voluntary mass pattern	Patient initiated mass movement
5	Selective with overlay of mass pattern	Slow volitional movement of individual joint. Stress results into mass action
6	Selective	Volitional control of individual joint

Identifying Functional Problems and Cause of the Problems

Treatment is most effective when functional problems are formulated and described in focal rather than diffuse terms. Treatment of focal problems lends itself well to surgical intervention, which can target particular muscles. Surgical lengthening, transfer, or release of targeted muscles can provide very effective solutions to problems of function that are clearly identified from the outset. The localizing approach is useful because it forces the clinician to indicate the desired outcome in advance. The outcome is based on an analysis that identifies the specific spastic muscles responsible for the problem. For example, if the clinical problem is an equinovarus foot that inhibits walking, surgically lengthening or transferring the tibialis posterior will not solve the problem if tibialis anterior and gastrocsoleus muscles are really the culprits responsible for the problem. Identifying the specific offending muscles is critically important to localized strategies of intervention.

MANAGEMENT OF SPASTICITY DURING THE PERIOD OF PHYSIOLOGIC RECOVERY

During this phase of recovery, limb flaccidity changes to spasticity. When spasticity becomes pronounced, temporary measures are used to prevent contracture formation. The treatment of spasticity depends on the time, since injury and the prognosis for further recovery. In the period of physiologic recovery, temporizing interventions are used because interventions which cause permanent changes may result in chronic imbalance of forces across joints.

Oral Agents

Oral antispastic agents may be used during this period. Antispastic agents that have sedating properties, such as baclofen, diazepam, and clonidine, may compromise patients with attention deficits or memory disorders. Even a drug such as dantrolene sodium, which has a peripheral mechanism of action, may also cause drowsiness. Other serious side effects such as hepatotoxicity can occur. Continuous infusion of intrathecal baclofen has been reported to be useful in managing spasticity secondary to spinal cord injury but its role in spasticity due to stroke is not very well studied.

Focal Treatments

Focal injection with neurolytic or chemodenervating agents is the most suitable approach for treating restricted motion secondary to spasticity. Neurolytic agents such as phenol and chemodenervation agents such as botulinum toxin A are used during this period because their effects are temporary, lasting only 3 to 5 months. These agents are used when restricted motion occurs as a result of focal spasticity. When these agents wear off the patient is re-evaluated to determine whether additional recovery has taken place and whether there is further indication for repeating the treatment.

Phenol Blocks

Phenol, a derivative of benzene, in aqueous concentrations of 5% or more denatures the protein membrane of peripheral nerves. When phenol is injected in or near a nerve bundle, its neurolytic action on the myelin sheath or the cell membranes of axons with which it makes contact serves to reduce neural traffic along the nerve. The onset of the destructive process with higher concentrations of phenol may begin to show effects several days after injection. The denaturing process induced by phenol extends biologically on the order of weeks but eventually regeneration occurs. A phenol block is used as a temporizing measure rather than a permanent intervention. The effect of a phenol block typically lasts 3 to 5 months.

It has been shown that phenol destroys axons of all sizes in a patchy distribution but more on the outer aspect of the nerve bundle onto which the phenol is dripped. When phenol is percutaneously injected, it is likely that the nerve block will be incomplete. This is especially useful in situations in which a spastic muscle also has volitional capacity, because under these circumstances, it is desirable to reduce spasticity while still preserving volitional capacity of a given muscle or muscle group.

The technique of phenol injection is based on electrical stimulation. Motor branches are injected close to the offending muscle or muscle group. These branches are referred to as motor points. A surface stimulator is briefly used to approximate the percutaneous stimulation site in advance. A 25-gauge Teflon-coated hypodermic needle is advanced toward the motor nerve. Electrical stimulation is adjusted by noting whether muscle contraction of the index muscle takes place. As the electrode gets closer to the motor nerve, less current intensity is required to produce a contractile response. The motor nerve is injected when minimal current produces a visible or palpable contraction of the muscle. Generally, 4 to 7 mL of 5% to 7% aqueous phenol is injected at each site. Care must be taken not to inject the agent into a blood vessel; this is done by aspirating before the injection.

Botulinum Neurotoxin A (BoNT-A)

BoNT-A is an agent used in the localized treatment of spasticity. Ordinarily, an action potential propagating along a motor nerve to the neuromuscular junction triggers the release of acetylcholine (ACh) into the synaptic space. The released ACh causes depolarization of the muscle membrane, activating a biochemical sequence that leads to muscle contraction. BoNT-A is a protein produced by *Clostridium botulinum* that inhibits this calcium-mediated release of ACh at the neuromuscular junctions. A 3–7 days delay between injections of BoNT-A and the onset of clinical effect is typical. Effects are not seen immediately by the patient, and usually a follow-up visit is arranged to check the result. The clinical benefit lasts 2 to 4 months but may be more variable. BoNT-A is injected directly into an offending muscle and, depending on the size of the muscle being injected; dosing has ranged between 10 and 200 units (U). Current practice is to wait at least 12 weeks before reinjection and not to administer a total of more than 400 U in a single treatment session.

Because this upper limit of 400 U may be reached rather quickly, a different strategy is needed for the limb requiring many proximal and distal injections. BoNT-A and phenol may be combined, with BoNT-A being injected into smaller distal muscles and phenol aimed at larger proximal ones. BoNT-A injections have gained much popularity in the past several years. The advantages of BoNT-A are its ease of injection and the lack of residual scarring after injection. The disadvantages of BoNT-A toxin are its high cost and antibody formation, which requires higher doses for repeated injections. Phenol, by contrast, requires more technical expertise to localize the nerve or motor points for injection. Phenol is caustic and causes localized scarring of the nerve and muscle. On the other hand, phenol is inexpensive and readily available.

Casting

A combination of peripheral nerve blocks and casting or splinting techniques are commonly used to give temporary relief of spasticity. Casting maintains muscle fibres length and diminishes muscle tone by decreasing sensory input. Local anesthetic nerve blocks are very helpful when they are administered before cast application because relieving the spasticity allows for easier limb positioning. Casts are used primarily for the correction of contractual deformities by applying a cast on a weekly basis. Serial casting is most successful when a contracture has been present for less than 6 months.

MANAGEMENT OF RESIDUAL DEFORMITIES

Neurological recovery reaches plateau within 6 months. Decisions can then be made regarding surgery to correct limb deformities and rebalance the muscle forces. This is the phase during which orthopedic surgery can made greatest contribution.

Rationale of Orthopedic Surgery

The orthopedic surgical techniques used to correct limb deformities from inappropriate muscle activity are release, denervation, lengthening, or transfer. Muscle or tendon release removes the deforming force of that muscle. Release is only used on muscles with no potential for function. A release corrects both active deformity and a static contracture. Denervation of a muscle removes the deforming force of that muscle and is useful when no fixed contracture is present.

Lengthening of a muscle-tendon unit diminishes the spastic response to quick stretch (spasticity) in a muscle that has volitional use. By removing the overactive stretch response of the muscle, its volitional use is significantly improved. Lengthening of a muscle tendon corrects both static and dynamic deformities. Lengthening is often performed exclusively to correct a dynamic deformity. When the patient is under general anesthesia and the muscles are relaxed, a purely dynamic deformity (e.g. an equinus foot deformity) appears corrected. Even then muscle is lengthened to decrease its activity during function. This is one situation where muscle is lengthened to decrease its activity even in the absence of a fixed contracture.

Transfer of a muscle-tendon unit redirects a muscle force. It is not necessary for the muscle to have normal control. It is critical that the transferred muscle has a predictable action to achieve the desired result.

Timing and Realistic Expectations of Orthopedic Surgery

When evaluating patients with CNS dysfunction, questions commonly arise regarding the indications for surgery, the cost, what outcome to expect, and the practicality of this approach. These issues should be considered on an individual basis for each patient. The following general principles can serve as guidelines for decision-making.

- *Operate early, before deformities are severe and fixed.* Orthopedic surgery is a powerful rehabilitation tool. It is often the only treatment that will correct a limb deformity or improve function. Surgery should not be considered a treatment of last resort when conservative measures have failed. Physical and occupational therapy cannot effect a permanent change in motor control. Drug therapy for increased muscle tone has generalized effects and cannot be targeted to specific offending muscles. Phenol blocks and botulinum toxin injections provide only temporary modulation of muscle tone. When a permanent treatment is needed to decrease muscle tone or redirect muscle force, consider surgery. The results of surgical intervention are improved when deformities are corrected early. Less muscle lengthening is needed when deformities are mild and there is little or no fixed contracture to overcome. Early surgery preserves maximum muscle strength, joint capsule and ligament flexibility, and articular cartilage integrity. In general, the patient will also be in better physiologic condition to undergo surgery if there has not been a period of several years of immobility.

■ *Better underlying motor control means better function for the extremity.* Orthopedic surgery cannot impart control to a muscle. Lengthening a spastic muscle can improve its function by diminishing the overactive stretch response and uncovering any control that is present. Successful surgery depends on a careful evaluation preoperatively to determine the amount of volitional control present in each individual muscle that is affecting limb posture and movement.

Surgery should not be reserved only for patients with severe impairment and deformity. Individuals with milder degrees of impairment can benefit greatly from relatively simple procedures such as lengthening of the Achilles tendon to regain a plantigrade foot for standing, transfers and ambulation. The amount of improvement correlates best with the degree of underlying motor control and not the severity of the deformity.

■ *Consider the cost of not correcting limb deformities.* The cost of performing a surgical procedure is likewise limited when compared with a lifetime of attendant care, spasticity medications, repeated blocks, orthotics to control limb position, complications such as skin ulceration, infection, fractures due to fall and lost productivity for the patient and caretakers.

■ No soft tissues surgery will be successful if there is an underlying bony restriction. Preoperative radiographs are essential to assess joint congruency, or to detect heterotopic bone or other deformity.

COMMONLY SEEN RESIDUAL DEFORMITIES AND THEIR MANAGEMENT

Shoulder

The paretic shoulder deserves special attention because it is a common source of pain. A variety of different factors contribute to the painful, immobile shoulder:

spasticity with adductors, internal rotation contracture, inferior subluxation and adhesive capsulitis.

Adducted and Internally Rotated Shoulder

The arm is adducted tightly against the lateral chest wall, and shoulder internal rotation causes the forearm to lie against the middle of the chest. The tendon of pectoralis major is often prominent when the examiner attempts to abduct and externally rotate the shoulder but other muscles contribute to the deformity. The glenohumeral joint normally functions as a universal joint, enabling the hand to reach an almost spherical volume of locations in three-dimensional space. When patients attempt to reach forward, spastic adductors and internal rotators can severely restrict acquisition of targets in the environment and on the body. The patient's ability to stabilize, push, or apply force to an object is also compromised. From the perspective of passive function goals such as skin care and axillary hygiene, spastic adductors and internal rotators hinder efforts of caregivers to gain access to the axilla to provide needed care. Restricted motion may impair dressing, washing and bathing, and promote skin irritation and maceration. Passive manipulation of the shoulder during personal care may cause pain and trigger spastic resistance in reactive muscles.

Muscles that contribute to spastic adduction and internal rotation dysfunction of the shoulder include latissimus dorsi, teres major, the clavicular and sternal heads of pectoralis major and subscapularis. Involvement of latissimus dorsi and teres major should be considered when hyperextension posturing of the shoulder is observed. Antagonistic activity in these muscles may be masking a patient's potential for active flexion. Diagnostic lidocaine block to the thoracodorsal nerve or the lower subscapular nerve may unmask that voluntary potential. When the pectoralis major is chronically spastic, the musculotendinous insertion of pectoralis major is prominent and tight. However, the two heads of this muscle may be differentially spastic, and EMG recordings from each or diagnostic lidocaine blocks to medial and lateral pectoral nerves may help to distinguish whether one or both heads are pathophysiologically active. Release of all four muscles may be required to relieve the deformity in a nonfunctional extremity. In patients who have evidence of underlying control of muscle function, despite the presence of dyssynergy, the pectoralis major, latissimus dorsi and teres major muscles can be fractionally lengthened at their muscle tendon junctions. Alternately, the teres major muscle can be partially released from its origin on the scapula and allowed to slide distally in the same manner as the supraspinatus slide.

Inferior Subluxation

Inferior subluxation of the shoulder is a common occurrence in patients with flaccid paralysis of the shoulder girdle. The subluxation is usually self-limiting, but occasionally, the shoulder will be chronically subluxated, causing pain. The patients typically have no functional use of the extremity. Patients complain of increased pain when upright. The pain may be due to chronic stretch on the shoulder capsule or from traction on the brachial plexus. Physical examination shows a positive sulcus sign, with little to no active motion of the involved shoulder. There is a prominence of the acromion and atrophy of the deltoid. There may be contracture of the shoulder in adduction and internal rotation. Radiographs show inferior subluxation of the humerus on the glenoid.

Conservative treatment may include electrical stimulation to the deltoid and supraspinatus muscles use of a sling. This relieves the symptoms by elevating the humeral head in the glenoid. Although, this technique is usually successful in the short run, this is frequently unacceptable to the patient as a permanent solution. A surgical solution to this problem of excessive laxity is the biceps suspension procedure. This procedure converts the long head of the biceps tendon to a proximally based suspensory ligament. This preserves passive shoulder motion while correcting the subluxation.

Spastic Abduction

Overactivity of the supraspinatus muscle can cause spastic abduction posturing. The deformity is usually dynamic, becoming more prominent with ambulation, transfers, or other attempted activities. The affected arm is held in an abducted posture, making balance while ambulating difficult. Patients complain that their balance is thrown off because of bumping into furniture, doorways, and people in crowds. Diagnosis requires examination of the patient at rest and during a variety of activities. It is also helpful to elicit from caretakers or family members any history of activities that trigger this posture.

Adhesive Capsulitis

Adhesive capsulitis is commonly seen in patients following stroke. They have a characteristically painful shoulder with limited glenohumeral motion. Three clinical and four arthroscopic stages have been identified. The treatment in this group of patients is similar to that for the general population. Nonsteroidal anti-inflammatory drugs, physical therapy, and intra-articular injections are all useful.

Elbow

Spastic Flexion

Upright posture favors hypertonia in the antigravity elbow flexors of the upper limb. In the patient without motor control, severe flexion posturing can lead to skin maceration in the antecubital fossa, malodor, and skin breakdown. In reality, a continuum of volitional control is seen. Many patients complain that their elbows persistently ride up when they stand up and walk. They also complain that their flexed elbow hooks door frames and other people, and that putting on a shirt or jacket is a struggle. Elbow flexion shortens the upper extremity. Consequently, reaching for objects is affected.

Functional Elbow Lengthening

Control of limb placement depends on both shoulder and elbow control. Smooth control of elbow flexion and extension is frequently impaired. The usual clinical picture is one of cogwheel motion on attempted extension of the elbow. Elbow extension range is often limited with a very prolonged period of extension. Elbow flexion is relatively normal. Dynamic EMG combined with electrogoniometric measurement of elbow motion of stroke patients has revealed a consistent pattern of muscle activity responsible for this clinical picture. The pattern most commonly seen is that all three heads of the triceps muscle are operating in a normal phasic pattern. The brachioradialis muscle most frequently shows continuous spastic activity. One or both heads of the biceps muscle are also spastic. Less spasticity is observed in the brachialis muscle. Armed with this information, a rational surgical plan can be devised to improve elbow control.

Fractional (myotendinous) lengthening is preferred whenever possible in spastic muscles. This allows the underlying tone and strength of the muscle to determine the amount of lengthening rather than having the surgeon estimate this elusive quantity. Lengthening over the muscle belly eliminates the need for suturing, and this diminishes the amount of scarring that occurs. A new tendon reforms and fills in the gap within several months. The fractional lengthening technique allows the patient to begin gentle active motion immediately after surgery because the muscle tendon unit remains intact. In contrast, a Z-lengthening technique requires immobilization for a minimum of 4 weeks to allow healing of the relatively avascular tendon and prevent inadvertent rupture.

Three methods are available to decrease tone in a spastic brachioradialis. Surgical lengthening of the brachioradialis can be used, if volitional control is demonstrated on EMG. If little or no control is demonstrated, release of the severely spastic brachioradialis muscle at the level of the elbow may be performed. Lengthening of the spastic biceps and brachialis muscles also improves elbow motion and hand placement.

Nonfunctional Elbow Release

Persistent spasticity of the elbow flexors causes a myostatic contracture and flexion deformity of the elbow. This results in skin maceration and breakdown of the antecubital space. This position of severe elbow flexion also predisposes the ulnar nerve to an acquired compression neuropathy by increasing the vulnerability to direct pressure and decreasing the cross sectional area of the cubital tunnel. In such case, surgical release of the biceps tendon and brachioradialis muscle combined with lengthening or release of the brachialis are performed. Gradual extension of the elbow with serial casting or physical therapy corrects the preoperative deformity and decreases the ulnar nerve compression. Anterior transposition of the ulnar nerve may be necessary to improve ulnar nerve function further.

Spastic Extension

Spastic extension of the elbow is much less common than spastic flexion. They complain of difficulty reaching their face for activities of daily living. When needed, surgical lengthening in the form of V-Y triceps plasty allows improved flexion range of motion, at the cost of decreased extension power and extensor lag. Use this procedure with caution in patients who rely on their arms to assist with ambulation or transfers because triceps strength is lost with lengthening procedure.

Forearm

Supination and pronation deformities are commonly associated with elbow spasticity, wrist spasticity, or both. Pronation deformities are much more common. These deformities are most often treated together with the associated deformities. They seldom require treatment individually.

Spastic Pronation

Pronation bias makes it difficult for a person to reach for a target underhand, whereas supination deformity impairs reaching for targets that require overhand reach. Many activities of daily living depend on active supination. The use of feeding and grooming utensils and clothes fasteners becomes problematic when spastic or contracted pronators which restrict supination. Physical examination reveals a fully pronated resting position of the forearm. When passive supination range of motion exceeds active supination range, the possibility of pronator muscle dyssynergy during active supination should be suspected. Muscles that contribute to this are pronator teres and pronator quadratus. During the period of functional recovery, phenol or botulinum toxin may be injected into either or both pronators. In the period of residual deficits, surgical lengthening of pronator teres and pronator quadratus may be performed depending on their individual voluntary capacities and the clinical goal is to improve active supination function by reducing pronator dyssynergy.

Spastic Supination

Spastic supination is a far less common deformity but is also associated with elbow flexion deformities. The biceps, supinator, or both may cause supination deformity. In the functional extremity, perform a biceps Z-lengthening. In a nonfunctional extremity, perform a distal biceps release. Often, at the conclusion of this procedure, the arm is able to achieve a functional range of pronation. If not, attention must be turned to the supinator.

Wrist

A flexed wrist is common after stroke but hyperextension deformity may also be seen. Patients complain of difficulty inserting their hand into shirts, jackets, and other narrow openings and they frequently have pain on passive motion. They may also have symptoms of carpal tunnel syndrome secondary to compression of the median nerve against the transverse carpal ligament by taut flexor tendons.

Spastic Flexion

Muscles that potentially contribute to wrist flexion include the flexor carpi radialis (FCR), flexor carpi ulnaris (FCU), palmaris longus (PL), flexor digitorum sublimis (FDS), and flexor digitorum profundus (FDP). Singly or in combination, these muscles may have variable features of spasticity, contracture, and voluntary control. Because they have a larger cross-sectional area, wrist flexor muscles are generally stronger than their extensor counterparts. Despite a net balance of forces favoring flexion, the extent to which a patient may have voluntary control over wrist extensors should be investigated by temporary diagnostic motor point blocks.

Begin clinical examination by observing resting posture of the wrist. FCR, FCU, or both may bowstring across the wrist, and radial or ulnar deviation suggests their respective involvement. A clenched fist points to extrinsic finger flexors as having a role. If finger nails dig into the palm, FDP is likely to be involved. If the proximal interphalangeal (PIP) joint is markedly flexed but the distal interphalangeal (DIP) joint is not, involvement of FDS is likely.

In an extremity with good volitional control, perform fractional lengthening of the appropriate wrist and extrinsic finger flexors.

When wrist flexion deformities are severe and there is little or no function seen in the hand, perform a release of the wrist flexors. Then stabilize the wrist with a wrist fusion to eliminate the need for a wrist orthosis after surgery. Gravity alone can cause a recurrence of the flexion deformity. Because the median nerve is compressed against the proximal transverse carpal ligament, causing a painful neuropathy, perform a carpal tunnel release as well.

Hand

Functional Procedures versus Procedures for Hygiene

Preoperative evaluation is performed to determine which extremities have sufficient volitional control of the muscles to allow surgical procedures aimed at restoring function to the hand. Often, severe deformities are present, but there is insufficient or no volitional activity in the muscles. In these cases, perform contracture releases to decrease pain, improve position and cosmesis of the hand, and to ease basic skin care and hygiene.

During the period of residual deficits, a variety of orthopedic options are available. When volitional control is demonstrated in the extrinsic flexor muscles, the fractional lengthening is indicated. In a hand with skin maceration and malodor from a clenched fist deformity in which no volitional movement is detected, more significant lengthening of the flexor tendons is required. In this situation, perform a superficialis-to-profundus (STP) tendon transfer.

Spastic Thumb-in-palm Deformity

The thumb-in-palm deformity may result from spastic activity in FPL, adductor pollicis (AP), or the thenar muscles, particularly flexor pollicis brevis. The thumb is held within the palm, the DIP joint of the thumb is commonly flexed, and the thumb is unable to function during key grasp. In addition, skin maceration and breakdown can occur if proper hygiene is prevented. Clinically, spasticity of the flexor pollicis longus is indicated by flexion of the interphalangeal joint. Some patients may be able to extend the thumb if the wrist is flexed. Adduction of the thumb metacarpal indicates spasticity of the AP muscle and possibly the first dorsal interosseous muscle. A quick stretch of the thumb into abduction often elicits a clonic response. An anesthetic block of the ulnar nerve in Guyon's canal at the wrist temporarily eliminates intrinsic tone. This will demonstrate the presence of any myostatic contracture and will also confirm that the AP was an offending muscle in the deformity. Contracture of the skin of the web space and interphalangeal joint contracture of the thumb may also develop over time. If some volitional potential in thumb extensors or thumb abductors is present, lengthening of the spastic FPL and AP will facilitate key grasp. In the period of residual deficits and remediable function, orthopedic treatment consists of fractional lengthening of the FPL at the myotendinous junction combined with a thenar muscle slide, in which the origins of the thenar muscles are detached from the transverse palmar ligament while preserving the neurovascular pedicle. Fractional lengthening of the FPL at the myotendinous junction will improve thumb extension. This is generally performed in conjunction with wrist or digital flexor lengthening. In order to provide a functional lateral pinch, it is desirable to stabilize the interphalangeal joint of the thumb. In those cases with a fixed adduction contracture, perform surgical lengthening of the thenar muscles.

Deformities from Intrinsic Spasticity

When spasticity of the extrinsic flexors is present, intrinsic spasticity should be expected. However, intrinsic spasticity and contracture are frequently masked by the presence of extrinsic flexor spasticity or contracture. Extension of the fingers at the metacarpophalangeal joints may be blocked by spasticity of the interossei and lumbrical muscles of the hand. Another manifestation of intrinsic spasticity is the tendency to swan-neck or boutonniere positioning of the fingers. These hand deformities can be painful and disfiguring. Such contractures often lead to maceration of the palmar skin and recurrent nail bed infections from poor hygiene.

The degree of tension caused by the intrinsic muscles can be demonstrated by comparing the amount of proximal interphalangeal joint flexion obtained with the metacarpophalangeal joints, both flexed and extended. If there is less proximal interphalangeal joint flexion with metacarpophalangeal joint extension, then the intrinsic tendons are tight. Perform this test, both before and after a lidocaine block of the ulnar nerve at the wrist, in order to distinguish between intrinsic tone and contracture.

Boutonniere deformities are commonly associated with intrinsic spasticity. They result from a combination of intrinsic spasticity combined with FDS tone. Swan-neck deformities may also result from increased intrinsic tone. The central extensor band is relatively shortened relative to the lateral bands because of tension exerted by the intrinsics and long extensor.

In the period of residual deficits, three treatment options are available. The procedure chosen is based on considerations of contracture and the presence or absence of volitional activity in the intrinsic muscles. When no significant intrinsic contracture is present and there is no volitional control in the intrinsic muscles, perform a neurectomy of the motor branches of the ulnar nerve in the palm When a contracture of the intrinsic muscles is present and no volitional activity, perform a release of the lateral bands of the extensor hood mechanism at the level of the proximal phalanx. In these cases, neurectomy of the motor branches of the ulnar nerve is performed simultaneously to prevent recurrence of the intrinsic plus deformity from spasticity of the interosseous muscles. When there is either a dynamic or static intrinsic plus deformity and volitional control, release the interossei from their proximal origins on the metacarpals and allow to slide distally. A static deformity is one in which a myostatic contracture is present. A dynamic deformity is one in which the deformity results mostly from increased tone with little or no fixed contracture.

Hip

Adduction Deformity

Scissoring of the legs in an ambulatory patient gives the patient a narrow base of support while standing and results in poor balance. A preoperative obturator nerve block eliminates the adductor spasticity and allows assessment of the adduction contracture. Alternatively, the patient can be examined at the time of surgery while under anesthesia, to determine if a fixed myostatic contracture is present. When no fixed adduction contracture is present, transection of the anterior branches of the obturator nerve will denervate the adductors and allow the patient a broader base of support. Commonly, a small contracture is found and the adductor longus muscle is released at the time of the obturator neurectomy.

A hip adduction contracture that interferes with nursing care and hygiene in a nonambulatory patient or excessive limb scissoring during attempted transfers and ambulation in a patient with active function are indications for surgical release. In a severely spastic patient, a flexion contracture of the hip and knee commonly occurs in conjunction with an adduction contracture.

Flexion Deformity

Spasticity of the hip flexors can result in a crouched gait with compensatory knee flexion to maintain balance. This is a very costly deformity because it requires constant use of the quadriceps, hip extensor, and calf muscles to maintain upright posture. The energy requirement for the continuous firing of these muscles is extremely high. Few patients are able to remain ambulatory with this deformity.

The hip flexor muscles are needed to advance the limb during gait. Avoid complete release of the hip flexors in any patient with the potential to ambulate.

Nonfunctional Release Complete Hip Release for Severe Contracture

A hip flexion contracture or severe spasticity in a nonambulatory patient that causes poor hygiene or pressure sores that cannot be healed secondary to limited positioning of the patient are indications for surgical release. An adduction contracture of the hip and a flexion deformity of the knee are commonly associated with a hip flexion contracture in the severely spastic patient. When a severe adduction contracture of the hip is present, it may be necessary to perform a percutaneous release of the adductor longus tendon in the groin in order to position the patient adequately and prepare for further surgery. Simultaneously, correct any flexion contracture of the knee to prevent the leg from positioning in flexion and causing a recurrent and more resistant contracture.

Knee

Flexion Deformity

A knee flexion deformity is caused by overactivity of the hamstring muscles. When the knee flexion deformity is less than 60° and the patient has documented volitional activity in the hamstring muscles, perform a lengthening procedure. This approach will correct the flexion deformity while preserving the function of the hamstrings.

In a nonambulatory patient with severe spasticity of the hamstring muscles or a knee flexion contracture of greater than 60° is present, attempts to correct the knee position with casting or bracing may result in posterior subluxation of the tibia. Distal release of the hamstring tendons does not prevent a patient from becoming ambulatory. If the hip flexion contracture or spasticity is not corrected at the same time as the hamstring release, a recurrent knee flexion contracture is likely to develop that is very resistant to surgical correction.

Dynamic Stiff-knee Gait

Patients with a stiff-knee gait are unable to flex the knee during the swing phase of gait. The deformity is a dynamic one, meaning that it only occurs during walking.

There is no restriction of passive knee motion, and the patient does not have difficulty sitting. Usually, the knee is maintained in extension throughout the gait cycle. Toe drag, which is likely in the early swing phase, may cause the patient to trip; thus balance and stability are also affected. The limb appears to be longer functionally. Circumduction of the involved limb, hiking of the pelvis, or contralateral limb vaulting may occur as compensatory maneuvers.

Abnormal activity is also common in the rectus or vastus intermedius muscle. If knee flexion is improved with a block of the rectus femoris or vastus intermedius muscle, the rationale for surgical intervention is strengthened. Any equinus deformity of the foot should be corrected before evaluation of a stiff-knee gait because equinus causes a knee extension force during stance.

Transfer of the rectus femoris to a hamstring tendon not only removes it as a deforming muscle force, it also converts the rectus into a corrective (flexion) force to facilitate knee flexion during swing.

Ankle

Equinus Deformity

Equinus is the most common spastic deformity that causes gait difficulty. Equinus results from the overactivity or premature activity of the gastrocnemius and soleus muscles. Surgical lengthening of the Achilles tendon is indicated when the patient's foot and ankle position is not adequately controlled by an orthosis or when attempting to make the patient brace free.

Varus

Varus deformities most commonly occur as the result of increased and inappropriate activity of the tibialis anterior muscle. This deformity can be corrected by a split anterior tibial tendon transfer (SPLATT). The SPLATT maintains the half of the tendon on the medial aspect of the foot and transfers the other half of the tibialis anterior tendon to the lateral side of the foot.

In approximately 10% of stroke patients, the tibialis posterior muscle is also spastic and can contribute to the varus deformity. Myotendinous lengthening, proximal to the medial malleolus, can correct this problem.

With the equinovarus deformity, the patient may also have a hitchhiker's great toe secondary to spasticity of the EHL tendon. The EHL also contributes to the varus deformity of the forefoot. Many patients with this condition complain of shoe wear problems from pressure of the hallux against the shoe. Most commonly, the EHL is lengthened in combination with a SPLATT procedure.

Cavus

A cavus deformity is defined as an elevated arch that does not flatten with weight-bearing. The deformity is probably a result of muscle imbalance of both the intrinsic and extrinsic muscles of the foot. If the foot is supple, plantar fascia is incised to correct the deformity. If the foot is rigid, a bony fusion must be performed.

Clawfoot

Toe clawing or curling is a common accompaniment of overactivity of the gastrocnemius muscles. Toe curling is caused by overactivity of the flexor hallucis longus and flexor digitorum muscle as well as the short toe flexor and occasionally the intrinsic muscles of the foot. Flexor tendons release can correct this deformity. This procedure is commonly performed in combination with an Achilles tendon lengthening because bringing the foot into a plantigrade position will worsen the toe curling.

Calf Weakness

Muscle paresis (weakness) is an integral part of UMN syndrome. Lengthening the Achilles tendon to correct an equinus deformity weakens the gastrocnemius-soleus muscle group, which was already weak as a consequence of the underlying UMN syndrome. This calf paresis generally results in the need for an AFO during ambulation. Thus, transfer of the FDL muscle can be done to augment calf strength. With this transfer, more patients eventually achieve brace-free ambulation. In prior study of treatment of a spastic equinovarus foot deformity, 30% of patients were able to walk safely without an AFO. When the strength of the gastrocsoleus is augmented by transfer of the FDL to the os calcis, 70% of patients achieve brace-free ambulation.

Foot Deformities in the Nonambulatory Patient

Severe deformities of the feet are common in patients with spasticity. Even in the nonambulatory patient, these deformities cause significant problems.

These complications include pressure sores, inability to wear shoes or protective footwear, and difficulty positioning the feet on wheelchair supports for improved sitting balance. Correct these deformities surgically to maintain a plantigrade foot.

The most common deformity is equinovarus with claw toes. As in the more functional patient, muscle balance must be achieved by performing the SPLATT, an Achilles tendon lengthening, and release of the toe flexor tendons, release of the plantar fascia to correct a cavus deformity.

AUTHOR'S PERSPECTIVE

Patients with stroke can initially be overwhelming to an orthopedic surgeon. However, the care of these patients follows standard, well-known orthopedic principles. Considering the specific limb problems individually and then constructing a prioritization list is the most effective method of dealing with patients who have multiple problems. As a starting point, it is helpful to consider problems in functional categories and next to consider whether or how correction of a specific limb deformity is likely to improve the function. Examples of functional categories include dressing, eating, transfers and walking.

Walking is a commonly desired goal for patients and their caregivers. A patient with a severe equinovarus foot deformity often is unable to walk. If the patient has some active hip flexion to provide limb advancement and good sitting balance, then correction of the foot deformity is likely to make the patient ambulatory. It may also be necessary to correct a hand contracture for the patient to use a cane or walker to achieve this goal. If the patient lacks active hip flexion and has poor trunk balance, then correction of the foot deformity will not allow walking. Correction of the foot may still be useful to allow shoe wear or to improve sitting balance with the foot resting on the leg support of a wheelchair.

By using a systematic approach and dividing problems into both functional and anatomic categories, it is easier to sort through the numerous musculoskeletal issues faced by persons with neurologic disorders. A major improvement in function and quality of life is achieved for many, giving both the surgeon and the patient a feeling of satisfaction and accomplishment.

Conclusion

INTRODUCTION

Physiotherapy and rehabilitation for the hemiplegic patients is a very complex process, and especially the patients suffering from a longer period of time demand lots of care, love, affection, proper treatment, understanding, apart from the technical know-how from the treatment provider. It is, therefore, of vital importance that the caregivers and those who are attached to the rehabilitation of the particular patient look after the entire aspect of a person's well-being rather than to look at their own individual field. This is the crux of any rehabilitation program be it orthopedic rehabilitation, sports rehabilitation, neurological rehabilitation or post-surgical rehabilitation.

India is a vast country with diverse culture, different languages, and of course, different individualistic needs of people. A lot has been said about the people living in developed countries, but still, people of developing countries and underdeveloped countries are somewhat neglected; more so with the patients. In the medical care, the purpose and application of the treatment sometimes differ with the country concerned. Therefore, not all the methods suggested and successfully applied in one country will hold the same ground and will deliver the similar result in another country. India is fast emerging as a global social and economical power and hence, it is important that the needs of people and the patients are looked upon in a different light focusing on the individualistic and holistic approach integrating the modern scientific procedures and ancient eastern wisdom.

Neurological rehabilitation is no different than the other fields of patient care. But, then also, there is a vast difference in terms of the time taken for the full recovery of the patient or the years of active life lost. This issue is taken up by the WHO even in India. Thus, there is an acute need of prompt and standardized neurological rehabilitation package for every patient of India according to their individual needs.

In India, there seems to be a gross lack of awareness about the rehabilitation team members amongst the patients and their relatives. Also, there is a generalized lack of rehabilitation specialists even in major cities across India. Patients are not aware that physiotherapy incorporates various advanced techniques, especially for hemiplegia patients who immensely benefit in the speedy and near normal recovery. Even in today's advanced world, many of the patients do not get services of qualified rehabilitation professionals. There seems to be lack of proper education of the patient regarding sexual functions post hemiplegia. The matter is more over complicated by the presence of the psychological disturbances and fear of non-acceptance in the society. Lack of vocational guidance above all does not help in reaching the ultimate goal of returning back to the full and satisfied life. Spirituality and faith helps the patients in fighting this dreadful disease and condition. Family support is the main pillar and family is the most important rehabilitation team member in Indian scenario. Strong cultural values and ethics combined with faith and dedication from the part of the treatment provider will ensure best results for the chronically suffering hemiplegia person.

The real heart of the treatment is to open up the eyes of the public at large towards the gross negligence these patients are facing and they do have a right to proper and best treatment combined with love, affection and care. If the reality is dawned on the people, they would find out ways to combat it with full force and then, a day will come when an ideal set up for a complete rehabilitation care for the hemiplegia sufferers is done in our country India, which is a pioneer in the field of medicine and has shown the world, the most effective system of holistic medicine namely `ayurveda', since thousands of years.

A study carried out by this author on 81 hemiplegia patients in Western India shows striking results which are given below.

PLACE WHERE INITIAL PHYSIOTHERAPY WAS CARRIED OUT

Ideally, it is assumed that the patients who are admitted to the hospitals start receiving the full rehabilitation treatment from the initial stages of their condition. The study suggests that only 65% of the patients received the physiotherapy treatment in the hospital where they were admitted. Twenty-five percent patients started with physiotherapy after they were discharged from the hospital, where the physiotherapist would go to them or home visits. Ten-percent patients started this treatment directly as OPD patients.

This suggests that even in a developed Western India where basic medical facilities are good, there are 35% of patients who are not receiving the treatment timely. It is a well-known fact that if physiotherapy is started earlier, the chances of recovery are far more beneficial than that of late treatment. An awareness program for the first-time patients should be incorporated. Medical and nursing staff should be educated towards the importance of early rehabilitation and care should be taken that proper measures are taken.

PHYSIOTHERAPY TO BE CARRIED OUT BY QUALIFIED PHYSIOTHERAPIST

Seventy-two percent patients received physiotherapy treatment by a qualified practitioner. Twenty-seven percent received treatment from unqualified practitioner and 1% did self-treatment initially after the hemiplegia. This is the genuine situation of our country where there are unqualified persons impersonating the doctors. That is the reason why 27% of educated patients fall prey to substandard rehabilitation program and in turn ruin their lives. The situation of such quacks is gruesome in the villages and towns where there are not enough qualified medical professionals. Young medical professionals do not wish to practice in villages and interiors due to lack of proper infrastructure and hence, the patient is the sufferer at the end. This situation needs to be addressed on a larger scale and the help of the government of India and the nongovernment organizations is equally important as that of the doctors. The patients and the people in general should be taught about the value of quality medical treatment and they should become aware about their right to proper treatment. The awareness of fundamental right of receiving good medical attention and treatment can make the patients and their relatives more demanding towards the treatment provider and thus, the problem of unqualified practitioners can be minimized.

INVOLVEMENT OF REHABILITATION PROFESSIONALS OTHER THAN PHYSIOTHERAPIST

As discussed earlier, apart from the primary caretaker like the family physician, neurophysician, neurosurgeon, and physiotherapist and nursing care, there are other team members of the rehabilitation team who are of vital importance in complete recovery of the patient. No team member is inferior to other in terms of the importance of the treatment application. All the patients should timely receive the services of all the members of the team and coordination of all the members with each other is advisable for the benefit of the patient.

Eighty-five percent patients received only physiotherapy and no other rehabilitation treatment (other than the primary caretakers). Only 15% patients received services of other members which included occupational therapist in 2 cases, orthotist in 2 cases, speech therapist in 5 cases and clinical psychologist in 1 case. This shows a sheer lack of understanding in the value of rehabilitation amongst doctors, relatives of patients as well as physiotherapists.

AWARENESS ABOUT HELPFULNESS OF REHABILITATION PROFESSIONALS

Sixty-four percent patients were aware that other than physiotherapists, there are different rehabilitation professionals who could propel their recovery and assist them in achieving full recovery. Thirty-three percent knew nothing about the rehabilitation team. Only 1% patient knew about all the members of the rehabilitation team.

When there is no awareness, the patients would not demand the services of the full team and hence, would remain in a traumatic state coordinating each aspect of recovery by themselves.

It is the duty of the treating doctor to guide and educate their patients regarding the value of each member of the team as it is long since the importance of the team is reported. In this study, 91.3% patients received information regarding the importance of physiotherapy from their treating doctors. Only 8.7% patients were informed through other sources like family and friends.

SATISFACTION WITH REHABILITATION

Seventy-four percent patients were satisfied with their rehab program and 26% were not satisfied with it; even when 33% were unaware about the total rehab care!! The other factor which influences the satisfaction is the faith of the patient in the treatment provider. In India, we have full faith in the doctor and we also put the medical professionals close to God. In such a situation, even if the unqualified or underqualified person is providing the treatment, the patients will be satisfied and will not look for other options till too late. It is a proven fact that all the treatment centers are not the same. The treatment provided at different clinics will be bound to be different and hence, the satisfaction level of the person would differ. Until and unless a standardized approach is taken for neurorehab, the patients will receive different treatment techniques and the resultant recovery will vary.

AWARENESS ABOUT DIFFERENT PHYSIO-THERAPY TECHNIQUES AMONGST PATIENTS

Neurological physiotherapeutic techniques differ from the conventional techniques of mobilization and strengthening. These treatment techniques are known as adjunct therapy. Bobath, NDT, neuromotor relearning, hydrotherapy, Rood's approach, proprioceptive neuromuscular rehabilitation, constraint therapy, etc. are different techniques which immensely benefit the hemiplegia patient rather than using only the conventional therapy by the physiotherapist Seventy-six and a half percent patients studied were not aware about any of the neurophysiotherapeutic techniques of treatment. Only 22.2% were aware about any of the two techniques. As the patients are unaware about the treatment techniques, they cannot know whether they are receiving proper treatment for their problems. This is demand and supply law. Only if there is a demand, there will be the supply. If patients are aware, they will demand full therapy program from the treatment provider and hence, complacency on the part of the treatment provider will have to reduce and they will try to be more sensitive towards the needs of the patient. As for an example, a patient starts taking physiotherapy treatment at a certain place under guidance of a certain practitioner. Now, it is possible that this practitioner may not be skillful enough to tackle every aspect of rehabilitation. In this scenario, the patient will receive treatment as per the level of understanding on the part of the practitioner and not as the treatment should be. The treatment becomes subjective and not objective. But, if the patient or the relatives of the patient are aware about the various physiotherapeutic techniques, they can monitor the quality of the treatment and demand the type of the treatment. It is obvious that in the society, now a day, people have become aware regarding the medical field. More and more numbers of people have started talking in medical terms and terms like angioplasty, angiography, bypass, root canal treatment, joint replacement, arthroscopy, laparotomy, antibiotics, antioxidants, CT scans, MRI, etc., are commonly used in a day-to-day life amongst the lesser educated people also. If terminology for the neurorehabilitation treatment techniques become famous and be used by the general populace, the overall quality of rehabilitation is bound to improve. This is the central idea of this study.

SEXUAL FUNCTIONS IN HEMIPLEGICS

In India, till today, the word 'sex' has got a taboo attached to it and people are not comfortable talking about it in general public or they are not ready to discuss their problems with anyone. Out of 81 hemiplegics which were interviewed, only 28, i.e., only 35% of patients were ready to share their experiences. Out of them, 14% of people were sexually inactive while 86% were active. All the patients who were active, faced positional problems during the act. While they could reach up to orgasm, they were not enjoying the act as before due to their physical disability status and the chief reason being the upper limb spasticity. Many of them had become sexually excited within few days of their problem, but they engaged in the sexual act or coitus after a few months. This time was as long as one year in some of the patients. The reason for the same was the skepticism regarding engaging in sexual act after the disease. Both the partners had fear and reservations whether to do or not to do. They also did not ask their doctors or neither did they discuss it with their friends due to embarrassment.

A few of the cooperative individuals in fact reported a decrease in spasticity and a feeling of relaxation post-coitus. Juha et al. found out after a study of 192 stroke patients that psychological and social implications were the main reasons for the decrease on libido and a fear of impotency post-stroke which impaired their sexual life. The right side brain damaged patients had more problems in arousal, vaginal lubrication and orgasm than the left side brain damage patients. A proper guidance to the spouse of the patient and the patient themselves will provide a good education regarding the problems associated with hemiplegia and their implications on the sexual life. This understanding will in turn help to normalize the sexual life of the patient and their spouses as it is of vital importance for the healthy social life and complete rehabilitation of the patient. Alternative positions during the act can be demonstrated to both the partners so that they can enjoy it without the feeling of inadequacy. The hemiplegic person can assume a position of lying on their back and their spouse can be on top to minimize the problems of spastic upper limb coming in way and also, the pelvic thrust movements will be done by the partner and hence, the intensity of the act will not be less.

Initially, during the more disability state, sexual arousal can be obtained by manually caressing the genitals of the patient by the partner after a soft talk. This can prepare the patient to overcome the fear and the patient will feel that he/she is sexually accepted and loved. Gradually, as the recovery comes, more and more active positions can be used and sexual satisfaction can be used as a moral boosting activity for the patients which will encourage them to become more and more normal in all aspects of life.

PSYCHOLOGICAL ASPECTS OF HEMIPLEGIA

Physiotherapists and all other clinicians who deal with the patients on a direct basis need to understand the patient and their problems effectively. This will ensure a healthy communication with the patient as well their relatives. Also, the rehabilitation team member should make themselves understood and hence, they all require a working knowledge about the psychology of a chronically ill patient. It is a proven fact that all the hemiplegic patients suffer from some or the other kind of psychological problem. This includes mood swings, depression, lack of concentration, decreased initiation, distortion of self-image, loss of confidence and totally giving up attitude for the recovery. Depression is more common after 6 to 8 months of the initiation of hemiplegia. Nevertheless, it is the duty of the treatment provider to diagnose the problem and help patient cope up with it or if it is absent then, to prevent it altogether.

Out of the 81 patients which were interviewed, 68% of people complained of mood swings at the end of six months of their problem; while, the numbers were as high as 85% in the initial stages. Thirty-two percent of patients had settled psychologically when the condition had become chronic. This suggests that as the time passes, more and more numbers of patients learn to cope up with their disability which was difficult initially. The distortion of the self-image was the biggest factor for such a kind of condition. The thought that when they would get full recovery bogged all the patients. The patients who had more frequent mood swings were the ones who had a negative thought process that they would never recover. The study shows that the actual motor recovery of the patient was no meter for the negative thought process. Seemingly recovered patients i.e., 90 to 100 on Barthel index also showed increased mood swings and negative thoughts.

It was a pleasant surprise to know that 88.88% patients had accepted their condition. The remaining 11% of the unfortunate ones had not still accepted the condition of their disability. The acceptance doesn't mean that the patients accepted the disability and did not want to do anything for that. In fact, they were the patients who were really motivated for trying out all the measures which will make them as normal as possible. The persons who did not accept the condition blamed many factors for their condition and hence, their concentration and zeal for carrying out physiotherapy was not as good. This, in turn, reduced the output of their therapy and they lagged behind in every aspect of their rehabilitation.

Twenty-four percent patients had a vague feeling of totally giving up every measure for their recovery due to frustration and longer time of the recovery. This type of feeling was not a constant one on many of them, but, was a passing feeling sometimes. It was commonly seen that the immediate relatives of the patient complained that the patient has become increasingly irritable and short-tempered. Though all of them take it lightly, this feeling should be curbed with proper counseling of the patient and the caretakers before it takes a definite form of some psychological condition. The irony is that, most of the patients denied of becoming irritable, clearly showing that they themselves were not happy about this feeling and were not, therefore, accepting it.

As the acceptance of the condition increases gradually, the frequency and intensity of mood swing decreases. The understanding of the pathogenesis of the disease and the education regarding the proper rehabilitation techniques reduces the anxiety levels of the patient and their relatives.

SOCIAL FUNCTIONS

Social functions and psychological functions are very closely associated with each other. Man is a social animal and a family being. No one loves to live an isolated life. Due to the physical disability, the person's efficiency of routine activities decreases and hence, there are a lot of chances that that person starts feeling isolated and dejected. He is unable to move out for the recreational activities as before and that multiplies the problem of social isolation. The closely knitted family system of our country gives a fillip to faster accommodation of the situation. Other way round the same system can prove to be very demanding on the patient if the family members are more expectant. But, overall, the family support system is a good tool and a very important part of complete rehabilitation.

Many patients have a feeling of fear of non-acceptance in the society due to the disability status. They feel inferior to the so called normal individuals and hence they feel low in their presence and hence, avoid going to places where they are not feeling absolutely comfortable. Out of 81 patients, 53% patients had a fear of non-acceptance. This feeling can be tackled by a sensitive approach towards the patient and proper counseling. The patients should be encouraged to move out of the house as early as possible, due to which, they would come in contact with the world, early in the rehabilitation process. The real life situations would put demands on them, and by successfully tackling them, they would feel confident and the fear would minimize. General public should be taught to be more sensitive towards the disabled or differently-abled persons and their behavior should be of helping and not ridiculing. It is commonly seen that if these patients are given too much of attention and if people feel too sorry for them, they do not like it and hence, such a type of behavior should be totally avoided. They should not be talked to as if talking to a child. This is a common mistake people make. One should remember that the patient is an adult and is differently-abled; not a child or a mentally challenged person.

The fear of non-acceptance may not always mean that the patients do not mingle with others easily. The study suggests that only a 26% of people have difficulty in mingling with others. The main reason is the feeling of inferiority and a fear of non-acceptance. The interaction of the environment and the response of the patient towards them influence this factor. Almost all the patients reported a significant increase in spasticity when they went to a newer place. The gait or the walking pattern also changed significantly. The apprehension and anxiety towards newer places increases manifold even in chronic cases. A positive attitude and self-suggestion or autosuggestions may minimize the problem to a greater extent.

All the patients had an excellent family support; which is evident from the study. Ninty-five percent patients reported of having a very good family support. This is very important because, when the patient is having disability and is dependent, there is an acute need of love and care which is provided best by the immediate family members and the friends. The affection which the family provides is not obtained by paid staffs which are available in India. The family support is indispensable and cannot be replaced by even rehab experts in the country like India. The family is one of the three pillars on which the entire recovery depends. The other two pillars are the rehab experts and the patient himself.

Seventy-three percent patients went for the recreational outing as before. This included the visits to relatives, restaurants, movie halls, shopping and others. This is a good index as a person will feel fit only if he can move out of the house for recreation and merry making. This kind of routine will ease out undue stress in the mind of the patient and he will become free and light. This will ensure an increased zeal in carrying out the required task for the recovery. The remaining 27% patients could not go out for recreation, mainly due to the physical status and the feeling that they were dependent and will have to take assistance from somebody for their recreation. In western developed countries, there are qualified recreational therapists who are associated with the rehabilitation team and who provide timely recreation to the patient right from their hospital stay. The rehabilitation hospitals are equipped with the gaming zones, gardens and libraries so that patients of all age groups get recreation of their choice. Physical activity of choice will facilitate the brain and in turn facilitate motor response to the limbs; thus increasing the chances of faster recovery. In our country, such kinds of recreational therapists are not possible to have due to budget constraints and lack of proper infrastructure. But, nevertheless, this work is done by patient's family and friends and rehabilitation specialists like the physiotherapists as they are the ones who spend more time with the patient than any other specialist.

It is usually seen that the sporting activity and life-like situation activities generate and facilitate quality motor movements from the brain. This fact can be utilized to a beneficial aspect in all the hemiplegic patients in all the stages. Even if they do not possess any motor recovery, they can indulge in such playing activity using their normal side. This will facilitate the activity from the brain. Playing cards, ball, simple games, should be started early. More advanced games and sports like ball catching and throwing, hitting the ball with clasped hands, hitting the ball with the affected hand, etc. can be extremely helpful. As the recovery progresses, ball catching and throwing can be progressed on the wobble or the balancing board. Playing indoor cricket, badminton, volleyball, basketball can be incorporated as soon as possible. This will ensure an increase in the motor function as well as provide recreation to the patient.

In our environment, government hospitals and some private hospitals do have a rehabilitation unit, where recreation facilities are available. But due to difficulty in handling and lack of proper attention, these units are existent merely on paper only and the actual work on the patients is still not up to the mark. Well, there are some exceptions but owing to the size of our country India and sheer numbers of our patients, these units are extremely less. The private physiotherapy clinics where most of the patients go for treatment do not have enough space and enough time to take care about this and hence, the patients are the sufferers in longer run.

SPIRITUALITY AND FAITH

All the patients, despite their faith and religion, told to have faith in the almighty. It was seen that 16% of the patients had increased faith in the god. The reason for the same was the fact that they had accepted their condition and saw the presence and will of the Lord in their condition. Seventy-nine percent of the patients did not find any change in their faith, and were as religious as before. Only 5% patients reported of having decreased faith. These patients had a grudge that why they were given this problem by the lord. They found it very difficult to accept their condition. Also, they had a higher chance of feeling of depression than others. It is a known fact that faith can heal and modify most of the problems. The religious faith can increase the acceptance of the condition and can prepare the patient to be patient and face the challenges which are posed by the disability. Faith induces an increase in inner strength of the person. It is a known fact that the positive thinking and autosuggestions along with the religious practices help in speedy recovery of the patient. Chanting of the Lord's name along with meditation can decrease spasticity by providing deep relaxation and increase in alpha rhythm activity in the brain.

WORK AND PROFESSION

According to the study, out of 81 examined chronic hemiplegia sufferers, 30% patients had never gone for any work. Either they were females as home makers or were students. Out of the remaining 57 patients, 61% patients had resumed their previous job or business, while 39% could not resume their duties again. Out of the home makers and students, all the students and 50% home makers had resumed their previous work.

The study clearly suggests that approximately 40% patients were unable to resume their work due to their physical disability status. Most of them had lack of confidence and inability to cope up with the work place. In India, most of the public places including the offices and the recreational areas are not accessible easily for the disabled or differently-abled individuals. The public transport system is not disabled person-friendly even in a developed cities. The towns and villages lack basic public transport altogether. Thus, for the patient, going to the workplace is difficult, if he/she is unable to drive their own vehicle. Otherwise, they have to utilize autorickshaw or taxi which is not economical for daily use and hence, such patients cannot resume their work.

When a person becomes disabled like in this case, hemiplegia, they are off from the work for a long period of time. When they resume walking and going out, they may not be using their affected upper limb effectively and the patients who have proprioception and perception problems do not feel confident in carrying out their duty. Due to this problem, they think that their work efficiency would be less, and sometimes even the employer discourages them from resuming duties. To add to the problem, we do not have a vocational guide as our rehabilitation team member. The vocational guide assesses the potential and disability of the patient and accordingly advices the patient for the type of the work they can attempt successfully. The young hemiplegia victims have entire professional life ahead of them and sometimes these patients are still in school or colleges and so, they need proper guidance regarding their future profession. Due to lack of this training, they feel frustrated and depressed and their problems increase rather than decrease as the time passes. Thus, a timely counseling with the vocational guide can ease out the worries of the patient and they can return to the work of premorbid state or can take up a new profession and earn and support themselves and their family.

In India, the patient spends most of the time with the physiotherapists. In cities and in midsize towns, physiotherapists are readily available. Apart from the big centers, most of the times, they are the only rehabilitation team members associated with the patient. Physiotherapist, therefore, should be equipped to deal with such a situation. Patients should not be deprived of the total rehab care and hence, physiotherapist should at least provide information regarding the importance of the other team members and should provide basic treatment.

Thus, it is not really surprising that some of the resourceful physiotherapists also provide vocational guidance to the patient and help the patient for complete rehabilitation. Active involvement of the rehabilitation team member and working in interdisciplinary manner becomes advisable in a country like India. Relatives of the patient are one of the most important team members and hence, their assistance should always be taken. Their assistance is readily available and is economically cheap. They can spend a lot of time with the patient and their services are invaluable.

It is a wish and dream of every chronic hemiplegia patient to have full recovery and lead a normal and a fulfilling life as soon as possible.

FUNCTIONAL RECOVERY

It is important that both the patient and the treating physiotherapist have a harmonious relationship regarding the treatment and its effect leading to recovery. Goals of both the parties should be the same. The road to recovery is long and tedious and always demands lot of mental strength and patience. The treatment of hemiplegia is a continuous process and should not be dependent upon discrete therapy sessions. The final outcome of recovery is dependent upon many factors. The site and extent of lesion in the brain is the most important of the factors. Then, the amount and quality of treatment including the physiotherapy and rehabilitation and participation of patient are other very important factors. Patients always want very speedy recovery. They may not be totally aware regarding the site and extent of the brain damage and so, they may not even estimate the time of recovery correctly. They should be told about the method of recovery and they should be educated that the recovery is a process and not a destination in this case. When the treatment provider and the patient are working harmoniously, their goal is same and the attitude is focused. When the harmony is distorted due to various reasons, even when the recovery of the patient is good enough for the brain injury they possess, they may not feel the same. Sometimes, only the maintenance of the condition and prevention of further deterioration may be the goal of the therapist. But, if the communication between the patient and the therapist is improper, patient may feel less or no recovery.

AN IDEAL REHABILITATION OF A PERSON SUFFERING FROM HEMIPLEGIA

A Vision and a Mission

In India, the rehabilitation of the hemiplegic patient can be bettered by using the resources already existent and incorporating more proactive approach towards the patient care. The ideal rehabilitation model is as follows.

- The patient is immediately admitted to the hospital on the first signs of motor weakness in any of the limbs or the face or any difficulty in speaking. In the case of an accident where there is any evidence of the head injury, the neurological examination is performed and signs for the brain damage are looked out for.
- Emergency medical treatment is carried out with immediate effect without any delay after the cause of the brain damage is confirmed using advanced imaging techniques.
- The relatives of the patients are informed about the condition of the patient and possible prognosis is explained.
- Nursing staff which is expert in neurological rehabilitation care is recruited.
- Physiotherapy in form of turning, posture maintenance, chest physiotherapy, passive movements, active movements wherever applicable is started immediately.
- Relatives of the patient and the nursing staff are taught the basic physiotherapeutic techniques so that it can be followed out from time to time and avoid complications like bed sore, deep vein thrombosis, chest complications, stiff joints and tight muscles. Early mobilization will help the brain to learn motor activities rapidly and the sensory system is also activated.
- Adjunct therapy like the PNF, Bobath techniques, etc. is started as soon as possible.

- Early weight-bearing on the lower limbs is started as soon as advised by the experts.
- Psychiatrist or clinical psychologist is called for a special session with the patient as well as the relatives of the patient. They are made to understand the problem and they are made ready to face the newer challenges.
- The rehabilitation professionals give the introduction of the entire team members to the patient and the relatives and their importance is laid down upon.
- Other team members like the orthotist and the occupational therapist take up their assessment sessions and the required things are done.
- The relatives of the patient are educated regarding the value of recreation for the patient as it will make the hospital stay for the patient easy. It will also make the hospital stay of the relatives fun-filled and stress-free.
- If the patient is fit for discharge from the hospital, they can be taken to patient's residence or a transient care unit.
- The transient care unit may be located in the hospital premises or can be at any other place. Here, the medical staff sees the patient say once a day or once in two days and the rehabilitation professionals take up the treatment charge.
- If the patient is shifted to one's own residence, then they are treated at home by the physiotherapist. The therapist usually coordinates the entire rehabilitation program and each other team member is referred time to time for expert advice.
- As soon as the patient is able to walk and come out of the house, he is encouraged to go to a rehabilitation clinic, as, he may meet several other hemiplegia sufferers and they may have a chance to interact with them. This will induce a feeling of confidence in them.
- All the advanced techniques of physiotherapy and rehabilitation are told to the patient and hence, best of the treatment can be availed by the patient timely.
- Time to time clinical psychologist's session is organized for the patient's mental health.
- Vocational guidance is given to the patient in a realistic manner but care is taken that it has a positive effect on the patient and patient's morale boosts up.
- Patients are told about the problems they may face on the social front and are taught the ways to tackle it.
- Assessment of all the functions is done by the experts on a regular basis and the therapy is modified as and when required.

- If need be, a video or still photographical data of the patient's initial symptoms is kept for comparison with the later stages.
- Patient is encouraged to carry out each and every activity of the premorbid state as and when the time comes and help is given where applicable and needed.
- The patient is taught to become independent in every aspect and is taught to become independent of the rehabilitation team, because they have to learn to manage their life on their own.
- Patient is educated regarding the prognosis in a realistic manner and realistic goals are set for the patient. These goals are the short term and the long term goals.
- The patient may be off therapy when the patient is fully rehabilitated in every aspect in a holistic manner.

The entire process of rehabilitation can be carried out in a more organized manner if the patient after taking discharge from the hospital is directly shifted to a rehabilitation hospital or a rehabilitation care center.

This rehabilitation hospital has to have all the rehabilitation services under one roof and hence, the patient will get all the consultations at one place only. The coordination between the rehabilitation team members would be excellent and the responsibilities are shared without any member becoming complacent.

The patient goes through the entire rehab process at one place which will save a lot of time and it would be extremely convenient. This rehab hospital may be a costly affair economically, but as they say, 'no amount of money is as important as one's health', and truly, 'health is wealth'.

Standardization of Treatment Techniques

Treatment protocol and the physiotherapy techniques used for the patients suffering from hemiplegia need to be standardized in India with an immediate effect. The treatment program is not standardized and hence, at various places, different techniques are used. This does not ensure a uniform approach and the patients get confused by this. The rate of recovery also differs and hence, discussion of prognosis with the patient becomes difficult. It is true that all the centers of treatment providers cannot have same protocol, as all the patients are different and need different way of approach. But, at the same time, presently, there is a complete lack of a proper protocol for the patients. This leads to a very vague treatment sessions at many places. Thus, patient has to totally depend upon the treating person and his power of discretion and dedication rather than patient having to depend upon the science of physiotherapy.

Standardization of treatment techniques will require some amount of ground work for the research fellows. It may be a difficult affair, but is not impossible. The best place to start the standardization is targeting the educational institutions. If physiotherapy students who are future torch bearers of the field of neuro-rehabilitation are trained from their colleges in the standardized protocol for hemiplegics, they are bound to implement these techniques in the practice. For professional physiotherapists, CME programs on a nationwide scale would ensure an insight into the standardization of the technique. If this is implemented, there would be evidence-based practice which is the order of the day and all the patients regardless of their geographical location, would receive the best rehabilitation treatment.

This author strongly supports the idea of standardization in all treatment approaches of physiotherapy and recommends the above mentioned steps towards achieving this goal together.

Ethics and Values in Treatment

In any field of patient care, the importance of the ethics and values is of paramount importance. Ethics are the moral principles or the moral values on which the human life is based upon. In India we call it 'dharma', the righteous action. As humans, we like others to behave in a certain manner with us; like no one should speak untruth with us, no one should cause harm to us, etc. If we behave in the manner which we like ourselves to be behaved with, it becomes ethical or moral conduct for us.

Patient care, especially in neurological cases, demands a great deal of ethical practice. The patients who come for the treatment come with lots of hope. At this time, it is the duty of the treatment provider to adhere to the basic values of the life and treat the patient truthfully. It is the duty of the care taker to explain the exact diagnosis, treatment program and prognosis to the patient. The treatment provider should first understand his or her own limitations and strengths and second, he or she should convey this to the patient concerned. If there are limitations in treating the patient, then, the patient should be referred to the expert without the delay.

A balance between the earning in terms of money and service to the society should be maintained for healthy system of healthcare. The clinician should refrain oneself from the glittering world of malpractice at all costs. He should not indulge in bogus referrals as this creates an everlasting ill impression in the minds of the patients for the entire medical and healthcare fraternity. Last but not the least, the patient should be seen as a human being and should not be treated as a case or a part of it.

Honesty towards the patient and the profession at large will make the society and the system of healthcare, readily acceptable to one and all, will provide comfort, care, love, support and compassion along with the treatment which is being administered.

Assessment Scores and Scales

ABCD SCORE

It is used to predict the risk of stroke during the first seven days after a TIA. Researchers found there to be over 30% risk of stroke in TIA patients with an 'ABCD score' of six, as compared to no strokes in those with a low ABCD score. Can be used in routine clinical practice to identify high-risk individuals who require emergency investigation and treatment.

	Risk factor	Category	Score
A	Age of patient	Age $\geq$60	1
		Age <60	
B	Blood pressure at assessment	SBP >140 or DBP $\geq$90	0
		other	
C	Clinical features presented with	Unilateral weakness	2
		Speech disturbances (no weakness)	1
		Other	0
D	Duration of TIA symptoms	$\geq$60 minutes	2
		10–59 minutes	1
		>10 minutes	0
		TOTAL	**6**

Reference

1. Rothwell P, Giles M, Flossmann E, Lovelock C, Redgrave J, Warlow C, et al. A simple tool to identify individuals at high early risk of stroke after a transient ischaemic attack: The ABCD score. The Lancet. 2005;366:29-36.

THE BARTHEL INDEX

Patient Name: ____

Rater Name:____

Date: ____

Activity   **Score**

Feeding

0 = unable
5 = needs help cutting, spreading butter, etc., or requires modified diet
10 = independent   _________

Bathing

0 = dependent
5 = independent (or in shower)   _________

Grooming

0 = needs to help with personal care
5 = independent face/hair/teeth/shaving (implements provided)   _________

Dressing

0 = dependent
5 = needs help but can do about half unaided
10 = independent (including buttons, zips, laces, etc.   _________

Bowels

0 = incontinent (or needs to be given enemas)
5 = occasional accident
10 = continent   _________

Bladder

0 = incontinent, or catheterized and unable to manage alone
5 = occasional accident
10 = continent   _________

Toilet Use

0 = dependent
5 = needs some help, but can do something alone
10 = independent (on and off, dressing, wiping)   ________

Transfers (bed to chair and back)

0 = unable, no sitting balance
5 = major help (one or two people, physical), can sit
10 = minor help (verbal or physical)
15 = independent   ________

Mobility (on level surfaces)

0 = immobile or >50 yards
5 = wheelchair independent, including corners, >50 yards
10 = walks with help of one person (verbal or physical) >50 yards
15 = independent (but may use any aid; for example, stick) >50 yards   ________

Stairs

0 = unable
5 = needs help (verbal, physical, carrying aid)
10 = independent   ________

TOTAL (0–100)   ________

The Barthel ADL Index: Guidelines

1. The index should be used as a record of what a patient does, not as a record of what a patient could do.
2. The main aim is to establish degree of independent from any help, physical or verbal, however, minor and for whatever reason.
3. The need for supervision renders the patient not independent.
4. A patient's performance should be established using the best available evidence. Asking the patient, friends/relatives and nurses are the usual sources, but direct observation and common senses are also important. However, direct testing is not needed.
5. Usually the patient's performance over the preceding 24–48 hours is important, but occasionally longer periods will be relevant.

6. Middle categories imply that the patient supplies over 50% of the effort.
7. Use of aids to be independent is allowed.

References

1. Mahoney FI, Barthel D. Functional evaluation: The Barthel Index. Maryland State Medical Journal. 1965;14:56-61. Used with permission.
2. Loewen SC, Anderson BA. Predictors of stroke outcome using objective measurement scales. Stoke. 1990;21:78-81.
3. Greshman GE, Philips TF, Labi ML. ADL status in stroke: Relative merits of three standard indexes. Arch Phys Med Rehabil. 1980;61:355-8.
4. Collin C, Wade DT, Davies S, Home V. The Barthel ADL Index: A reliability study. Int Disability study. 1988;10:61-3.

BECK'S DEPRESSION INVENTORY

This depression inventory can be self-scored. The scoring scale is at the end of the questionnaire.

1. 0   I do not feel sad.
   1   I feed sad.
   2   I am sad all the time and I cannot snap out of it.
   3   I am so sad and unhappy that I cannot stand it.
2. 0   I am not particularly discouraged about the future.
   1   I feel discouraged about the future.
   2   I feel I have nothing to look forward to.
   3   I feel the future is hopeless and that things cannot improve.
3. 0   I do not feel like a failure.
   1   I feel I have failed more than the average person.
   2   As I look back on my life, all I can see is a lot of failures.
   3   I feel I am a complete failure as a person.
4. 0   I get as much satisfaction out of things as I used to.
   1   I do not enjoy things the way I used to.
   2   I do not get real satisfaction out of anything anymore.
   3   I am dissatisfied or bored with everything.
5. 0   I do not feel particularly guilty.
   1   I feel guilty a good part of the time.
   2   I feel quite guilty most of the time.
   3   I feel guilty all the time.
6. 0   I do not feel I am being punished.
   1   I feel I may be punished.
   2   I expect to be punished.
   3   I feel I am being punished.

7. 0 I do not feel disappointed in myself.
   1 I am disappointed in myself.
   2 I am disgusted with myself.
   3 I hate myself.
8. 0 I do not feel I am any worse than anybody else.
   1 I am critical of myself for my weaknesses or mistakes.
   2 I blame myself all the time for my faults.
   3 I blame myself for everything bad that happens.
9. 0 I do not have any thoughts of killing myself.
   1 I have thoughts of killing myself, but I would not carry them out.
   2 I would like to kill myself.
   3 I would kill myself if I had the chance.
10. 0 I do not cry any more than usual.
    1 I cry more now than I used to.
    2 I cry all the time now.
    3 I used to be able to cry, but now I cannot cry even though I want to.
11. 0 I am no more irritated by things than I ever was.
    1 I am slightly more irritated now than usual.
    2 I am quite annoyed or irritated a good deal of the time.
    3 I feel irritated all the time.
12. 0 I have not lost interest in other people.
    1 I am less interested in other people than I used to be.
    2 I have lost most of my interest in other people.
    3 I have lost all of my interest in other people.
13. 0 I make decision about as well as I ever could.
    1 I put off making decisions more than I used to.
    2 I have greater difficulty in making decisions more than I used to.
    3 I cannot make decisions at all anymore.
14. 0 I do not feel that I look any worse than I used to.
    1 I am worried that I am looking old or unattractive.
    2 I feel there are permanent changes in my appearance that make me look unattractive.
    3 I believe that I look ugly.
15. 0 I can work about as well as before.
    1 It takes an extra effort to get started at doing something.
    2 I have to push myself very hard to do anything.
    3 I cannot do any work at all.

16. 0   I can sleep as well as usual.
     1   I do not sleep as well as I used to.
     2   I wake up 1–2 hours earlier than usual and find it hard to get back to sleep.
     3   I wake up several hours earlier than I used and cannot get back to sleep.
17. 0   I do not get more tired than usual.
     1   It takes an extra effort to get started at doing something.
     2   I have to push myself very hard to do anything.
     3   I am too tired to do anything.
18. 0   My appetite is no worse than usual.
     1   My appetite is not as good as it used to be.
     2   My appetite is much worse now.
     3   I have no appetite at all anymore.
19. 0   I have not lost much weight, if any, lately.
     1   I have lost more than five pounds.
     2   I have lost more than ten pounds.
     3   I have lost more than fifteen pounds.
20. 0   I am no more worried about my health than usual.
     1   I am worried about physical problems like aches, pains, upset stomach, or constipation.
     2   I am very worried about physical problems and it is hard to think of much else.
     3   I am so worried about my physical problems that I cannot think of anything else.
21. 0   I have not noticed any recent change in my interest in sex.
     1   I am less interested in sex than I used to be.
     2   I have almost no interest in sex.
     3   I have lost interest in sex completely.

Interpreting the Beck's Depression Inventory

Now that you have completed the questionnaire, add up the score for each of the twenty-one questions by counting the number of right of each question you marked. The highest possible total for the whole test would be sixty-three. This would mean you circled number three on all twenty-one questions. Since the lowest possible score for each question is zero, the lowest possible score for the test would be zero. This would mean you circles zero on each question.

Total score	**Levels of depression**
1–10	These ups and downs are considered normal
11–16	Mild mood disturbances
17–20	Borderline clinical depression
21–30	Moderate depression
31–40	Severe depression
Over 40	Extreme depression

A persistent score of 17 or above indicates that you may need medical treatment.

BERG BALANCE SCALE

Patient Name:
Rater Name:
Date:

Balance item

Score (0–4)

1. Sitting unsupported
2. Change of position: Sitting to standing __________
3. Change of position: Standing to sitting __________
4. Transfers __________
5. Standing unsupported __________
6. Standing with eyes closed __________
7. Standing with feet together __________
8. Tandem standing __________
9. Standing on one leg __________
10. Turning trunk (feet fixed) __________
11. Retrieving objects from floor __________
12. Turning 360 degrees __________
13. Stool stepping __________
14. Reaching forward while standing __________
    TOTAL (0–56): __________

Interpretation

0–20, wheelchair bound
21–40, walking with assistance
41–56, independent

References

1. Berg K, Wood-Dauphinee S, Williams JI, Maki, B. Measuring balance in the elderly: Validation of an instrument. Can J Pub Health, July/August supplements 1992;2:57-11.
2. Berg K, Wood-Dauphinee S, Williams JI, Gsyton. Measuring balance in the elderly: Preliminary development of an instrument: Physiotherapy. Canada.1989;41:304-11.

CANADIAN NEUROLOGICAL SCALE

Patient Name: ____

Rater Name:____

Date: ____

Mentation Score

Level consciousness		Alert	3.0
		Drowsy	1.5
Orientation		Oriented	1.0
		Disoriented/NA	0.0
Speech		Normal	1.0
		Expressive Deficit	0.5
		Receptive Deficit	0.0
		TOTAL:	

Section A1	Motor Functions	Weakness	Score
NO	**Face**	None	0.5
COMPREHENSIVE		Present	0.0
DEFICIT	**Arm: Proximal**	None	1.5
		Mild	1.0
		Significant	0.5
		Total	0
	Arm: Distal	None	1.5
		Mild	1.0
		Significant	0.5
		Total	0
	Leg: Proximal	None	1.5

Section A1	Motor Functions	Weakness	Score
		Mild	1.0
		Significant	0.5
		Total	0

	Leg: Distal	None	1.5
		Mild	1.0
		Significant	0.5
		Total	0
		TOTAL:	_______

Section A2	Motor Functions	Weakness	Score
NO	**Face**	Symmetrical	0.5
COMPREHENSIVE		Asymmetrical	0.0
DEFICIT	**Arm**	Equal	1.5
		Unequal	0.0
	Leg	Equal	1.5
		Unequal	0.0

References

1. CoteR, Hachinski VC, Shurvell BL, Norris JW, Wolfson C. The Canadian Neurological: Scale A preliminary study in acute stoke. Stroke. 1986;17:731–37.
2. Cote R, Battista RN, Wolfson C, Bouncher J, Hachinski VC. The Canadian Neurological: Scale Validation and reliability assessment. Neurology. 1989;39:638–43.

CINCINNATI PREHOSPITAL STROKE SCALE

Facial Drop

Normal: Both sides of the face move equally

Abnormally: One side of face does not move at all

Arm Drift

Normal: Both arms move equally or not at all

Abnormally: One arm drifts compared to the other

Speech

Normal: Patient uses correct words with no slurring

Abnormally: Slurred or inappropriate words or mute

References

1. Kothari RU, Pancioli A, Liu T, Brott T, Broderick J. Cincinnati Prehospital Stroke Scale: Reproducibility and validity. Ann Emerg Med. 1999;33(4):373-8.

THE EUROPEAN STROKE SCALE

Overview

The European stroke scale can be used to assess a patient who has recently had a stroke involving the distribution of a middle cerebral artery. This can be used to measure therapeutic efficacy and to match patients for comparison.

Parameters

1. Level of consciousness.
2. Comprehension: The patient is asked to follow these commands: (a) Stick out tongue, (b) put a figure from the (unaffected) side to the nose, (c) close the eyelids, the examiner must not demonstrate the action.
3. Speech: The examiner makes general conversation with the patient.
4. Visual field: The examiner stands at the arm's length and compares the patient's field of vision by advancing a moving finger from the periphery inwards. The patient is asked to fixate on the examiner's pupil. The test is done first with one eye open and other closed, then the opposite.
5. Gaze: The examiner steadies the patient's head and asks the patient to follow the examiner's finger. The examiner observes the resting eye position and subsequently, the full range of movements by moving the finger from the left to the right, then vice versa.
6. Facial movements: The patient's face is examined while talking and smiling, with any asymmetries noted. Only the muscles in the lower half of the face are assessed.
7. Arm in outstretched position: The patient is asked to close the eyes. The patient's arms are actively lifted into a 45° position relative to the horizontal plane, with both hands in mid-position facing each other. The patient is asked to maintain this position for 5 seconds after the examiner withdraws the support. Only the affected side is evaluated.
8. Arm raising: The patient's arm is rested next to the leg with the hand in mid-position. The patient is asked to raise the arm outstretched to 90° (vertical).
9. Extension of wrist: The patient is tested with the forearm supported. The hand is unsupported but relaxed in pronation. The patient is to extend the hand.
10. Fingers: The patient is asked to form a pinch grip with the thumb and forefinger and to resist a weak pull. The examiner assesses the strength of the pinch grip by pulling on the pinched fingers using one finger.

11. Leg maintained in position: The examiner actively lifts the patient's affected leg into position, with the thigh perpendicular to the bed and the lower leg parallel to the bed, the patient is asked to close the eyes and to maintain the leg in position for five seconds without support.
12. Leg flexing: The patient is supine with the leg outstretched. The patient is asked to flex the hip and knee.
13. Dorsiflexion of foot: The patient's leg is outstretched, with the patient asked to dorsiflex the foot.
14. Gait.

Parameter	Findings	Points
Level of consciousness	Alert, keenly responsive	10
	Drowsy but can be aroused by minor stimulation to obey, answer or respond	8
	Requires repeated stimulation to attend, or is lethargic or obtunded, requiring strong or painful stimulation to make movements	6
	Cannot be roused by any stimulation, does react purposefully to painful stimuli	4
	Cannot be roused by any stimulation, does react with decerebration to painful stimuli	2
	Cannot be roused by any stimulation, does not react to painful stimuli	0
Comprehension	Patients perform 3 commands	8
	Patients perform 1 or 2 commands	4
	Patient does not perform any command	0
Speech	Normal speech	8
	Slight word-finding difficulty, conversation is possible	6
	Severe word-finding difficulties, conversation is difficult	4
	Only yes or no	2
	Mute	0

Visual field	Normal	8
	Deficit	0
Gaze	Normal	8
	Median eye position, deviation to one side impossible	4
	Later eye position, return to midline possible	2
	Later eye position, return to midline impossible	0
Facial movement	Normal	8
	Paresis	4
	Paralysis	0
Arm (ability to maintain out-stretched position)	Arm maintaining position for 5 seconds	4
	Arm maintained position for 5 seconds but affected hand pronates	3
	Arm drifts before 5 seconds pass and maintains lower position	2
	Arm cannot maintain position but attempts to oppose gravity	1
	Arm falls	0
Arm (raising)	Normal	4
	Straight arm, movement not full	3
	Flexed arm	2
	Trace movements	1
	No movements	0
Extension of the wrist	Normal (full isolated movement, no decrease in strength)	8
	Full isolated movement, reduced strength	6
	Movement not isolated and/or full	4
	Trace movements	2
	No movement	0
Fingers	Equal strength	8
	Reduced strength on affected side	4
	Pinch grip impossible on affected side	0

Leg (maintain position)	Leg maintains position for 5 seconds	4
	Leg drifts to intermediate position by the end of 5 seconds	2
	Leg drifts to bed within 5 seconds but not immediately	1
	Leg falls to bed immediately	0
Leg (flexing)	Normal	4
	Movement against resistance, reduced strength	3
	Movement against gravity	2
	Trace movements	1
	No movements	0
Dorsiflexion of foot	Normal (leg outstretched, full movement, no decrease in strength)	8
	Leg outstretched, full movement, reduced strength	6
	Leg outstretched, movement not full or knee flexed or foot in supination	4
	Trace movements	2
	No movement	0
Gait	Normal	10
	Gait has abnormal aspect and/or distance limited and/or speed limited	8
	Patient can walk with aid	6
	Patient can walk with physical assistance of one or more persons	4
	Patient cannot walk but can stand unsupported	2
	Patient cannot stand nor walk	0

European stroke score = SUM (points for all 14 parameters)

Interpretation:

- Minimum score: 0
- Maximum score: 100
- A completely normal person would have a score of 100.
- The maximum affected person has a score of 0.

Reference

1. Hanston L, De Weerdt W, et al. The European Stroke Scale. Stroke. 1994;25:2215-19.

FAMILY ASSESSMENT DEVICE

1. Nathan B, Epstein, MD; Lawrence M Baldwin, PhD; Duane S Bishop, MD.

Instructions

This assessment contains a number of statements about families. Read each statement carefully and decide how well it describes your own family. You should answer according to how you see your family.

For each statement are four (4) possible responses:

Strongly agree (SA)	Check SA if you feel that the statement describes your family very accurately.
Agree (A)	Check A if you feel that the statement describes your family for the most part.
Disagree (D)	Check D if you feel that the statement does not describes your family for the most part.
Strongly disagree (SD)	Check SD if you feel that the statement does not describe your family at all.

For each statement, there is an answer space below. Do not pay attention to the blanks at the far right-hand side of each space.

Try not to spend too much time thinking about each statement, but respond as quickly and as honestly as you can. If you have difficulty, answer with your first reaction. Please be sure to answer *every* statement and mark all your answers in the space provided *below* each statement.

1. Planning family activities is difficult because we misunderstand each other.

    _______ SA_______A_______D_______SD_______

2. We resolve most everyday problems around the house.

    _______ SA_______A_______D_______SD_______

3. When someone is upset the other knows why.

    _______ SA_______A_______D_______SD_______

4. When you ask someone to do something, you have to check that they did it.

_______ SA_______A_______D_______SD_______

5. If someone is in trouble, the others become too involved.

_______ SA_______A_______D_______SD_______

6. In times of crisis, we can turn each other for the support.

_______ SA_______A_______D_______SD_______

7. We don't know what to do when an emergency comes up.

_______ SA_______A_______D_______SD_______

8. We sometimes run out of the things that we need.

_______ SA_______A_______D_______SD_______

9. We are reluctant to show our affection for each other.

_______ SA_______A_______D_______SD_______

10. We make sure members meet their family responsibilities.

_______ SA_______A_______D_______SD_______

11. We cannot talk to each other about the sadness we feel.

_______ SA_______A_______D_______SD_______

12. We usually act on our decisions regarding problems.

_______ SA_______A_______D_______SD_______

13. You only get the interest of others when something is important to them.

_______ SA_______A_______D_______SD_______

14. You can't tell how a person is feeling from what they are saying.

_______ SA_______A_______D _______SD_______

15. Family tasks don't get spread around enough.

_______ SA_______A_______D_______SD_______

16. Individuals are accepted for what they are.

_______ SA_______A_______D_______SD_______

17. You can easily get away with breaking the rules.

_______ SA_______A_______D_______SD_______

18. People come right out and say things instead of hinting at them.

_______ SA_______A_______D_______SD_______

19. Some of us just don't respond emotionally.

_______ SA_______A_______D_______SD_______

20. We know what to do in an emergency.

_______ SA_______A_______D_______SD_______

21. We avoid discussing our fears and concerns.

_______ SA_______A_______D_______SD_______

22. It is difficult to talk to each other about tender feelings.

_______ SA_______A_______D_______SD_______

23. We have trouble meeting our financial obligations.

_______ SA_______A_______D_______SD_______

24. After our family to solve a problem, we usually discuss whether it worked or not.

_______ SA_______A_______D_______SD_______

25. We are too self-centered.

_______ SA_______A_______D_______SD_______

26. We can express feelings to each other.

_______ SA_______A_______D_______SD_______

27. We have no clear expectations about toilet habits.

_______ SA_______A_______D_______SD_______

28. We do not show our love for each other.

_______ SA_______A_______D_______SD_______

29. We talk to people directly rather than through go-betweens.

_______ SA_______A_______D_______SD_______

30. Each of us has particular duties and responsibilities.

______ SA______A________D________SD__________

31. There are lots of bad feelings in the family.

______ SA______A________D________SD__________

32. We have rules about hitting people.

______ SA______A________D________SD__________

33. We get involved with each other only when something interests us.

______ SA______A________D________SD__________

34. There is little time to explore personal interests.

______ SA______A________D________SD__________

35. We often don't say what we mean.

______ SA______A________D________SD__________

36. We feel accepted for what we are.

______ SA______A________D________SD__________

37. We show interest in each other when we can get something out of it personally.

______ SA______A________D________SD__________

38. We resolve most emotional upset that come up.

______ SA______A________D________SD__________

39. Tenderness takes second place to other things in our family.

______ SA______A________D________SD__________

40. We discuss who are responsible for household jobs.

______ SA______A________D________SD __________

41. Making decisions is a problem for our family.

______ SA______A________D________SD __________

42. Our family shows interest in each other only when they can get something out of it.

______ SA______A________D________SD __________

43. We are frank (direct, straightforward) with each other.

_______ SA_______A_______D_______SD _________

44. We don't hold to any rules or standards.

_______ SA_______A_______D_______SD _________

45. If people are asked to do something, they need reminding.

_______ SA_______A_______D_______SD _________

46. We are able to make decisions about how to solve problems.

_______ SA_______A_______D_______SD _________

47. If the rules are broken, we don't know what to expect.

_______ SA_______A_______D_______SD _________

48. Anything goes in our family.

_______ SA_______A_______D_______SD _________

49. We express tenderness.

_______ SA_______A_______D_______SD _________

50. We confront problems involving feelings.

_______ SA_______A_______D_______SD _________

51. We don't get along well together.

_______ SA_______A_______D_______SD _________

52. We don't talk to each other when we are angry.

_______ SA_______A_______D_______SD _________

53. We are generally dissatisfied with the family duties assigned to us.

_______ SA_______A_______D_______SD_________

54. Even though we mean well, we intrude too much into each other's lives.

_______ SA_______A_______D_______SD_________

55. There are rules in our family about dangerous situations.

_______ SA_______A_______D_______SD_________

56. We confide in each other.

_______ SA_______A_______D_______SD_________

57. We cry openly.

_______ SA_______A_______D_______SD_______

58. We do not have reasonable transport.

_______ SA_______A_______D_______SD_______

59. When we do not like what someone has done, we tell them.

_______ SA_______A_______D_______SD_______

60. We try to think of different ways to solve problems.

_______ SA_______A_______D_______SD_______

Suggested Terminology for Objective Data (Evaluation Criteria)

Levels of Assistance	Functional Skills
Complete independence (FIM 7)	All of the tasks described as making up the activity are typically performed safely, without modification, assistive devices, or aids, and within a reasonable time; no assistance required. Performs activity safely alone and feels secure.
Modified Independence (FIM 6)	One or more of the following may be true: the activity requires an assistive device; the activity takes more than reasonable time, or these are safety (risk) considerations; not manual assistance/helper required.
Supervision or Setup (FIM 5)	Patient requires no more help than standby, cueing or coaxing, without physical contact, or, someone is needed to set up needed items or apply orthoses; requires supervision and/or verbal cues to complete activity (may not always be done safely or correctly).
Contact Guarding	A variation of minimal assist where patient requires occasional contact to maintain balance or dynamic stability; requires hand contact because of occasional loss of balance (protective safeguard)
Minimal (contact) assistance (FIM 4)	Patient requires small amount of help accomplish activity; patient requires no more help than touching, and expends 75% or more of the effort. Patient is able to assume all of his body weight, but requires guidance for initiation, balance, and/or stability during the activity.
Moderate Assistance (FIM3)	Patient requires more help than touching; expands half (50%) or more (up to 75%) of the effort. Patient is able to assume part of his body weight in initiating and performing the activity.

Maximal Assistance (FIM 2)	Patient contributes little or nothing towards execution of activity; patient expands less than 50% of the effort, but at least 25%.
Total Assistance (FIM1)	Patient lacks the necessary strength or mental capability to perform any part of the activity or performance is impractical; patient expends less than 25% of the effort. Patient is unable to safely initiate and/or perform any part of the activity on his own.

References

1. Definitions were partially taken from guide for the uniform data set for medical rehabilitation (adult functional independence measure (FIM). Version 4.0. Buffalo, NY 14214: State University of New York at Buffalo. 1993.
2. O' Sullivan, Schmitz. Physical Rehabilitation: Assessment and Treatment (4th edn). Philadelphia: FA Davis Company, 2001.pp. 5-6.

Regarding Assistance:

The patient may require more than person and varying amounts of assistance (for example, maximum assist and minimum assist of one). Always document the type of activity, number of people required for assistance, and the amount of assistance given by those assisting.

THE FRENCHAY ACTIVITIES INDEX

Items   **Code**

In the last 3 months

■ preparing main meals   1 = never

■ washing up $2\leq$ time per week

                                                               3 = 1–2 times per week

                                                               4 = most days

■ Washing clothes   1 = never

■ Light housework   2 = 1–2 times in 3 months

■ Heavy housework   3 = 3-12 times in 3 months

■ Local shopping $4\geq1$ time per week

■ Social outings

■ Walking outside >15 minutes

■ Actively pursuing hobby

■ Driving car/bus travel

In the last 6 months

■ Outings/car rides   1 = never

                                                               2 = 1–2 times in 6 months

	3 = 3–12 times in 6 months
	4 = 0.1 time per week
■ Gardening	1 = never
■ Household/car maintenance	2 = light
	3 = moderate
	4 = all necessary
■ Reading books	1 = none
	2 = 1 in 6 months
	3≥ in 2 weeks
	4≤ 1 in 2 weeks
■ Gainful work	1 = none
	2≥10 hour/week
	3 = 10–30 hour/week
	4≤30 hour/week

GERIATRIC DEPRESSION SCALE (SHORT FORM)

Patient's name: _________________________ Date: _____________

Instructions: Choose the best answer for how you feel over the past week.

No.	Question	Answer	Score
1.	Are you basically satisfied with your life?	Yes/No	–
2.	Have you dropped many of your activities and interests?	Yes/No	
3.	Do you feel that life is empty?	Yes/No	–
4.	Do you often get bored?	Yes/No	–
5.	Are you in good spirits most of the time?	Yes/No	–
6.	Are you afraid that something bad is going to happen to you?	Yes/No	–
7.	Do you feel happy most of the time?	Yes/No	–
8.	Do you often feel helpless?	Yes/No	–
9.	Do you prefer to stay at home, rather than going out and doing new things?	Yes/No	–
10.	Do you feel you have more problems with memory than most?	Yes/No	–
11.	Do you think it is wonderful to be alive?	Yes/No	–
12.	Do you feel pretty worthless the way you are now?	Yes/No	–
13.	Do you feel full of energy?	Yes/No	–
14.	Do you feel that your situation is hopeless?	Yes/No	–

15. Do you think that most people are better
    off than you are?   Yes/No   –

                                                                TOTAL

Scoring

Assign one point for each of these answers:

1. No	4. Yes	7. No	10. Yes	13. No
2. Yes	5. No	8. Yes	11. No	14. Yes
3. Yes	6. No	9. Yes	12. Yes	15. Yes

A score of 0 to 5 is normal. A score above 5 suggests depression.

References

1. Yesavage JA, Brink TL, et al. Development and validation of a geriatric depression screening scale: A preliminary report. J Psychiatr Res. 1983;17:37-49.

GLASGOW COMA SCALE

Patient Name: ____

Rater Name: ____

Date: ____

Activity   Score

Eye Opening

None	1 = Even to supraorbital pressure	_______
To pain	2 = Pain from sternum/limb/supraorbital pressure	_______
To speech	3 = Nonspecific response, not necessarily to command	_______
Spontaneous	4 = Eyes open, not necessarily aware	_______

Motor Response

None	1 = To any pain; limbs remain flaccid	_______
Extension	2 = Shoulder adducted and shoulder and forearm internally rotated	_______
Flexor response	3 = Withdrawal response or assumption of hemiplegic posture	_______

Withdrawal   4 = Arm withdraws to pain, shoulder abducts   __________

Localizes pain   5 = Arm attempts to remove supra-orbital/chest pressure   __________

Obeys commands 6 = Follows simple commands   __________

Verbal Response

None   1 = No verbalization of any type

Incomprehensible   2 = Moans/groans, no speech

Inappropriate   3 = Intelligible, no sustained sentences

Confused   4 = Converses but confused, disoriented

Oriented   5 = Converses and oriented.   __________

TOTAL (3–15):   __________

References

1. Teasdale G, Jennett B. Assessment of coma and impaired consciousness. A practical scale. The Lancet. 1974;13;2(7872):81-4.

HEMISPHERIC STROKE SCALE

Patient Name: ____

Rater Name: ____

Date: ____

Scored to give 0 (good) to 100 (bad)

Levels of Consciousness   Score

15-Glasgow Coma Scale Score   __________

Language

Comprehension

Give three commands:
- 'Stick out your tongue' *or* 'close your eyes'
- 'Point to the door'

- 'Place left/right hand on left/right ear and then on left/right knee (using unaffected side)

Score on number correctly followed:
>   0 = 5
>   1 = 4
>   2 = 2
>   3 = 0

Naming

Ask patient to name the following items:
- Watch or belt
- Watch strap or belt buckle
- Index finger or ring finger

Score on number correctly named:
>   0 = 5
>   1 = 4
>   2 = 2
>   3 = 0

Repetition

Ask the patient to repeat the following:
- A single word, such as 'dog' or 'cat'
- 'The president lives in Washington'
- 'No ifs, ands, or buts'

Score on number repeated:
>   0 = 5
>   1 = 4
>   2 = 2
>   3 = 0

Fluency

Score according to patient's spontaneous speech fluency,
or
Ask patient to name as many words as he can within one minute beginning with the letter 'A' (excluding proper names)

Score as:

    5 = Essentially no verbal output

    3 = Moderately loss; inability to recognize stationary finger, sees moving finger

    1 = Mild loss; defect to double simultaneous stimulation

    0 = Normal

        Page 1 TOTAL _________

Other Cortical Functions and Cranial Nerves

Visual Fields _________

Test clinically and score hemi-field loss as:

    3 = Severe loss; inability to recognize moving hand, no response to threat

    2 = Moderate loss; inability to recognize stationary finger, sees moving finger

    1 = Mild loss: Defect to double simultaneous stimulation

    0 = Normal

Gaze

Score eye movements:

    2 = Gaze play, or persistent deviation

    1 = Gaze preference, or difficulty with far lateral gaze

    0 = Normal

Facial expression _________

Score movements:

    3 = Severe weakness; drooling

    2 = Moderate loss; asymmetry at rest

    1 = Mild weakness; asymmetry on smiling

    0 = Normal

Dysarthia _________

Score talking:

    2 = Severe dysarthria

1 = Moderate dysarthria
0 = Normal
    Page 2 TOTAL: _______

Neglect Syndrome

Ask about weak limbs, and ask to bisect a line 20 cm long on piece of paper in visual midline
Score:
    2 = Anosagnosia, or denial of body part
    1 = Consistently bisects line towards 'good' side of body
    0 = Bisects line in middle

Visual Construction _______

Ask patient to copy three figure given, and score:
    3 =   Unable to copy any finger
    2 =   Can copy a square
    1 =   Can copy a 'Greek Cross' (Cross of St. George)
    0 =   Can copy 3D drawing of cube

Motor Fuction

Arm, proximal _______
Arm, distal _______
Leg, proximal _______
Leg, distal _______

All scored 0–7 as:
       7 =   No movement (MRC 0)
       6 =   Trace movement only (MRC 1)
       5 =   Motion without gravity only (MRC 2)
       4 =   Moves against gravity but not against
             resistance (MRC 3)
       3 =   Moderate weakness (MRC 4)
       2 =   Mild weakness (MRC 4)
    Page TOTAL: _______
       1 = Positive drift of arm/leg (MRC 4+)
       0 = Normal (MRC 5)

Deep Tendon Reflexes ______

2 = Hypoactive or hyperactive
0 = Normal

Pathological Reflexes ______

2 = Babinski (plantar) and another abnormal
1 = Babinski (plantar) and another abnormal
0 = Normal

Muscle Tone ______

2 = Increased or decreased
0 = Normal

Gait ______

Test ability to stand and walk, and score:
6 = Unable to stand unsupported or cannot evaluate
5 = Can stand with support but cannot walk
4 = Severe abnormal; walking distance limited even
   with support (from aid or person)
3 = Moderately abnormal; no assistance required
   (apart from a stick/cane), but distance limited
2 = mildly abnormal (weak, uncoordinated); can walk
   independently but slowly
1 = Minimally abnormal, no reduction in speed or distance
0 = Normal
   Page 3 TOTAL: ______

Sensory

Primary Modalities (of affected side only), Arm ______
Test touch, pain and score as:
4 = Anesthesia
3 = Severe hyperesthesia
2 = Moderate hyperesthesia or deficit only; or
      extinction to double simultaneous stimulation
1 = Mild hyperaesthesia or dysaesthesia
0 = Normal

Stereognosis

Test ability to distinguish two coins and a key, and score:

    3 = Unable to achieve any distinctions

    2 = Can distinguish a coin from a key

    1 = Can distinguish between two very different sized coins

       (penny and ten-pence piece, penny and quarter)

    0 = Can distinguish between two similar sized coins

       (penny and nickel, or two-pence piece and ten-pence piece)

Page 4 TOTAL : _____________

OVERALL TOTAL: _____________

References

1. Adams RJ, Meador KJ, Sethi KD, Grotta JC, Thomson DS. Graded neurologic scale for use in acute hemispheric stroke treatment protocols. Stroke. 1987;18:665-9.

HUNT AND HESS SCALE

Patient Name: ____

Rater Name:____

Date: ____

For non-traumatic sub-arachnoid hemorrhage patients (Choose single most appropriate grade)

Description

Description	Grade
Asymptomatic, mild headache, slight nuchal rigidity	1
Moderate to severe headache, nuchal rigidity, no neurologic deficit other than cranial nerve palsy	2
Drowsiness/ confusion, mild focal neurologic deficit	3
Stupor, moderate-severe hemiparesis	4
Coma, decerebrate posturing	5

      GRADE (1-5):

References

1. Hunt WE, Hess RM. Surgical risk as related to time of intervention in the repair of intracranial aneurysms. J. Neurosurg. 1968;28(1):14-20.

2. Hunt WE, Meagher JN, Hess RM. Intracranial aneurysm. A nine-year study.
3. Ohio State Med J 1966 Nov;62(11):1168-71.

MATHEW STROKE SCALE

Patient Name: ____

Rater Name:____

Date: ____

Activity　　　　　　　　　　　　　　　　　　　　　　　Score

Mentation

Level of consciousness

    8 = Fully conscious

    6 = Lethargic but mentally intact

    4 = Obtunded

    2 = Stuporous

    0 = Comatose

Oriented (time, place, person)

    6 = Oriented × 3

    4 = Oriented × 2

    2 = Oriented × 1

    0 = Disoriented

Speech

    0–23, according to Halstead-Reitan test　　　　　__________

Cranial nerves

Homonymous hemianopsia

    3 = Intact

    2 = Mild

    1 = Moderate

    0 = Severe

Conjugate deviation of eyes

    3 = Intact

    2 = Mild

    1 = Moderate

    0 = Severe

Facial Weakness

3 = Intact

2 = Mild

1 = Moderate

0 = Severe

Motor Power

Right arm ___________

Right leg ___________

Left arm ___________

Left leg ___________

5 = Normal strength

4 = Contracts against resistance

3 = Elevates against gravity

2 = Gravity eliminated

1 = Flicker

0 = No movements

Performance, or disability status scale

28 = Normal

21 = Mild impairment

14 = Moderate impairment

7 = Severe impairment

0 = Death

Reflexes

3 = Normal

2 = Asymmetrical or pathological reflexes

1 = Clonus

0 = No reflexes elicited

Sensation

3 = Normal

2 = Mild

1 = Severe sensory abnormality
0 = No response to pain
TOTAL ___________

Reference

1. Mathew NT, Rivera VM, Meyer JS, Charney JZ, Hartmann A. Double-blind evaluation of glycerol therapy in acute cerebral infarction. Lancet.1972;2:1327-9.

MINI-MENTAL STATE EXAMINATION (MMSE)

Patient's name: ________________________ Date___________

Instructions: Score one point for each correct response within each question or activity.

Maximum Score	Patient's Score	Questions
5		"What is the year? Season? Date? Day? Month?"
5		"Where are we now? State? Country? Town/city? Hospital? Floor?"
3		The examiner names three unrelated objects clearly and slowly, then the instructor asks the patient to name all three of them. The patient's response is used for scoring. The examiner repeats them until patient learns all of them, if possible.
5		"I would like you to count backward from 100 by sevens" (93, 86, 79, 72, 65,.....); Alternative: "Spell WORLD backwards." (D-L-R-O-W)
3		"Earlier I told you the names of three things. Can you tell me what those were?"
2		Show the patient two simple objects, such as a wristwatch and a pencil, and ask the patient to name them.
1		"Repeat the phrase: 'No ifs, ands, or buts."
3		"Take the paper in your right hand, fold it in half, and put it on the floor" (The examiner gives the patient a piece of blank paper).
1		"Please read this and do what it says." (Written instruction is "Close your eyes").

1	"Make up and write a sentence about anything." (This sentence must contain a noun and a verb).
1	"Please copy this picture" (The examiner gives the patient a blank piece of paper and asks him/her to draw the symbol below. All 10 angels must be present and two must intersects).

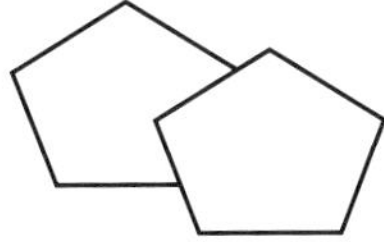

30	**TOTAL**

Interpretation of the MMSE:

Method	Score	Interpretation
Single Cut off	>24	Abnormal
Range	>21	Increased odds of dementia
	>25	Decreased odds of dementia
Education	>21	Abnormal for 8th grade education
	>23	Abnormal for high school education
	>24	Abnormal for college education
Severity	24–30	No cognitive impairment
	18–23	Mild cognitive impairment
	0–17	Severe cognitive impairment

Interpretation of the MMSE Scores

Score	Degree of Impairment	Formal Psychometric Assessment	Day-to-Day Functioning
25–30	Questionably significant	If clinical signs of cognitive impairment are present, formal assessment of cognition may be valuable	May have clinically significant but mild deficits. Likely to affect only most demanding activities of daily living
20–25	Mild	Formal assessment may be helpful to better determine pattern and extent of deficits	Significant effect. May require some supervision, support and assistance
10–20	Moderate	Formal assessment may be helpful if there are specific clinical indications	Clear impairment. May require 24-hour supervision

| 0–10 | Severe | Patient not likely to be testable | Marked impairment. Likely to require 24-hour supervision and assistance with ADL |

References

1. Folstein MF, Folstein SE, McHug PR. Mini-mental state: A practical method for grading the cognitive state of patients for the clinician. J Psychiatry Res. 1975;12:189-98.

MODIFIED RANKIN SCALE (MRS)

Patient Name: ____

Rater Name: ____

Date: ____

Score	Description
0	No symptoms at all
1	No significant disability despite symptoms; able to carry out all usual duties and activities
2	Slightly disability; unable to carry out all previous activities, but able to look after own affairs without assistance
3	Moderate disability; requiring some help, but able to walk without assistance
4	Moderately severe disability; unable to walk without assistance and unable to attend to own bodily needs without assistance
5	Severe disability; bedridden, incontinent and requiring constant nursing care and attention
6	Dead.

TOTAL (0–6): ______________

References

1. Rankin J. Cerebral vascular accidents in patients over the age of 60. Scott Med J. 1957;2:200-15
2. Bonita R, Beaglehole R. Modification of Rankin Scale: Recovery of motor function after stroke. Stroke. 1998;19(12):1497-500.
3. van Swieten JC, Koudstaal PJ, Visser MC, Schouten HJ, van Gijin J. Interobserver agreement for the assessment of handicap in stroke patients. Stroke. 1988;19(5): 604-7.

MOTOR ASSESSMENT SCALE

Agency: _______________ PID#: _____________ Date: ________ CPT#:________

Patient's name: _____________________ Therapist: __________________

If the patient cannot complete any part of a section score a zero (0) for that section. There are 9 sections in all.

Supine to Side-lying onto Intact Side (Starting position: Supine with knees straight)

1. Uses intact arm to pull body towards intact side. Uses intact leg to hook impaired leg to pull it over.
2. Actively moves impaired leg across body to roll but leaves impaired arm behind.
3. Impaired arm is lifted across body with other arm. Impaired leg moves actively and body follows as a block.
4. Actively moves impaired arm across body. The rest of the moves as a block.
5. Actively moves impaired arm and leg rolling to intact side but overbalances.
6. Rolls to intact side in 3 seconds without use of hands.

Supine to Sitting over side of bed

1. Assisted to the side-lying position: Patient lifts head sideways but can't sit up.
2. May be assisted to side-lying and is assisted to sitting but has head control throughout.
3. May be assisted to side-lying and is assisted with lowering Les off bed to assume sitting.
4. May be assisted to side-lying but is able to sit up without help.
5. Able to move from supine to sitting without help.
6. Able to move from supine to sitting without help in 10 seconds.

Balance Sitting

1. Assisted to sitting and needs support to remain sitting.
2. Sits unsupported for 10 seconds with arms folded, knees and feet together and feet on the floor.
3. Sits unsupported with weight shifted forward and evenly disturbed over both hips/legs. Head and thoracic spine extended.

4. Sits unsupported with feet together on the floor. Hands resting on thighs. Without moving the legs the patient turns the head and trunk to look behind the right and left shoulders.
5. Sits unsupported with feet together on the floor. Without allowing the legs or feet to move and without holding on, the patient must reach forward to touch the floor (10 cm or 4 inches in front of them); the affected arm may be supported if necessary.
6. Sits on stool unsupported with feet on the floor. Patient reaches sideways without moving the legs or holding on and returns to sitting position. Support affected arm if needed.

Sitting to Standing
1. Assisted to standing—any method.
2. Assisted to standing. The patient's weight is unevenly distributed and may use hands for support.
3. Stands up. The patient's weight is evenly distributed but hips and knees are flexed—no use of hands for support.
4. Stands up. Remains standing for 5 seconds with hip and knees extended with weight evenly distributed.
5. Stands up and sits down again. When standing hips and knees are extended with weight evenly distributed.
6. Stands up and sits down again three times in 10 seconds with hip and knees extended and weight evenly distributed.

Walking

1. With assistance, the patient stands on affected leg with the affected weight bearing hip extended and steps forward with the intact leg.
2. Walks with the assistance of one person.
3. Walks 10 feet or 3 meters without assistance but with an assistive device.
4. Walks 16 feet or 5 meters without a device or assistance in 15 seconds.
5. Walks 33 feet or 10 meters without assistance or a device. Is able to pick up a small object from the floor with either hand walk back in 25 seconds.
6. Walks up and down 4 steps with or without a device but without holding onto a rail three times in 35 seconds.

Upper Arm Function

1. Supine: Therapist places affected arm in 90 degrees shoulder flexion and holds elbow in extension—hand toward ceiling. The patient protracts the affected shoulder actively.

2. Supine: Therapist places affected arm in above position. The patient must maintain the position for 2 seconds with some external rotation and with the elbow in at least 20 degrees of full extension.
3. Supine: Patient assumes above position and brings hand to forehead and extends again. (flexion and extension of elbow). Therapist may assist with supination of forearm.
4. Sitting: Therapist places affected arm in 90 degrees of forward flexion. Patient must hold affected arm in position for 2 seconds with some shoulder external rotation and forearm supination. No excessive shoulder elevation or pronation.
5. Sitting: Patient lifts affected arm to 90 degrees forward flexion—holds it there for 10 seconds and then lowers it with some shoulder external rotation and forearm supination. No pronation.
6. Standing: Have patient's affected arm abducted to 90 degrees with palm flat against wall. Patient must maintain arm position while turning body towards the wall.

Hand Movements

1. Sitting at a table (wrist extension): Affected forearm resting on table. Place cylindrical object in palm of patient's hand. Patient asked to lift object off the table by extending the wrist—no elbow flexion allowed.
2. Sitting at a table (radial deviation of wrist): Therapist should place forearm with ulnar side on table in mid-pronation/supination position. Thumb in line with forearm and wrist in extension. Fingers around cylindrical object. Patient is asked to lift hand off table. No wrist flexion or extension.
3. Sitting (pronation/supination): Affected arm on table with elbow unsupported at side. Patient asked to supinate and pronate forearm (3/4 range acceptable).
4. Place a 5 inch ball on the table so that the patient has to reach forearm with arm extended to reach it. Have the patient reach forward with shoulder protracted, elbow extended, wrist in neutral or extended, pick up the ball with both hands and put it back down in the same spot.
5. Have the patient pick up a polystyrene cup with their affected hand and put it on the table on the other side of their body without any alteration to the cup.
6. Continuous opposition of thumb to each finger fourteen times in 10 seconds. Each in turn taps the thumb, starting with the index finger. Do not allow thumb to slide from one finger to the other or go backwards.

Advanced Hand Activities

1. Have the patient reach forward to pick up the top of a pen with their affected hand, bring the affected arm back to their side and put the pen cap down in front of them.
2. Place eight jellybeans, (beans), in a teacup an arm's length away on the affected side. Place another teacup an arm's length away on the intact side. Have the patient pick up one jellybean with their affected hand and place the jellybean in the cup on the intact side.
3. Draw a vertical line on a piece of paper. Have the patient draw horizontal lines to touch the vertical line. The goal is 10 lines in 20 seconds with at least 5 lines stopping at the vertical.
4. Have the patient pick up a pen/pencil with their affected hand, hold the pen as for writing, and position it without assistance and make rapid consecutive dots (not strokes) on a sheet of paper. Goal: At least 2 dots a second for 5 seconds.
5. Have the patient take a dessert spoon of liquid to their mouth with their affected hand without lowering the head toward the spoon or spilling.
6. Have the patient hold a comb and comb the back of their head with the affected arm in abduction and external rotation, forearm in supination.

General Tonus (check one—add "6" to score if tone on affected side is normal)

______ Flaccid, limp, no resistance when body parts are handled.
______ Some resistance felt as body parts are moved.
______ Variable, sometimes flaccid, sometimes good tone, sometimes hypertonic.
______ Hypertonic 50% of the time.
______ Hypertonic all of the time.
6 = Consistently normal response

This test is designed to assess the return of function, a stroke or other neurological impairment. The test looks at a patient's ability to move with low tone or in a synergic pattern and finally move actively out of that patient into normal movement.

The higher the score, the higher the functioning; the patient is on the affected side.

High score: 54

Low score: 0

MOTRICITY INDEX

The Motricity Index for motor Impairment after Stroke

Overview: The Motricity Index can be used to assess the motor impairment in a patient who has a stroke.

Tests for Each Arm:
1. Pinch grip: Using a 2.5 cm cube between the thumb and forefinger
   * 19 points are given if able to grip cube but not hold it against gravity
   * 22 points are given if able to hold cube against gravity but not against a week pull
   * 26 points are given if able to hold the cube against a weak pull strength is weaker than normal.
2. Elbow flexion from 90° so that the arm touches the shoulder
   * 14 points are given if movement is seen with elbow out the arm horizontal.
3. Shoulder abduction moving the flexed elbow from off the chest
   * 19 points are given when shoulder is abducted to more than 90° beyond the horizontal against gravity but not against resistance.

Test for each Leg:
1. Ankle dorsiflexion with foot in a foot in a plantar flexed position
   * 14 points are given if there is less than a full range of dorsiflexion.
2. Knee extension with the foot unsupported and the knee at 90°
   * 14 points are given for less than 50% of full extension.
   * 19 points are given for full extension.
3. Hip flexion with the hip bent at 90° moving the knee towards the chin
   * 14 points are given if there is less than a full range of passive motion
   * 19 points are given if the hip is fully flexed yet it can be easily pushed down.

MRC grade	MRC score	Points for pinch grip	Points for other tests
No movement	0	0	0
Palpable flicker but no movement	1	11	9
Movement but not against gravity	2	19	14
Movement against gravity	3	22	19
Movement against resistance	4	26	25
Normal	5	33	33

Arm score for each side = SUM (points for the 3 arm tests) + 1
Leg score for each side = SUM (points for the 3 leg tests) + 1
Side score for each side = [(arm score for side) + (leg score for side)]/2

Interpretation:
- Minimum score: 0
- Maximum score: 100

References

1. Collin C, Wade D. Assessing motor impairment after stroke: A pilot reliability study. J Neurology Neurosurg Psychiatry. 1990;53:576-9.

NIH STROKE SCALE

Patient identification: __ __ __ __ __ __ __

Pt. Date of birth: __ __ /__ __/__ __ __ __

Hospital: _______________(__ __-__ __)

Date of examination: __ __ /__ __/__ __ __

Interval: [ ] Baseline [ ] 2 hours post-treatment [ ] 24 hours post onset of symptoms ± 20 minutes   [ ] 7–10 days [ ] 3 months [ ] Other _____________(__ __)

Time:__ __:__ __   [ ]am [ ]pm

Person Administering Scale_________________________________

Administer stroke scale items in the order listed. Record performance in each category after each subscale exam. Do not go back and change score. Follow directions provided for each exam technique. Score should reflect what the patient does, not what the clinician thinks the patients can do. The clinician should record answer while administering the exam and work quickly. Expect where indicated, the patient should not be coached (i.e., repeated requests to patient to make a special effort).

Instructions	Scale definition	Score
1a. Level of consciousness	0 = **alert;** keenly responsive. 1 = **Not alert;** but arousable by minor stimulation to obey, answer, or respond. 2 = **Not alert;** requires repeated stimulation to attend, or is obtunded and requires strong or painful stimulation to make movements (not stereotyped). 3 = Responds only with reflex motor or automatic effects or totally unresponsive, flaccid, and are flexic.	_________

1b. LOC **Questions:**	0 = **Answers** both questions correctly. 1 = **Answers** one question correctly. 2 = **Answers** neither question correctly.	__________
1c. LOC **Commands**	0 = **Performs** both tasks correctly. 1 = **Performs** one task correctly. 2 = **Performs** neither task correctly.	__________

2. Best Gaze

0 = **Normal.**   __________

1 = **Partial gaze palsy;** gaze is abnormal in one or both eyes, but forced deviation or total gaze paresis is not present.

2 = **Forced deviation,** or total gaze paresis not overcome by the oculocephalic maneuver.

3. Visual

0 = **No visual loss.**   __________

1 = **Partial hemianopia.**

3 = **Bilateral hemianopia** (blind including cortical blindness)

4. Facial palsy

0 = **Normal** symmetrical movements.   __________

1 = **Minor paralysis** (flattened nasolabial fold, asymmetry on smiling).

2 = **Partial paralysis** (total or near-total paralysis of lower face).

3 = **Complete paralysis** of one or both sides (absence of facial movements in the upper and lower face).

5. Motor Arm

0 = **No drift;** limb holds 90 (or 45) degrees for full 10 seconds.   __________

1 = **Drift;** limb holds (or 45) degrees, but drifts down before full 10 seconds; does not hit bed or other support.

2 = **Some effort against gravity;** limb cannot get to or maintain (if cued) 90 (or 45) degrees, drift down to bed, but has some effort against gravity.

3 = **No effort against gravity;** limb falls.

4 = **No movement.**

UN = **Amputation** or joint fusion, explain: __________

5a. Left Arm   __________

5b. Right Arm   __________

6. Motor Leg

0 = **No drift;** leg holds 30-degrees position for full 5 seconds.   __________

1 = **Drift;** leg falls by the end of the 5-seconds period but does not hit bed.

2 = **Some effort against gravity;** leg falls to bed by 5 seconds, but has some effort against gravity.

3 = **No effort against gravity;** leg falls to bed immediately.

4 = **No movement.**

UN= **Amputation** or joint fusion, explain: __________

6a. Left Leg __________

6b. Right Leg __________

7. Limb Ataxia 0 = **Absent.** __________

1 = **Present in one limb.**

2 = **Present in two limbs.**

UN = **Amputation** or joint fusion, explain: __________

8. Sensory 0 = **Normal;** no sensory loss. __________

1 = **Mild-to-moderate sensory loss;** patient feels pinprick is less sharp or is dull on the affected side; or there is a loss of superficial pain with pinprick, but patient is aware of being touched.

2 = **Severe to total sensory loss;** patient is not aware of being touched in the face, arm, and leg.

9.Best Language 0 = **No aphasia;** normal. __________

1 = **Mild-to-moderate aphasia;** some obvious loss of fluency or facility of comprehension, without significant limitation on ideas expressed or form of expression. Reduction of speech and/or comprehension, however, makes conversation about provided materials difficult or impossible. For example, in conversation about provided materials, examiner can identify picture or naming card content from patient's response.

2 = **Severe aphasia;** all communication is through fragmentary expression; great need for inference, questioning, and guessing by the listener. Range of information that can be exchanged is limited; listener carries burden of communication. Examiner cannot identify materials provided from patient's response.

3 = **Mute, global aphasia;** no usable speech or auditory comprehension.

10. Dysarthria 0 = **Normal.**

    1 = **Mild-to-moderate dysarthria;** patient slurs at least some words and, at worst, can be understood with some difficulty.

    2 = **Severe dysarthria;** patient's speech is so slurred as to be unintelligible in the absence of or out of proportion to any dysphasia, or is mute/anarthric.

    UN= **Intubated** or other physical barrier, explain: __________

11. Extinction and inatten- tion (formerly neglect)

    0 = **No abnormally.**

    1 = **Visual, tactile, auditory, spatial, or personal inattention** or extinction to bilateral simultaneous stimulation in one of the sensory modalities.

    2 = **Profound hemi-inattention or extinction to more than one modality;** does not recognize own hand or orients to only one side of space.

ORGOGOZO STROKE SCALE

Patient Name: ____

Rater Name: ________________________________ ______________________

Date: ____

Activity   **Score**

Score

Consciousness

  0 = Coma

  5 = Stupor

10 = Drowsiness

15 = Normal __________

Verbal Communication

  0 = Impossible

  5 = Difficult

10 = Normal __________

Eyes and Head Shift

    0 = Forced
    5 = Gaze failure
    10 = None

Facial Movements

    0 = Paralysis
    5 = Normal   __________

Arm Raising

    0 = Impossible
    5 = Incomplete
    10 = Possible   __________

Hand Movements

    0 = Useless
    5 = Useful
    10 = Skilled
    15 = Normal   __________

Upper Limb Tone

    0 = Increased or decreased
    5 = Normal   __________

Leg Raising

    0 = Impossible
    5 = Gravity
    10 = Resistance
    15 = Normal   __________

Foot Dorsiflexion

    0 = Foot drop
    5 = Gravity
    10 = Resistance or normal   __________

Lower Limb Tone

0 =   Increased or decreased

5 =   Normal   ___________

TOTAL (0–100):   ___________

Reference

1. Orgogozo JM, Capildeo R. Development of neurological score for clinical evaluation of infarctions in the Sylvian territory Presse Med. 1983:12(48):3039-44.

RIVERMEAD MOBILITY INDEX

Overview: The Rivermead Mobility Index is a measure of disability related to bodily mobility. It demonstrates the patient's ability to move her or his own body. It does not measure the effective use of a wheelchair or the mobility when aided by someone else. It was developed for patients who had suffered a head injury or stroke at the Rivermead Rehabilitation Center in Oxford, England.

Rivermead Motor Index

No.	Parameter	Question
1	Turning over in bed	Do you turn over from your back to side without help?
2	Lying to sitting	From lying in bed, do you get up to sit on the edge of the bed on your own?
3	Sitting balance	Do you sit on the edge of the bed without holding on for 10 seconds?
4	Sitting to standing	Do you stand up (from any chair) in less than 15 seconds and stands there for 15 seconds (using hands and with an aid if necessary)?
5	Standing unsupported	Observe standing for 10 seconds without any aid or support.
6	Transfer	Do you manage to move from bed to chair and back without any help?
7	Walking inside with an aid if needed	Do you walk 10 meters with an aid or furniture if necessary but with no standby help?
8	Stairs	Do you manage a flight of stairs without help?
9	Walking inside (even ground)	Do you walk around outside on pavements without help?
10	Walking inside with no aid	Do you walk 10 meters inside with no caliper splint aid or use of furniture and no standby help?
11	Picking off floor	If you drop something on the floor, do you manage to walk 5 meters pick it up and even then walk back?
12	Walking outside (uneven ground)	Do you walk over uneven ground (grass, gravel, dirt, snow, ice, etc.) without help?
13	Bathing	Do you get in and out of bath or shower unsupervised and wash self?
14	Up and down 4 steps	Do you manage to go up and down 4 steps with no rail and without help but using an aid if necessary?
15	Running	Do you run 10 meters without limping in 4 seconds (a fast walk is acceptable)?

Response   Points
Yes   1
No   0

Rivermead motor index = SUM (points for all 15 questions)

Interpretation:

Minimum score = 0

Maximum score = 1

The higher the score, the better the mobility.

Reference

1. Collen FM, Wade DT, et al. The Rivermead mobility index: A further development of the Rivermead motor assessment. Int Disabil Studies. 1991;13:50-54.

SCANDINAVIAN STROKE SCALE

Patient Name: _______________________________

Rater Name: _______________________________

Date: _______________________________

Function

	Score	Prognostic score	Long-term score
Consciousness:			
Fully conscious	6	_______	
Somnolent, can be walked to full consciousness	4		
Reacts to verbal commands, but is not fully conscious	2		
Eye movement:			
No gaze palsy	4	_______	
Gaze palsy present	2		
Conjugate eye deviation	0		
Arm, motor power*:			
Raises arm with normal strength	6		
Raises arm with reduced strength	5	_______	
Raises arm with flexion in elbow	4		
Can move, but not against gravity	2		
Paralysis	0		
Hand, motor power*:			
Normal strength	6	_______	
Reduced strength in full range	4		
Some movements, fingertips do not reach palm	2		
Paralysis	0		
Leg motor power*:			
Normal strength	6	_______	
Raises straight leg with reduced strength	5		
Raises leg with flexion of knee	4		
Can move, but not against gravity	2		
Paralysis	0		
Orientation:			
Correct for time, place and person	6	_______	
Two of these	4		
One of these	2		
Completely disoriented	0		

Speech:

No aphasia	10	________
Limited vocabulary or incoherent speech	6	
More than yes/no, but no longer sentences	3	
Only yes/no or less	0	

Facial palsy:

None/dubious	2	________
Present	0	

Gait

Walks 5 m without aids	12	________
Walks with aids	9	
Walks with help of another person	6	
Sits without support	3	
Bedridden/wheelchair	0	

Maximal Score　　　　________　　22　　48

* Motor power is assessed only on the affected side.

Reference

1. Multicenter trial of hemodilution is ischemic stroke—background and study protocol. Scandinavian Stroke Study Group. Stroke. 1985;16(5):885-90.

TINETTI BALANCE ASSESSMENT TOOL

Patient's Name: _________________ DOB: _________ Ward: ______

Balance Section

Patient is seated in hard, armless chair;

Sitting balance	Leans or slides in chair	=	0
	Steady, safe	=	1
Rises from chair	Unable to, without help	=	0
	Able, uses arms to help	=	1
	Able, without use of arms	=	2
Attempts to rise	Unable to without help	=	0
	Able, requires >1 attempt	=	1
	Able, to rise, 1 attempt	=	2
Immediate standing balance (first 5 seconds)	Unsteady (strangers, moves feet, trunk sway)	=	0
	Steady but uses walker or other support	=	1
	Steady without walker or other support	=	2
Standing balance	Unsteady	=	0
	Steady but wide stance and uses support	=	1
	Narrow stance without support	=	2
Nudged	Begins to fall	=	0
	Staggers, grabs, catches self	=	1
	Steady	=	2
Eyes closed	Unsteady	=	0
	Steady	=	1
Turning 360 degrees	Discontinuous steps	=	0
	Continuous	=	1
	Unsteady (grabs, staggery)	=	0
	Steady	=	1
Sitting down	Unsafe (misjudged distance, falls into chair)	=	0
	Uses arms or not a smooth motion	=	1
	Safe, smooth motion	=	2
	Balance score		**/16 /16**

Gait Section

Patients stands with therapist, walks across room (+/–aids), first at usual pace, then at rapid pace.

Indication of gait (immediately after told to 'go'.)	Any hesitancy or multiple attempts	= 0
	No hesitancy	= 1
Step length and height	Step to	= 0
	Step through R	= 1
	Step through L	= 1
Foot clearance	Foot drop	= 0
	L foot clears floor	= 1
	R foot clears floor	= 1
Step symmetry	Right and left step length not equal	= 0
	Right and left step length appear equal	= 1
Step continuity	Stopping or discontinuing between steps	= 0
	Steps appear continuous	= 1
Path	Marked deviation	= 0
	Mild/moderate deviation or uses walking aid	= 1
	Straight without walking aid	= 2
Trunk	Marked sway or uses walking aid	= 0
	No sway but flex knees or back or uses arms for stability	= 1
	No sway, flex, use of arms or walking aid	= 2
Walking time	Heels apart	= 0
	Heels almost touching while walking	= 1

Gait score	/12	/12
Balanced score carried forward	/16	/16
Total score = Balance score + Gait score	/28	/28

Risk Indicators:

Tinetti Tool Score	**Risk of falls**
≥18	High
19–23	Moderate
/24	Low

THE TRUNK CONTROL TEST FOR MOTOR IMPAIRMENT AFTER STROKE

Overview

The trunk control test can be used to assess the motor impairment in a patient who has had a stroke. It correlates with eventually walking ability.

Testing done by patient lying on bed

1. Roll to weak side
2. Roll to strong side
3. Balance in sitting position on the edge of the bed with the feet off the ground for at least 30 seconds
4. Sit up from lying down

Scoring each test	Points
Unable to do without assistance	0
Able to do so using nonmuscular help or in an abnormal style	12
Able to complete task normally	25

Trunk control test = SUM (points for all 4 tests)

Interpretation

- Minimum score: 0
- Maximum score: 100
- If the test is done at 6 weeks after stroke, a score more than 50 predicts recovery of the ability to walk by 18 weeks.

Reference

1. Tinetti ME, Williams TF, Mayewski R. Fall risk index for elderly patients based on number of chronic disabilities. Am J Med. 1986:80:429-34
2. Collin C, Wade D. Assessing motor impairment after stroke: A pilot reliability study. J Neurol. Neurosurg Psychiatry. 1990;53:576-9.

STROKE IMPACT SCALE

The purpose of this questionnaire is to evaluate how stroke has impacted your health and life. We want to know from Your point of view how stroke has affected you. We will ask you questions about impairments and disabilities caused by your stroke, as well as how stroke has affected your quality of life. Finally, we will ask you to rate how much you think you have recovered from your stroke:

These questions are about the physical problems that may have occurred as a result of your stroke:

1. In the past week, how would you rate the strength of you.......	A lot of strength	Quite a bit of strength	Some strength	A little strength	No strength at all
a. Arm that was most affected by your stroke?	5	4	3	2	1
b. Grip of your hand that was most affected by your stroke?	5	4	3	2	1
c. Leg that was most affected by your stroke?	5	4	3	2	1
d. Foot/ankle that was most affected by your stroke?	5	4	3	2	1

These questions are about your memory and thinking:

2. In the past week, how difficult was it to	Not difficult at all	A little difficult	Somewhat difficult	Very difficult	Extremely difficult
a. Remember things that people just told you?	5	4	3	2	1
b. Remember things that happened yesterday?	5	4	3	2	1
c. Remember to do things (e.g., keep scheduled appointments or take medication)?	5	4	3	2	1
d. Remember the day of the week?	5	4	3	2	1
e. Add and subtract numbers?	5	4	3	2	1
f. Concentrate?	5	4	3	2	1
g. Think quickly?	5	4	3	2	1
h. Solve problems?	5	4	3	2	1

These questions are about how you feel, about changes in your mood and about your ability to control your emotions since your stroke.

3. In the past week, how often did you	None of the time	A little of the time	Some of the time	Most of the time	All of the time
a. Feel sad?	5	4	3	2	1
b. Feel that there is nobody you are close to?	5	4	3	2	1
c. Feel that you are a burden to others?	5	4	3	2	1
d. Feel that you have nothing to look forward to?	5	4	3	2	1
e. Blame yourself for mistakes?	5	4	3	2	1
f. Enjoy things as much as you ever have?	5	4	3	2	1
g. Feel quite nervous?	5	4	3	2	1
h. Feel that life is worth living?	5	4	3	2	1
i. Smile and laugh at least once a day?	5	4	3	2	1

The following items are about your ability to communicate with other people, as well as your ability to understand what you read and what you hear in a conversation:

4. In the past, how difficult was it to	Not difficult at all	A little difficult	Somewhat difficult	Very difficult	Extremely difficult
a. Say the name of someone whose face was in front of you?	5	4	3	2	1
b. Understand what was being said to you in a conversation?	5	4	3	2	1
c. Reply to questions?	5	4	3	2	1
d. Correctly name objects?	5	4	3	1	
e. Participate in a conversation with a group of people?	5	4	3	2	1
f. Have a conversation on the telephone?	5	4	3	2	1
g. Call another person on the telephone (select the correct phone number and dial)?	5	4	3	2	1

The following items ask about activities you might do during a typical day:

5. In the past two weeks, how difficult was it to ……	Not difficult at all	A little difficult	Somewhat difficult	Very difficult	Cannot do at all
a. Cut your food with a knife and fork?	5	4	3	2	1
b. Dress the top part (waist up) of your body?	5	4	3	2	1
c. Bathe yourself?	5	4	3	2	1
d. Clip your toenails?	5	4	3	2	1
e. Get to the toilet on time?	5	4	3	2	1
f. Control your bladder (not have an accident)?	5	4	3	2	1
g. Control your bowels (not have an accident)?	5	4	3	2	1
h. Do light household task/chores (e.g. dust, make a bed, take out garbage, do the dishes)?	5	4	3	2	1
i. Go shopping?	5	4	3	2	1
j. Handle money (e.g. pay monthly bills, manage checking account)?	5	4	3	2	1
k. Do heavy household chores (e.g. vacuum, laundry or yard work)?	5	4	3	2	1

The following questions are about your ability to be mobile, at home and in the community:

6. In the past 2 weeks, how difficult was it to ……	Not difficulty at all	A little difficulty	Somewhat difficult	Very difficult	Cannot do at all
a. Sit without losing your balance?	5	4	3	2	1
b. Stand without losing your balance?	5	4	3	2	1
c. Walk without losing your balance?	5	4	3	2	1
d. Move from a bed to a chair?	5	4	3	2	1
e. Get out of a chair without using your hands for support?	5	4	3	2	1
f. Walk one block?	5	4	3	2	1
g. Walk fast?	5	4	3	2	1
h. Climb one flight of stairs?	5	4	3	2	1
i. Climb several flights of stairs?	5	4	3	2	1
j. Get in and out of a car?	5	4	3	2	1

The following questions are about your ability to use your hand that was most affected by your stroke.

7. In the past 2 weeks, how difficult was it to use your hand that was most affected by your stroke to ……	Not difficulty at all	A little difficulty	Somewhat difficult	Very difficult	Cannot do at all
a. Carry heavy objects (e.g. bag of groceries)?	5	4	3	2	1
b. Turn a doorknob?	5	4	3	2	1
c. Open a can or jar?	5	4	3	2	1
d. Tie a shoelace?	5	4	3	2	1
e. Pick up a dime?	5	4	3	2	1

The following questions are about how stroke has affected your ability to participate in the activities that you usually do, things that are meaningful to you and help you to find purpose in life:

8. During the past 4 weeks, how much of the time have you been limited in ……	None of the time	A little of the time	Some of the time	Most of the time	All of the time
a. Your work, volunteer or other activities?	5	4	3	2	11
b. Your social activities?	5	4	3	2	1
c. Quite recreation (crafts, reading)?	5	4	3	2	1
d. Active reaction (sports, outings, travel)?	5	4	3	2	1
e. Your role as a family member and/or friend?	5	4	3	2	1
f. Your participation in spiritual or religious activities?	5	4	3	2	1
g. Your ability to feel emotionally connected to another person?	5	4	3	2	1
h. Your ability to control your life as you wish?	5	4	3	2	1
i. Your ability to help others in need?	5	4	3	2	1

On a scale of 0 to 100 representing full recovery and 0 representing no recovery, how much have you recovered from your stroke?

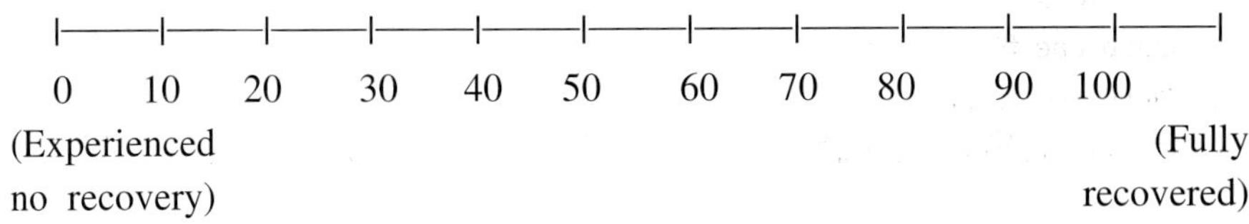

FUNCTIONAL INDEPENDENCE MEASURE (FIM)

Category	Measure
Self-care	Feeding
	Grooming
	Bathing
	Dressing upper body
	Dressing lower body
	Toileting
Sphincter Control	Bladder
	Bowel
Transfers	Bed, chair, wheelchair
Mobility	Toilet
	Tub or shower
Locomotion	Walker or wheelchair
	Stairs
Communication and Cognition	Comprehension
	Expression
	Social interaction
	Problem solving
	Memory
Total	18 measures

For each measure	Score
Complete independence, unaided	7
Modified independence, with device	6
Can perform with supervision	5
Able to complete 75% of activity; needs minimal assistance	4
Able to complete 50% of activity; needs moderate assistance	3
Able to complete 25% of activity; needs significant assistance	2
Unable to complete limited activity; requires total assistance	1

FIM score = Summation of score for each measure

Interpretation:
- Maximum FIM score = 18 * 7 = 126
- The higher the FIM score, the better the patient outcomes.

BERG BALANCE

Patient Name: _______________________________

Rater Name:_______________________________

Date: _______________________________

Balance Item	**Score (0–4)**

1. Sitting unsupported   _______
2. Change of position: Sitting to standing   _______
3. Change of position: Standing to sitting   _______
4. Transfers   _______
5. Standing unsupported   _______
6. Standing with eyes closed   _______
7. Standing with feet together   _______
8. Tandem standing   _______
9. Standing on one leg   _______
10. Turning trunk (feet fixed)   _______
11. Retrieving objects from floor   _______
12. Turning 360 degrees   _______
13. Stool stepping   _______
14. Reaching forward while standing   _______

TOTAL (0–56):   _______

Interpretation
  0–20: Wheelchair bound
  21–40: Walking with assistance
  41–56: Independent

THE REHABILITATION INDEX

Overview: The rehabilitation index is a measure of the resources that a person has to aid in his or her response to injury and to be rehabilitated as much as possible.

Factors measured:
  1. Impairment from injury
  2. Chronicity

3. Expected response
4. Intelligence quotient
5. Past performance in work and school
6. Emotional stability (poor to good)
7. Personality (poor to good)
8. Influence of socioeconomic status (bad to good)
9. Influence of other physical defects (marked to none)
10. Motivation.

Scoring:

- Points assigned from 1 to 10
- The higher the score, the better the resource (1 = worst; 10 = best)

Rehabilitation index = SUM (points for all 10 factors)

Interpretation:

- Minimum score: 10
- Maximum score: 100
- An index $\leq$ = 48 indicates that the patient is at poor risk for rehabilitation.

Limitations:

- All factors are graded equally but factors such as intelligence emotional stability and motivation can help some patients overcome adversity despite poor scores in other areas.

Bibliography

1. Actherberg S, Kappelle L, Algra A. Prognostic Modelling in Ischaemic Stroke Study, Additional Value of Genetic Characteristics Rationale and Design. Eur Neurol. 2008);59(5):243-52.
2. Allison R, Dennett R. Pilot randomized controlled trial to assess the impact of additional supported standing practice on functional ability post stroke. Clin Rehabil. 2007; 21(7):614-9.
3. Brahmachari I. Rehabilitation of stroke patients in Indian scenario: Activity and participation perspective. Ind J Phys Ther. 2013;1(2):47-51.
4. Bolpe B, Lynch D, Berland A. Intensive Sensorimotor Arm Training Mediated by Therapist or Robot Improves Hemiparesis in Patients with Chronic Stroke. Neurorehabil Neural Repair. 2008;22(3):305-10.
5. Brogardh C, Sjoulund B. Constraint-induced movement therapy in patients with stroke: A pilot study on effects of small group training and of extended mitt use. Clin Rehabil. 2006;20(3):218-27.
6. Burnhardt J, Chitravas N, Meslo I. Not All Stroke Units are the Same: A Comparison of Physical Activity Patterns in Melbourne, Australia, and Trondheim, Norway. Stroke. 2008;39:2059-65.
7. Burns A, Burridge J, Pickering R. Does the use of a constraint mitten to encourage use of the hemiplegic upper limb improve arm function in adults with subacute stroke? Clin Rehabil. 2007;20(10):895-904.
8. Byl N, Roderick J, Mohamed O. Effectiveness of Sensory and Motor Rehabilitation of the Upper Limb Following the Principles of Neuroplasticity: Patients Stable Poststroke. Neurorehabil Neural Repair. 2003;17(3):171-6.
9. Canning C, Ada L, Adams R. Loss of strength contributes more to physical disability after stroke than loss of dexterity. Clin Rehabil. 2004;18(3):300-08.
10. Casadio M. A proof of concept study for the integration of robot therapy with physiotherapy in the treatment of stroke patients. Clin Rehabil. 2003;23(3): 217-28.
11. Chae J, Hart R. Intramuscular Hand Neuroprosthesis for Chronic Stroke Survivors. Neurorehabil Neural Repair. 2003;17(2):109-17.
12. Chae J, Ng A, Yu D. Intramuscular Electrical Stimulation for Shoulder Pain in Hemiplegia: Does Time From Stroke Onset Predict Treatment Success? Neurorehabil Neural Repair. 2007;21(6):561-7.

13. Chan J, Liang C, Shaw F. Facilitation of Sensory and Motor Recovery by Thermal Intervention for the Hemiplegic Upper Limb in Acute Stroke Patients. Stroke. 2005;36(255):2665.

14. Church C, Price C, Pandyan A. Randomized Controlled Trial to Evaluate the Effect of Surface Neuromuscular Electrical Stimulation to the Shoulder after Acute Stroke. Stroke. 2006;37:2995-3001.

15. Dong K, Lim J, Shin H. The effect of aquatic therapy on postural balance and muscle strength in stroke survivors — a randomized controlled pilot trial. Clin Rehabil. 2008;22(10-11):966-76.

16. Duncan P, Zorowitz R, Dates B. Management of adult stroke rehabilitation care. Stroke. 2005;36:e100-e143.

17. Fang Y, Chen X, Li H. A study on additional early physiotherapy after stroke and factors affecting functional recovery. Clin Rehabil. 2003;17(6):608-17.

18. Feys H, Weerdt W, Verbeke G. Early and Repetitive Stimulation of the Arm can Substantially Improve the Long-term Outcome after Stroke: A 5-year Follow-up Study of a Randomized Trial. Stroke 2004;35:924-9.

19. Giaquinto S, Spiridigliozzi C. Religious faith eases post-stroke distress, may aid recovery: American heart Association, 2007.

20. Goodwin N, Sunderland A. Intensive, time-series measurement of upper limb recovery in the subacute phase following stroke. Clin Rehabil. 2003;17(1):69-82.

21. Green J, Young J, Forster A. Combined analysis of two randomized trials of community physiotherapy for patients more than one year post stroke. Clin Rehabil. 2004;18(3):249-52.

22. Han SW, Kim SH, Lee JY. A New Subtype Classification of Ischemic Stroke Based on Treatment and Etiologic Mechanism. Eur Neurol. 2007;57(2).

23. Harris J, Eng J. Individuals with the Dominant Hand Affected following Stroke Demonstrate Less Impairment than Those with the Nondominant Hand Affected. Neurorehabil Neural Repair. 2006;20(3):380-9.

24. Hesse S, Werner C, Pohl M. Computerized Arm Training Improves the Motor Control of the Severely Affected Arm after Stroke. Stroke. 2005;36:1960.

25. Higgins J, Salbach N, Wood S. The effect of a task-oriented intervention on arm function in people with stroke: A randomized controlled trial. Clin Rehabil. 2006;20(4):296-310.

26. Howe T, Taylor Y, Finn P. Lateral weight transference exercises following acute stroke: A preliminary study of clinical effectiveness. Clin Rehabil. 2005;19(1):45-53.

27. Jehkonen M, Laihosalo M, Koivisto A. Fluctuation in Spontaneous Recovery of Left Visual Neglect: A 1-year Follow-up. Eur Neurol. 2007;58:210-14.

28. Juha K, Neiminen P, Myllyla V. Sexual Functioning Among Stroke Patients and Their Spouses. Stroke. 1999;30:715-9.

29. Kalra L, Perez I, Gupta S. The Influence of Visual Neglect on Stroke Rehabilitation. Stroke. 1997;28:1386-91.

30. Kalra L, Ratan R. Advances in Stroke Regenerative Medicine. Stroke. 2007;39:273-5.

31. Kalra. Faith Under the Microscope. Stroke. 2007;38:848.

32. Kjendahl A. A one year follow-up study on the effects of acupuncture in the treatment of stroke patients in the subacute stage: A randomized, controlled study. Clin Rehabil. 1997;11(3):192-200.

33. Kroon J, Ijzerman M. Electrical stimulation of the upper extremity in stroke: Cyclic versus EMG-triggered stimulation. Clin Rehabil. 2008;22(8):690-7.

34. Kwakel G, Peppen R, Waggener R. Effects of Augmented Exercise Therapy Time after Stroke. Stroke. 2004;35(25):2529-39 .

35. Kwakel G, Waggener R, Koelman T. Effects of Intensity of Rehabilitation after Stroke: A Research Synthesis. Stroke. 1997;28:1550-6.

36. Lackner E, Hummelshein H. Motor-evoked potentials are facilitated during perceptual identification of hand position in healthy subjects and stroke patients. Clin Rehabil. 2003;17(6):648-55.

37. Lamina S, Hanif S, Darnley I. Effect of Cerebrovascular Accident on Sexual Function of Male Hemiplegic Patients. J Med Rehabil. 2007;1(1).

38. Langhorne P, Wagennar R, Partridge C. Physiotherapy after stroke: More is better? Physiotherapy Res Int. 1996;1(2):75-88.

39. Lettinga A, Reynders A, Mulder T. Pitfalls in effectiveness research: A comparative analysis of treatment goals and outcome measures in stroke rehabilitation. Clin Rehabil. 2002;16(2):174-81.

40. Leung J, Moseley A, Fereday S. The prevalence and characteristics of shoulder pain after traumatic brain injury. Clin Rehabil. 2007;21(2):171-81.

41. Lincoln N, Parry R, Vas C. Randomized, Controlled Trial to Evaluate Increased Intensity of Physiotherapy Treatment of Arm Function after Stroke. Stroke. 1999;30:573-9.

42. Luke C, Dod K, Brock K. Outcomes of the Bobath concept on upper limb recovery following stroke. Clin Rehabil. 2004;18(8): 888-98.

43. Margaret R, Turner S. Effectiveness of brain injury rehabilitation. Clin Rehabil. 1999;13(1):7-24.

44. Merians A, Jack D, Tremaine M. Virtual Reality–Augmented Rehabilitation for Patients Following Stroke. Phys Ther. 2002;82(9):898-915.

45. Ozcakir S, Siviroghu K. Botulinium toxin in post stroke spasticity, clinical medicine and research. 2007;5(2):132-8.

46. Page S, Levine P, Sisto S. Mental Practice Combined With Physical Practice for Upper Limb Motor Deficit in Subacute Stroke. Phys Ther 2001;81(8):1455-62.

47. Parry R, Lincoln N, Vass C. Effect of severity of arm impairment on response to additional physiotherapy early after stroke. Clin Rehabil. 1999;13(3):187-98.

48. Platz T, Eickhof C, Kaick S. Impairment-oriented training or Bobath therapy for severe arm paresis after stroke: A single-blind, multicentre randomized controlled trial. Clin rehabil. 2005;19(7):714-24.

49. Pohl M, Werner C, Holzgraefe M. Repetitive locomotor training and physiotherapy improve walking and basic activities of daily living after stroke: A single-blind, randomized multicentre trial. Clin Rehabil. 2007;21(1):17-27.

50. Pollock A, Baer G, Pomeroy P. Physiotherapy treatment approaches for the recovery of postural control and lower limb function following stroke. Cochrane Database Syst Rev 1 (2007) , CD 001920.

51. Rodgers H, Mackintosh J, Price C. Does an early increased-intensity interdisciplinary upper limb therapy programme following acute stroke improve outcome? Clin Rehabil. 2003;17(6):579-89.

52. Rosales R, Kong K, Goh K. Botulinium toxin injection for hypertonicity of upper extremity within 12 weeks after stroke. Neurorehab Neural Repair. 2012;26(7):812-21.

53. Ryan T, Enderby P, Rigby A. A randomized controlled trial to evaluate intensity of community-based rehabilitation provision following stroke or hip fracture in old age. Clin Rehabil. 2006;20(2):123-31.

54. Sacco S, Toni T, Angelo A. Acute Stroke Admission and Diagnostic Procedures According to the Hour and Day of Onset. Eur Neurol. 2009;61(2):100-06.

55. Seelen H, Hemmen B. Effects of movement imagery and electromyography-triggered feedback on arm-hand function in stroke patients in the subacute phase. Clin Rehabil. 2007;21(7):587-94.

56. Sheffler L, Hennessey M, Naples G. Improvement in Functional Ambulation as a Therapeutic Effect of Peroneal Nerve Stimulation in Hemiplegia: Two Case Reports. Neurorehabil Neural Repair. 2007;21(4):366-9.

57. Stinear J, Byblow W. Rhythmic bilateral movement training modulates corticomotor excitability and enhances upper limb motricity poststroke: A pilot study. J Clin Neurophysiol. 2004;21(2):124-31.

58. Sullivan JE, and Hedman LD. A Home Program of Sensory and Neuromuscular Electrical Stimulation with Upper-limb Task Practice in a Patient 5 Years after a Stroke. Phys Ther. November 2004;84 (11):1045-54.

59. Ter zoudi A, Vorvolakos T, Heliopoulos I. Sleep Architecture in Stroke and Relation to Outcome. Eur Neurol. 2009;61(1).

60. The Glasgow Augmented Physiotherapy Study (GAPS) group. Can augmented physiotherapy input enhance recovery of mobility after stroke? A randomized controlled trial. Clin Rehabil. 2004;18(5):529-37.

61. Turton AJ. A multiple case design experiment to investigate the performance and neural effects of a programme for training hand function after stroke. Clin Rehabil. 2004;18(7):754-63.

62. Van der Lee J, Snels I, Beckerman H. Exercise therapy for arm function in stroke patients: A systematic review of randomized controlled trials. Clin Rehabil. 2001;15(1):20-31.

63. Varona J, Guerra J, Bermajo F. Causes of Ischemic Stroke in Young Adults, and Evolution of the Etiological Diagnosis over the Long Term. Clin Neurol. 2007;57(4):212-8.

64. Verheyden G, Nieuwboer A, Winckel A. Clinical tools to measure trunk performance after stroke: A systematic review of the literature. Clin Rehabil. 2007;21(5):387-94.

65. Vliet P, Lincoln N, Foxall A. Comparison of Bobath based and movement science based treatment for stroke: A randomised controlled trial. J Neurol Neurosurg Psychiatry. 2005;76:503-08.

66. Volpe B, Krebs H, Hogan N. Robot training enhanced motor outcome in patients with stroke maintained over 3 years. Neurology. 1999;53:1874.

67. Volpe BT, Krebs HI, Hogan N. A novel approach to stroke rehabilitation: Robot-aided sensorimotor stimulation. Neurol. 2000;54:1938-44.

68. Wade D, Collen F, Robb G. Physiotherapy intervention late after stroke and mobility. BMJ. 1992;304:6827.

69. WHO Infobase Ref. #: S00753a1.

70. Wiles R, Ashburn A, Payne S. Discharge from physiotherapy following stroke: The management of disappointment. Soc Sci Med. September 2004;59(6):1263-73.

71. Winckel A, Feys H, Lincoln N. Assessment of arm function in stroke patients: Rivermead Motor Assessment arm section revised with Rasch analysis. Clin Rehabil. 2007;21(5):471-5.

72. Woldag H, Waldmann G, Heuschkel G. Is the repetitive training of complex hand and arm movements beneficial for motor recovery in stroke patients? Clin Rehabil. 2003;17(7):723-30.

73. Yozbatian N, Donmez B, Kayak N. Electrical stimulation of wrist and fingers for sensory and functional recovery in acute hemiplegia. Clin Rehabil. 2006;20(1):4-11.

RECOMMENDED BOOKS FOR FURTHER READING

1. The Principles of Exercise Therapy by M. Dena Gardiner, CBS Publishers & Distributors Pvt Ltd, 2005.
2. Adult Hemiplegia Evaluation and Treatment by Berta Bobath, 1990.
3. Steps to Follow: The Comprehensive Treatment of Patients with Hemiplegia by Patricia M. Davies, Springer, 2000.
4. Right in the Middle: Selective Trunk Activity in the Treatment of Adult Hemiplegia by Patricia M. Davies, Springer, 1990.
5. Cash's Textbook of Neurology for Physiotherapists by Patricia A. Downie, Jaypee Brothers Medical Publishers (P) Ltd, 1993.
6. Practical Exercise Therapy, Margaret Hollis, Phyllis Fletcher Cook (Ed), Wiley–Blackwell, 1999.
7. Physical Rehabilitation by Susan B. O'Sullivan and Thomas J. Schmitz, F. Davis Company, 2014.
8. Tidy's Physiotherapy, Stuart Porter, Churchill Livingstone, 2013.
9. Treatment for Hemiplegia by Sarah Johnstone.
10. PNF in Practice: An Illustrated Guide by Susan Adler, Springer, 2007.
11. A Motor Relearning Programme for Stroke by Janet H. Carr and Roberta B. Shepherd, Aspen Publishers, 1987.
12. Clayton's Electrotherapy (Physiotherapy Essentials) by Sheila Kitchen and Sarah Bazin, Bailliere Tindall, 1995.
13. BD Chaurasia's Human Anatomy by BD Chaurasia, CBS Publishers, 2013.
14. Guyton and Hall Textbook of Medical Physiology by John E. Hall, Elsevier Health Science, 2013.
15. Harrison's Principles of Internal Medicine by Dan Longo, Anthony Fauci, Dennis Kasper, Stephen Hauser, J Jameson, Joseph Loscalzo, McGraw-Hill, 2011.

Index

Page numbers followed by *t* refer to table, *f* refer to figure and *b* refer to box.